Lecture Notes in Statistics

Edited by P. Bickel, P. Diggle, S. Fienberg, K. Krickeberg, I. Olkin, N. Wermuth, S. Zeger

Springer
*New York
Berlin
Heidelberg
Barcelona
Hong Kong
London
Milan
Paris
Singapore
Tokyo*

Geert Verbeke
Geert Molenberghs

Linear Mixed Models in Practice
A SAS-Oriented Approach

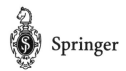 Springer

Geert Verbeke
Biostatistical Centre for Clinical Trials
Katholieke Universiteit Leuven
U.Z. Sint-Rafael
Kapucijnenvoer 35
B-3000 Leuven
Belgium

Geert Molenberghs
Biostatistics
Limburgs Universitair Centrum
Universitaire Campus, Building D
B-3590 Diepenbeek
Belgium

SAS® is a registered trademark of SAS Institute, Inc. in the USA and other countries.

Verbeke, Geert.
    Linear mixed models in practice: a SAS-oriented approach/Geert
Verbeke, Geert Molenberghs.
      p. cm.—(Lecture notes in statistics; 88)
    Includes bibliographical references and index.
    ISBN 0-387-98222-1 (softcover: alk. paper)
    1. Linear models (Statistics)—Data processing. 2. SAS (Computer
file) I. Molenberghs, Geert. II. Title III. Series: Lecture
notes in statistics (Springer-Verlag); v. 88.
    QA279.V46 1997
    519.5´35—dc21   97-15705

Printed on acid-free paper.

Camera-ready copy provided by the authors.
Printed and bound by Sheridan Books, Inc., Ann Arbor, MI.
Printed in the United States of America.

9 8 7 6 5 4 3

ISBN 0-387-98222-1 Springer-Verlag New York Berlin Heidelberg SPIN 10747620

To Godewina and Lien

To Conny and An

Preface

The dissemination of the MIXED procedure in SAS has provided a whole class of statistical models for routine use. We believe that both the ideas behind the techniques and their implementation in SAS are not at all straightforward and users from various applied backgrounds, including the pharmaceutical industry, have experienced difficulties in using the procedure effectively. Courses and consultancy on PROC MIXED have been in great demand in recent years, illustrating the clear need for resource material to aid the user. This book is intended as a contribution to bridging this gap.

We hope the book will be of value to a wide audience, including applied statisticians and many biomedical researchers, particularly in the pharmaceutical industry, medical and public health research organizations, contract research organizations, and academic departments. This implies that our book is explanatory rather than research oriented and that it emphasizes practice rather than mathematical rigor. In this respect, clear guidance and advice on practical issues are the main focus of the text. Nevertheless, this does not imply that more advanced topics have been avoided. Sections containing material of a deeper level have been sign posted by means of an asterisk.

The text grew out of two short courses for which the initiative was taken in 1995 and 1996 by the Biopharmaceutical Section of the Belgian Statistical Society. They took place at the Limburgs Universitair Centrum (Diepenbeek). Each of these two-day courses devoted one session to an example-based introduction of the linear mixed model (Luc Duchateau and Paul Janssen) where various types of applications were explored, two sessions to longitudinal data analysis with the linear mixed model (Geert Verbeke), and one session to missing data issues (Geert Molenberghs, Luc Bijnens, and David Shaw). This structure is directly reflected in the structure of this book. While this text is strictly speaking an edited volume, editors and authors have devoted a lot of attention to streamlining the treatment. In particular, we aimed for a single notational convention and for a clear delineation between the treatment of topics. For a couple of reasons there is a little residual overlap. First, the earlier chapters introduce concepts with emphasis on examples and simple derivations, while a broader treatment is given in later chapters. Secondly, we have chosen not to introduce new concepts until their first place of natural occurrence. Thirdly, different data structures require different choices at analysis time.

The various chapters have benefited from exposure to students in various situations, such as the European Course of Advanced Statistics (Milton-Keynes, September 1995) where Chapter 3 was used in a session on missing data. Most of the material has been used in the Analysis of Variance and Longitudinal Data Analysis courses at the Master of Science in Biostatistics Programme of the Limburgs Universitair Centrum and in the Topics in Biostatistics course of the Universiteit Antwerpen.

The first chapter provides a general introduction. Chapter 2 is an example-based treatment to statistical inference for mixed models. In Chapter 3, we discuss the analysis of longitudinal data using linear mixed models, from a practical point of view. Chapter 4 is devoted to four longitudinal case studies. The concluding chapter considers the ubiquitous problem of missing and incomplete longitudinal data.

It will be clear that we have placed a strong emphasis on the SAS procedure MIXED. This should not discourage the non-SAS users from consulting this book. We have put considerable effort in treating data analysis issues in a generic fashion, instead of making them fully software dependent. Therefore, a research question is first translated into a statistical model by means of algebraic notation. In a number of cases, such a model is then implemented using SAS code. Similarly, SAS output is in the majority of cases avoided, even though most parts of a typical SAS PROC MIXED output are discussed at least once. In general, we have opted to present relevant results of model fit (such as parameter estimates, standard errors, maximized log-likelihoods, etc.) in figures and tables that do not necessarily reflect the structure of the output. In Section 5.11, we give a brief treatment of the S-Plus set of functions termed OSWALD (Version 2.6).

Throughout this book we used SAS Versions 6.11 and 6.12. For the MIXED procedure, the differences between both versions are minor. They include different tabular output and a few new covariance structures. Selected macros for model checks, diagnostic tools, and for multiple imputation are available from Springer-Verlag's URL: `www.springer-ny.com`.

Luc Duchateau (ILRI, Nairobi)

Paul Janssen (LUC, Diepenbeek)

Geert Molenberghs (LUC, Diepenbeek)

Geert Verbeke (KUL, Leuven)

Contents

Acknowledgements

We are indebted to the board members of the Biopharmaceutical Section of the Belgian Statistical Society, Annick Leroy (Bristol-Myers Squibb, Waterloo), William Malbecq (Merck Sharpe and Dohme, Brussels), and Linda Ritter (ID2, Brussels) on the one hand, and to Paul Janssen (Limburgs Universitair Centrum, Diepenbeek) on the other hand who jointly took the initiative to organize a couple of workshops on "Linear Mixed Models in SAS". We gratefully acknowledge the help we had from the other members of the initial working group that was formed in preparation of these courses, Luc Wouters and Tony Vangeneugden (Janssen Pharmaceutica, Beerse), Luc Duchateau (ILRI, Nairobi), Luc Bijnens (EORTC, Brussels) and David Shaw (Shaw Statistics Ltd, Bucks). We thank Peter Diggle and Dave Smith (Lancaster University) for valuable support and stimulating discussions, not in the least on OSWALD. We appreciate input from Russell Wolfinger (SAS Institute, Cary) on SAS related matters. Several sections in the book are based on joint research: with Emmanuel Lesaffre (Katholieke Universiteit Leuven), Larry Brant (Gerontology Research Center and The Johns Hopkins University, Baltimore), Mike Kenward (University of Kent, Canterbury), and Stuart Lipsitz (Dana-Farber Cancer Institute and Harvard School of Public Health, Boston). Interesting sets of data were provided by Luc Wouters, Tony Vangeneugden, and Larry Brant. We are very grateful to Viviane Mebis (Limburgs Universitair Centrum) and Bart Spiessens (Katholieke Universiteit Leuven) for their invaluable secretarial and technical support. We apologize to our wives and daughters for the time we did not spend with them during the preparation of this book and we are very grateful for their understanding. The preparation of this book has been a period of close and stimulating collaboration, to which we will keep good memories.

Geert and Geert

Kessel-Lo, April 1997

1

Introduction

Geert Molenberghs
Geert Verbeke

In applied sciences one is often confronted with the collection of *correlated data*. This generic term embraces a multitude of data structures, such as multivariate observations, clustered data, repeated measurements, longitudinal data, and spatially correlated data.

Among those, multivariate data have received most attention in the statistical literature (e.g., Seber 1984, Krzanowski 1988, Johnson and Wichern 1992). Techniques devised for this situation include multivariate regression and multivariate analysis of variance, which have been implemented in the SAS procedure GLM for general linear models. In addition, SAS contains a battery of relatively specialized procedures for principal components analysis, canonical correlation analysis, discriminant analysis, factor analysis, cluster analysis, etc.

As an example of a simple multivariate study, assume that a subject's systolic and diastolic blood pressure are measured simultaneously. This is different from a *clustered setting*, where for example, for a number of families, diastolic blood pressure is measured for all of their members. A design where for each subject diastolic blood pressure is recorded under several experimental conditions is often termed a *repeated measures* study. In case diastolic blood pressure is measured repeatedly over time for each subject, we are dealing with *longitudinal data*. Although one could view all of these data structures as special cases of multivariate designs, we believe there are many fundamental differences, thoroughly affecting the mode of analysis. First, certain multivariate techniques, such as principal components, are hardly useful for the other designs. Secondly, in a truly multivariate set of outcomes, the variance-covariance structure is usually unstructured, in contrast to, for example, longitudinal data. Therefore, the methodology of the general linear model is too restrictive to perform satisfactory data analyses of these more complex data. In contrast, the *general linear mixed model*, as implemented in the SAS procedure MIXED, is much more flexible.

Replacing the time dimension in a longitudinal setting with one or more spatial dimensions, leads naturally to spatial data. While ideas in the longitudinal and spatial areas have developed relatively independently, more efforts have recently been spent in bridging the gap between both disciplines. In 1996, a workshop was devoted to this idea: "The Nantucket Conference on Modeling Longitudinal and Spatially Correlated Data: Methods, Applications, and Future Directions" (Gregoire 1997).

Still, restricting attention to the correlated data settings described earlier is too limited to fully grasp the wide applicability of the general linear mixed model. In designed experiments, such as ANOVA or nested factorial designs, the variance structure has to reflect the design and thus elaborate structures will be needed. A good mode of analysis should be able to account for various sources of variability. Chapter 2 is intended to give the reader some insight in the versatility of experimental data modeling.

Among the clustered data settings, longitudinal data perhaps require the most elaborate modeling of the random variability. Diggle, Liang, and Zeger (1994) distinguish between three components of variability. The first one groups traditional random effects (as in a random-effects ANOVA model) and random coefficients (Longford 1993). It stems from inter-individual variability, i.e., heterogeneity between individual profiles. The second component, serial association, is present when residuals close to each other in time are more similar than residuals further apart. This notion is well-known from the time-series literature (Ripley 1981, Diggle 1983, Cressie 1991). Finally, on top of the other two components, there is potentially also measurement error. This results from the fact that for delicate measurements (e.g., laboratory assays), even immediate replication will not be able to avoid considerable variation. In longitudinal data, these three components of variability can be distinguished by virtue of both *replication* as well as a clear *distance* concept (time), one of which is lacking in classical spatial and time series analysis, and in clustered data. This implies that adapting models for longitudinal data to other data structures is in many cases relatively straightforward. For example, clustered data could be analyzed by leaving out all aspects of the model that refer to time. Therefore, in addition to the designed experiments in Chapter 2, Chapters 3 to 5 illustrate the practical application of linear mixed models in the context of longitudinal data.

A very important characteristic of the data to be analyzed is the type of outcome. Methods for continuous data form the best developed and most advanced body of research, while the same is true for software implementation. This is natural, since the special status and the elegant properties of the normal distribution simplify model building and ease software development. It is in this area that the general linear mixed model and the SAS procedure MIXED is situated. However, also categorical (nominal, ordinal, and binary) and discrete outcomes are very prominent in statistical practice. For example, quality of life outcomes are often scored on ordinal scales.

Two fairly different views can be adopted. The first one, supported by large-sample results, states that normal theory should be applied as much as possible, even to non-normal data such as ordinal scores and counts. A different view is that each type of outcome should be analyzed using instruments that exploit the nature of the data. We will adopt the second standpoint. In addition, since the statistical community has been familiarized with generalized linear models (GLIM, McCullagh and Nelder 1989), some have taken the view that the normal model for continuous data is but one type of GLIM. Although this is correct in principle, it fails to acknowledge the fact that normal models are much further developed than any other GLIM (e.g., model checks and diagnostic tools), and that it enjoys unique properties (e.g., the existence of closed form solutions, exact distributions of test statistics, unbiased estimators). Extensions of GLIM to the longitudinal case are discussed in Diggle, Liang, and Zeger (1994), where the main emphasis is on generalized estimating equations (Liang and Zeger 1986). Generalized linear mixed models have been proposed by, for example, Breslow and Clayton (1993). Fahrmeir and Tutz (1994) discuss GLIM for multivariate settings.

In longitudinal settings each individual typically has a *vector* Y of responses with a natural (time) ordering among the components. This leads to several, generally non-equivalent, extensions of univariate models. In a *marginal model*, marginal distributions are used to describe the outcome vector Y, given a set X of predictor variables. The correlation among the components of Y can then be captured either by adopting a fully parametric approach or by means of working assumptions, such as in the semi-parametric approach of Liang and Zeger (1986). Alternatively, in a *random-effects model*, the predictor variables X are supplemented with a vector U of random effects, conditional upon which the components of Y are usually assumed to be independent. This does not preclude that more elaborate models are possible if residual dependence is detected (Longford 1993). Finally, a *conditional model* describes the distribution of the components of Y, conditional on X but also conditional on (a subset of) the other components of Y. In a longitudinal context, a particular relevant class of conditional models describes a component of Y given the ones recorded earlier in time. Well-known members of this class of *transition models* are *Markov type* models. Several examples are given in Diggle, Liang, and Zeger (1994).

For normally distributed data, marginal models can easily be fitted with PROC MIXED. For such data, integrating a random-effects model over the random effects produces a marginal model, in which the regression parameters retain their meaning and the random effects contribute in a simple way to the variance-covariance structure. For example, the marginal model corresponding to a random-intercepts model is a compound symmetry model that can be fitted without explicitly acknowledging the random-intercepts structure. In the same vein, certain types of transition models induce simple marginal covariance structures. For example, some first-order stationary auto-regressive models imply an exponential or AR(1) covariance structure. As a consequence, many marginal models derived from random-effects and transition models, can be fitted with PROC MIXED as well.

It should be emphasized that the above elegant properties of normal models do not extend to the general GLIM case. For example, opting for a marginal model for longitudinal binary data, precludes the researcher of answering conditional and transitional questions in terms of simple model parameters. This implies that each model family requires its own specific software tools. A few examples are the function for generalized estimating equations as included in the S-Plus set of functions termed OSWALD (Smith, Robertson, and Diggle 1996), and the GLIMMIX macro, described in Littell *et al* (1996). Both of these are very useful and promising additions to the existing software collection.

Motivated by the above discussion we have restricted the scope of this book to linear mixed models for continuous outcomes. Fahrmeir and Tutz (1994) discuss generalized linear (mixed) models for multivariate outcomes, while longitudinal versions are treated in Diggle, Liang, and Zeger (1994). Nonlinear models for repeated measurement data are discussed by Davidian and Giltinan (1995).

The second chapter of this book provides a gentle introduction to statistical inference for mixed models by means of five typical applications, which are described in Section 2.1. Selected models are given and their components (fixed effects, random effects, and variance-covariance parameters) are spelled out explicitly. First, a pharmaceutical quality control example is used to contrast a fixed-effects and a random-effects ANOVA model. The second example is concerned with the effect of a blood pressure lowering drug. Since this study was conducted in 9 different countries, an appropriate model should allow for country effect. Thus, the use of random-effects ideas to analyze multicenter studies in a broad sense is exemplified. Next, the potential of the linear mixed model to analyze cross-over trials is explored by means of a simple two-period two-treatment design. The classical fixed effects such as the overall mean, treatment effect, and period effect, are supplemented with a random patient effect. The fourth example consists of longitudinal data previously studied by Potthof and Roy (1964) and Jennrich and Schluchter (1986). By means of these data, the *time* dimension is introduced, which distinguishes longitudinal data from other applications of the ANOVA, clustered, or spatial data type. The final set of data, the cell proliferation data, includes three sources of variability: a stratum effect, a sub-stratum effect, and finally measurement error due to replication within each sub-stratum. This particular instance of a designed biological experiment enhances insight in how several error levels can be accommodated. Further, the ideas in these examples can easily be transported to other fields of application. One such example is a survey where nested strata (e.g., state and county effects) are of potential interest.

In Section 2.2, the proposed models are expressed in matrix form. For several cases, the matrices involved are spelled out explicitly. It is also shown how different but equivalent parameterizations can be used and how progress is still possible, even if such a parameterization is overspecified.

The parameters in mixed models include variance components and fixed-effects parameters. By means of a couple of well-known examples (a univariate normal sample with unknown mean and variance, and the classical one-way ANOVA model) it is illustrated how conventional maximum likelihood fails to provide an unbiased variance component estimator. In these simple cases, a bias correction is straightforward and intimately linked to estimation of the mean parameters. The so-obtained unbiased estimators, which can also be derived from standard least squares and ANOVA principles, are then reformulated in order to introduce *error contrasts*, a fundamental concept in the definition of *restricted maximum likelihood* (REML). As such, Section 2.3.1 facilitates the more formal REML discussion of Section 3.4.3. It is clear that variance components, while important, do not tell the full story behind random effects, since one may be interested in estimating the individual random effects, rather than merely the associated variance components. To this end, best linear unbiased prediction is discussed in Section 2.3.2. These ideas are taken up, from a more rigorous Bayesian perspective, in Section 3.11.

Section 2.4 is devoted to an informal, example-based treatment of inference for fixed effects. A more systematic overview of the principal ideas is given in Appendix A. Several issues, related to the occurrence of unknown variance-covariance parameters in the estimator for the fixed effects are discussed. These include the choice of approximate t- and F-distributions, with appropriate degrees of freedom. Several worked examples are given, in which point and interval estimation, as well as hypothesis testing is treated. By means of these examples, the reader is given a feel for how the Satterthwaite degrees of freedom approximation works. In both Sections 2.3 and 2.4, the SAS procedure MIXED is exemplified by means of the pharmaceutical quality control and the cell proliferation data.

To further illustrate the concepts introduced so far, the concluding Section

2.5 presents more elaborate data analyses for three examples of Section 2.1: the cell proliferation data, the cross-over experiment, and the multi-centric blood pressure reduction trial.

Chapter 3 is devoted to the analysis of longitudinal data from an applied point of view. A study of the natural history of prostate disease, introduced in Section 3.2, will be used throughout the chapter. These data consist of repeated measures of prostate specific antigen in men with prostate cancer, benign prostatic hyperplasia, or no evidence at all of prostate disease. The highly unbalanced character of the data set and the presence of multiple diagnostic classes makes it sufficiently versatile to illustrate a wide range of aspects of good modeling practice.

Laird and Ware (1982) present a two-stage formulation, which is particularly useful to provide intuition into the linear mixed model. In contrast to these authors, who merely use this formulation to develop the general linear mixed model theory, we borrow these ideas in Section 3.3 to explicitly perform a two-stage analysis of the prostate cancer data. The first stage summarizes individual profiles in terms of their proper regression coefficients. In the second stage, regression models are fitted to these subject-specific quantities, leading to population averaged parameters such as age or diagnostic group effects.

Section 3.4 contains a formal definition of the general class of linear mixed models. Maximum likelihood and restricted maximum likelihood are discussed and insight is given in the differences and similarities between both approaches. Several model fitting techniques are reviewed. In Section 3.5 the model corresponding to the two-stage analysis of Section 3.3 is fitted with the SAS procedure MIXED. By means of this worked example, we discuss most aspects of fitting linear mixed models in SAS to longitudinal data. The program as well as the output are discussed in full detail.

In principle, the SAS procedure MIXED uses distinct statements to specify random-effects models (the RANDOM statement) and marginal models (the REPEATED statement). However, the aforementioned connection between a random-intercepts model and a (marginal) compound symmetry model is taken up in Section 3.6 to illustrate that in many situations the use of these two statements is not without ambiguity.

In Section 3.7, the techniques for fixed-effects parameter estimation and testing of general linear hypotheses, described in Appendix A, are illustrated in the context of longitudinal data by means of the prostate cancer study. Emphasis is placed on the parameterization of the marginal mean structure, and its implications for the interpretation of the parameter estimates and resulting hypothesis tests. Some repeated measures analyses can be obtained with both PROC GLM and PROC MIXED. In Section

3.8 the relative merits of both procedures are contrasted.

Random effects describe how subject-specific profiles deviate systematically from the average profile. In order to obtain a clear picture of how random effects might be operating it is important to first find a parsimonious description of the random-effects structure. Technically, this involves testing for variance components. In Section 3.9 it is shown that testing for the need of random effects cannot be based on standard asymptotic testing theory since the null hypotheses lie on the boundary of the parameter space. Hence, an alternative, more complicated testing framework has to be adopted.

While testing for the need of random effects comes down to comparing *nested* covariance structures, situations can be envisaged where the comparison between non-nested covariance matrices is required. Section 3.10 describes some informal information criteria that have been proposed in the statistical literature and included in PROC MIXED.

If belief is granted to the selected random-effects structure, it might be of interest to estimate the subject-specific profiles. Since this involves the estimation of the *random* effects, it is most natural to adopt Bayesian techniques. The use and interpretation of the so-called *empirical Bayes* estimators is presented in Section 3.11.

A linear mixed model requires not only the specification of an adequate mean structure, but also the description of a covariance structure which can involve the three components of variability previously discussed. Misspecifying the mean structure will affect the covariance structure and vice versa. Therefore, in Section 3.12 some guidelines are offered which will aid the practicing statistician to streamline model selection.

When a candidate model has been selected, it is desirable to assess the quality of the fit. Even though a whole battery of model checking and diagnostic tools is available for classical multiple regression of which the linear mixed model is an extension, these techniques do not carry over in a straightforward fashion. An overview of recent developments in this area, illustrated by means of the prostate cancer data, is given in Section 3.13. These include an assessment of the distributional assumptions for the random effects, the detection of influential subjects, and a check on the residual covariance structure. For some of these tools, SAS macros have been developed which are available from the Web page listed in the Preface.

The linear mixed models methodology is applied to four longitudinal case studies in Chapter 4. The first three examples are intended to illustrate the general guidelines of Section 3.12. The first one is an unbalanced data set, drawn from a randomized clinical study. The aim of the study was to investigate the effect of administering an experimental drug (terlipressin) on variceal pressure. In the second example, the evolution of height of twenty school girls is related to their mothers' adulthood height. This set of data is balanced, with 5 measurements for each subject. In the third study a bivariate outcome (systolic and diastolic blood pressure) is measured twice (before and after treatment with captopril) for each participant. The fourth example, introduced already in Section 2.1, is on growth measurements for 11 girls and 16 boys. Specifically, for each subject the distance from the center of the pituitary to the maxillary fissure was recorded at the ages 8, 10, 12, and 14. Little and Rubin (1987) artificially deleted a subset of the measurements to illustrate the use of the EM algorithm. Therefore, this data set allows us to contrast the complete data analysis discussed in Section 4.4 with a number of incomplete data analyses, which will be conducted in Chapter 5.

Chapter 5 considers the ubiquitous problem of missing and incomplete longitudinal data. The main emphasis is on balanced designs, where missing data can be identified without ambiguity. A general missing data framework, mainly due to Rubin (1976) is sketched in Section 5.2. The classical taxonomy of missingness (missing completely at random, missing at random, informative) is reviewed and contrasted with the concept of ignorable non-response. The remainder of the chapter is devoted to various techniques for handling incomplete sets of data, roughly ordered by increasing level of complexity. The growth data introduced in Section 4.4 are used as a running example. Most of the analyses are conducted using the SAS procedure MIXED.

First, several simple methods to analyze incomplete data are discussed, including complete case analysis (Section 5.4), simple forms of imputation (Section 5.5), and available case analysis (Section 5.6). Even though most of these methods have been criticized in the scientific literature for their poor performance, some of them are still commonly used in applied research. A notorious example in this respect is *last observation carried forward*. For this reason we have considered it useful to show how these methods distort the estimation of fixed effects and/or variance-covariance parameters.

It is shown in Section 5.7 that when the missing data are missing at random (MAR), a valid likelihood-based analysis can be obtained using the SAS procedure MIXED, provided scientific interest is restricted to the measurement model. Some cautionary remarks are issued with respect to the way in which incomplete measurement sequences have to be passed to PROC MIXED. Two other methods to maximize an incomplete data likelihood, valid under MAR, are discussed: the EM algorithm (Section 5.9) and multiple imputation (Section 5.10). The latter can be performed using PROC MIXED in combination with an appropriate IML macro. Such a macro is available from the Web page listed in the Preface.

In Section 5.11 it is shown how both PROC MIXED and the OSWALD software (Smith, Robertson, and Diggle 1996) can be used to fit linear mixed models under the MAR assumption. OSWALD has the added advantage of providing means to fit models under the assumption of informative dropout. Such an analysis couples a linear mixed model for the measurement process with a logistic regression model for the dropout process. A balanced data set with dropout is used to exemplify these ideas.

Appendix A is devoted to a systematic overview of some important aspects of inference for fixed effects. In Appendix A.1 estimation is considered while hypothesis testing is treated in Appendix A.2. A short overview of several methods to determine approximate degrees of freedom is given in Appendix A.3, while more detail on Satterthwaite's (1941, 1946) procedure is given in Appendix A.4. Some issues with the use and interpretation of standard errors for covariance parameters, as well as with associated Z-statistics, are discussed in Appendix B. Finally, Appendices C and D contain background material, related to Chapter 2.

2

An Example-Based Tour in Linear Mixed Models

Luc Duchateau
Paul Janssen

2.1 Fixed Effects and Random Effects in Mixed Models

Linear models provide an appropriate framework for studying the relation between a continuous dependent variable (response) and one or more independent variables (factors or covariates). For analysis of variance models an independent variable typically takes as value a *level* of some factor, e.g., the independent variable can be a specific treatment from a given number of possible treatments. We therefore could think about the independent variable as a discrete variable. For regression models we typically interpret the covariate as a continuous variable. In this chapter the focus is on ANOVA models, except for Example 2.4 where we model a linear trend. If interest is restricted to the factor levels included in the study we call the ANOVA model a *fixed*-effects model. In many situations however the factor levels in the study can be considered as randomly selected from a population of all possible factor levels. If all factors in the model have this interpretation we call the ANOVA model a *random*-effects model. If some factors are fixed and other factors are random we say that the ANOVA model is a *mixed*-effects model. For fixed-, random-, and mixed-effects models we assume that the relation between the dependent variable and the factors is linear in the parameters. This collection of models is referred to as the class of general linear mixed models. Such models are extremely relevant in applied statistics. Applications in clinical trials, agriculture, economy, ... are numerous. Before we give a formal description of general linear mixed models we discuss in more detail the difference between fixed and random effects. Our discussion will be example-based. In statistical analysis fixed and random effects are handled in a different way, therefore a clear understanding of differences and similarities is needed for good modeling practice.

TABLE 2.1. *The concentration of active substance of antibiotic.*

BATCH							
1	2	3	4	5	6	7	8
40	33	46	55	63	35	56	34
42	34	47	52	59	38	56	29

For a fixed-effects factor we assume that there is a finite set of levels, that contains all levels of interest for the study. Let us consider a simple example: a clinical trial is set up to compare a new drug with a standard drug. Also the gender effect is of interest in the trial. We propose a fixed-effects model with 'drug' and 'gender' as the two fixed-effects factors. Each factor has two levels: 'drug' has the levels 'new drug' and 'standard drug'; 'gender' has 'female' and 'male' as levels.

For a random-effects factor we assume that there is an infinite set of levels (a population of levels) and we think about the levels present in the study as a sample from that population. The interest is in drawing inferences that are valid for the complete population of levels. A simple example: in a clinical trial we could think about the hospitals in the study as a sample from a larger population of hospitals and in each of the selected hospitals a drug is compared with a placebo. The appropriate model is a mixed-effects model with 'drug' as fixed-effects factor (two levels) and 'hospital' as random-effects factor.

To illustrate the wide scope of linear mixed models we now give five selected examples.

EXAMPLE 2.1: BATCHES OF ANTIBIOTIC AND QUALITY CONTROL

The efficiency an antibiotic still has after it has been stored for two years is of scientific interest. Eight batches of the drug are selected at random from a population of available batches. From each batch we take a sample of size two. For the sample elements the concentration of the active component is assessed. The concentrations are given in Table 2.1. Based on this experiment we want to determine (to estimate) the (overall) mean concentration. A further question is whether or not the random batch has a significant effect on the variability of the responses. To formalize these objectives we introduce a random-effects model

$$Y_{ij} = \mu + b_i + \varepsilon_{ij}, \tag{2.1}$$

where, for $j = 1, 2$; $i = 1, \ldots, 8$,
    Y_{ij} is the response of observation j in batch i,

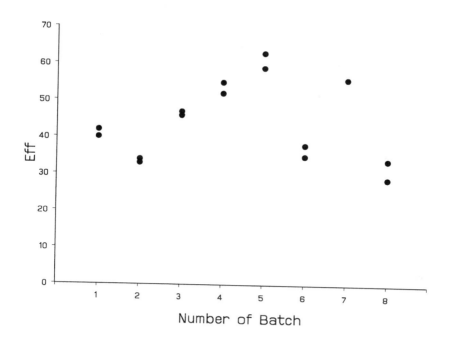

FIGURE 2.1. *The concentration of active substance of antibiotic.*

μ is the overall mean (a fixed parameter),
b_i is the random effect associated with batch i,
ε_{ij} is the random error for observation j in batch i.
The assumptions for the random elements are:
the b_i are i.i.d. $N(0, \sigma_b^2)$,
the ε_{ij} are i.i.d. $N(0, \sigma^2)$,
the b_i and ε_{ij} are independent.
In words: the b_i are independent random variables with common underlying normal distribution having mean zero and variance σ_b^2, etc.

From the model assumptions it is clear that the variability of the response can be expressed in terms of the *variance components* σ_b^2 and σ^2; we have

$$
\begin{aligned}
E(Y_{ij}) &= \mu, \\
\mathrm{Var}(Y_{ij}) &= \sigma_b^2 + \sigma^2.
\end{aligned}
$$

Recall from the above discussion that the study of the overall mean μ and the study of the importance of σ_b^2 are our objectives. To get a better feeling for the variability in the data it is instructive to present Table 2.1 in a graphical way. From Figure 2.1 it is clear that the within batch variability (σ^2) is much smaller than the between batch variability (σ_b^2).

Now assume that the eight batches are the complete stock. In that case the factor batch becomes a fixed effect. We then can use the fixed-effects model

$$Y_{ij} = \mu + \beta_i + \varepsilon_{ij}, \qquad (2.2)$$

where, for $j = 1, 2$; $i = 1, \dots, 8$,

Y_{ij}, μ, ε_{ij} are as in the model given above,
β_i is the main effect parameter for batch i.

We now have

$$
\begin{aligned}
E(Y_{ij}) &= \mu + \beta_i, \\
\operatorname{Var}(Y_{ij}) &= \sigma^2.
\end{aligned}
$$

This is quite different from the random-effects model considered above. Now each batch has its specific mean and the only source of variability comes from the random error.

This simple example provides a good illustration of how statistical modeling is determined by the interpretation of batch as either a random or a fixed effect.

EXAMPLE 2.2: DRUG EFFECT ON BLOOD PRESSURE

In a small study a new drug to decrease blood pressure has been proven to be effective. In a next phase the drug has been tested on a larger scale. Nine different countries have taken part in the trial. We consider the nine countries in the study as a random selection from the set of all possible countries. For each country a group of individuals (eligible for the trial) was available. There were different group sizes for different countries. In each group, each person is randomly assigned to drug or placebo. The response variable (=difbp) is the measurement of **difference** in **blood pressure** before and after treatment. The main objective of the study is to see whether the conclusions of the small study can be confirmed. In this study the treatment (drug or placebo) is a fixed effect and the country is a random effect. The data are given in Table 2.2 and they are represented graphically in Figure 2.2 (note that country is a nominal categorical variable, i.e., the ordering on the horizontal axis has no physical meaning).

A possible statistical model for this experiment is the following mixed-effects model

$$Y_{ijk} = \mu + \tau_i + c_j + \varepsilon_{ijk}, \qquad (2.3)$$

where, for $k = 1, \dots, n_{ij}$; $j = 1, \dots, 9$; $i = 1, 2$,

Y_{ijk} is the difbp of person k assigned to treatment i and from country j,

TABLE 2.2. *Drug effect on blood pressure.*

COUNTRY	TREATMENT	DIFBP (= difference in blood pressure)							
Australia	drug	44	5	17	17	40	39	22	11
		75	12						
(A)	placebo	61	23	5	14	-4	15		
Belgium	drug	52	-23	26	1	50	58	36	52
(B)	placebo	51	-2	32	75	65	37	0	33
Canada	drug	37	21	47	34	14	52	47	34
		43							
(C)	placebo	54	-3	51	40	37	65	10	48
France	drug	34	91	43	56				
(F)	placebo	42	27	37					
Germany	drug	43	0	44	10	0	0	-57	16
(G)		50	10	1	17	47	32		
	placebo	30	68	34	68	28	9	67	0
		18	52						
Great Britain	drug	14	0	19	-6	13	6	64	24
(GB)		42	40	28	0	22	-16	2	39
		56	25						
	placebo	-6	-9	-16	59	21	14	4	16
		32	21	17	54	20			
Korea	drug	47	16	13	83	57	50	80	63
		9	38	49					
(K)	placebo	43	10	6	0	24	42	-16	18
		46	13	-2	51	72			
South Africa	drug	67	33	0	37	46	9	43	64
(SA)		12	80	40	31	35	28	48	44
		42	50	37	19	28	3		
	placebo	19	0	97	38	23	48	46	27
		31	61	37	-1	16	8	21	-6
		68	53	63	13	17			
Sweden	drug	24	31						
(SE)	placebo	2							

μ is the overall mean,

τ_i is the main effect parameter for treatment i,

c_j is the random effect of country j,

ε_{ijk} is the random error of person k assigned to treatment i and from country j.

The assumptions for the random elements are

the c_j are i.i.d. $N(0, \sigma_c^2)$,

the ε_{ijk} are i.i.d. $N(0, \sigma^2)$,

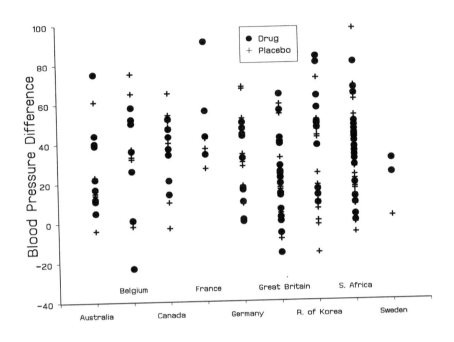

FIGURE 2.2. *Drug effect on blood pressure.*

the c_j and ε_{ijk} are independent.

Relevant questions for this study include the comparison of $\mu + \tau_1$ and $\mu + \tau_2$, i.e., a comparison of the mean difbp for drug and placebo; and the study of σ_c^2, i.e., the variability in the response induced by the countries. In Section 2.5 we consider in detail more general models for this multicenter trial.

EXAMPLE 2.3: A CROSS-OVER EXPERIMENT

In a small study, two drugs A and B are compared for their effect on the diastolic blood pressure (dbp). Each patient in the study receives the two treatments in a random order and separated in time so that one treatment does not influence the blood pressure measurement obtained after administering the other treatment (i.e., to rule out carry-over effect). In this experiment, the patient effect is random and the treatment effect is fixed. The data are given in Table 2.3. Note that Patient #4 has only the measurement for drug A and that Patient #16 has only the measurement for B. It can be seen (Figure 2.3) that after the application of drug A the

TABLE 2.3. *The diastolic blood pressure (DBP) data.*

Patient	Period			
	1		2	
	Drug	DBP	Drug	DBP
1	A	100	B	112
2	B	116	A	114
3	A	108	B	110
4	B	.	A	104
5	B	114	A	114
6	A	98	B	116
7	B	102	A	100
8	A	96	B	103
9	A	92	B	89
10	B	103	A	96
11	B	116	A	78
12	A	127	B	131
13	A	129	B	124
14	A	106	B	128
15	B	133	A	118
16	A	.	B	108
17	A	91	B	109
18	B	113	A	98
19	B	118	A	112

diastolic blood pressure is lower than after the application of drug B for almost all the patients (except Patients #9 and #13). This within patient comparison of the two drugs is exactly the type of comparison that should be made in a cross-over trial. Also note that for Patients #4 and #16 no such within comparison can be made. It will be shown however, when we revisit this example in Section 2.4, that the data for these two patients contribute information to the statistical analysis.

A possible model for this data set is

$$Y_{ijk} = \mu + \tau_i + \pi_j + p_k + \varepsilon_{ijk}, \qquad (2.4)$$

where, for $k = 1, \ldots, 19$; $j = 1, 2$; $i = 1, 2$,

Y_{ijk} is the dbp for patient k assigned to drug i in period j,

μ is the overall mean,

τ_i is the main effect parameter of treatment i,

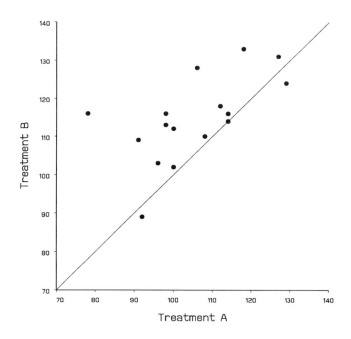

FIGURE 2.3. *The diastolic blood pressure data.*

π_j is the main effect parameter of period j,

p_k is the random error for patient k,

ε_{ijk} is the random error for patient k assigned to drug i in period j.

The assumptions for the random elements are

the p_k are i.i.d. $N(0, \sigma_p^2)$,

the ε_{ijk} are i.i.d. $N(0, \sigma^2)$,

the p_k and ε_{ijk} are independent.

Relevant questions include the study of $\tau_1 - \tau_2$ (the comparison of the mean responses of the two drugs); and the study of σ_p^2, i.e., the variability due to the random selection of the patient. In Section 2.5.2 we discuss how the model can be fitted to this set of data, while a simplified version is considered in Section 2.4.1.

EXAMPLE 2.4: GROWTH DATA

The Potthof and Roy (1964) data set contains growth measurements for 16 boys and 11 girls. For each subject the distance from the center of the pituitary to the maxillary fissure was recorded at the ages 8, 10, 12, and 14. The complete data set is given in Table 4.11 of Section 4.4, where the data are modeled in detail. Here, we propose a model that postulates, within each sex group a linear trend in the growth-time relation. We consider two alternative model specifications.

MODEL REPRESENTATION 1

$$Y_{ijk} = \beta_{i0} + \beta_{i1}t_j + c_{ik} + \varepsilon_{ijk}, \tag{2.5}$$

where $j = 1, \ldots, 4$ for each (i, k) with $k = 1, \ldots, n_i$ and $i = 1, 2$. The index i is the gender index ($i = 1$ for boys and $i = 2$ for girls); $t_1 = 8$, $t_2 = 10$, $t_3 = 12$ and $t_4 = 14$ and k is the subject index. Further, $n_1 = 16$ and $n_2 = 11$. The meaning of the model elements is as follows:

Y_{ijk} is the distance of interest for child k in sex group i at time t_j,
β_{i0} is the intercept for the linear trend for gender i,
β_{i1} is the slope for the linear trend for gender i,
c_{ik} is the random effect of child k in sex group i,
ε_{ijk} is the random error for child k in sex group i at time t_j.

The assumptions for the random elements are:

the c_{ik} are i.i.d. $N(0, \sigma_c^2)$,
the ε_{ijk} are i.i.d. $N(0, \sigma^2)$,
the c_{ik} and ε_{ijk} are independent.

From this model structure it follows that

$$\text{Var}(Y_{ijk}) = \text{Var}(c_k) + \text{Var}(\varepsilon_{ijk}) = \sigma_c^2 + \sigma^2,$$
$$\text{Cov}(Y_{ijk}, Y_{ij'k}) = \text{Var}(c_k) = \sigma_c^2,$$
$$\text{Cov}(Y_{ijk}, Y_{i'j'k'}) = 0 \qquad \text{for } i \neq i',$$
$$\text{Cov}(Y_{ijk}, Y_{ij'k'}) = 0 \qquad \text{for } k \neq k'.$$

The variance-covariance matrix for $\boldsymbol{Y}_{ik} = (Y_{i1k}, Y_{i2k}, Y_{i3k}, Y_{i4k})'$, therefore has the compound symmetry structure

$$\sigma^2 I_4 + \sigma_c^2 J_4 = \begin{pmatrix} \sigma^2 + \sigma_c^2 & \sigma_c^2 & \sigma_c^2 & \sigma_c^2 \\ \sigma_c^2 & \sigma^2 + \sigma_c^2 & \sigma_c^2 & \sigma_c^2 \\ \sigma_c^2 & \sigma_c^2 & \sigma^2 + \sigma_c^2 & \sigma_c^2 \\ \sigma_c^2 & \sigma_c^2 & \sigma_c^2 & \sigma^2 + \sigma_c^2 \end{pmatrix}.$$

Here I_4 is the (4×4) identity matrix and J_4 is the (4×4) matrix with all entries equal to one.

MODEL REPRESENTATION 2

An alternative model representation is given by

$$Y_{ijk} = \beta_{i0} + \beta_{i1}t_j + \varepsilon_{ijk},$$

where Y_{ijk}, β_{i0}, β_{i1} and t_j are as in Model Representation 1 and where ε_{ijk} is the random error for child k in sex group i at time t_j.

The within-subject dependencies, described in Model Representation 1 by the random-effects factor c_{ik}, are now modeled by specifying a more complex variance-covariance matrix for $\boldsymbol{\varepsilon}_{ik}$, with $\boldsymbol{\varepsilon}'_{ik} = (\varepsilon_{i1k}, \varepsilon_{i2k}, \varepsilon_{i3k}, \varepsilon_{i4k})$. To model a (common) intra-individual correlation it is natural to assume that

$$\boldsymbol{\varepsilon}_{ik} \sim N(\mathbf{0}, \sigma^2 I_4 + \sigma_c^2 J_4).$$

The specific feature of this approach is that modeling the association structure is done directly in terms of the variance-covariance matrix of $\boldsymbol{\varepsilon}_{ik}$.

For the data set in this example alternative variance-covariance structures are considered in Section 4.4. In that discussion, the compound symmetry structure considered here is referred to as Model 7. A possible advantage of Model Representation 1 is that one can think in terms of random effects rather than in terms of the structure of the variance-covariance matrix of the vector of random errors (as in Model Representation 2).

EXAMPLE 2.5: DRUG AND GROWTH STIMULATOR EFFECT ON CELL PROLIFERATION

Two drugs, A and B, are tested in vitro for their ability to enhance cell proliferation. The ability is tested in the presence and absence of a growth stimulating factor (gsf+ and gsf−). The factor combinations for the factor 'gsf' and the factor 'drug' are (gsf−, A), (gsf+, A), (gsf−, B) and (gsf+, B). The experiment is set up in the following way. Nine plates are used for the experiment. The plates are randomly selected from a population of plates. Each plate has two compartments and each compartment has two wells. We first assign in a random way gsf+ and gsf− to the two compartments of a given plate. Within a compartment the drugs A and B are randomly assigned to the two wells. The structure of the design is summarized in Figure 2.4. All wells contain a cell culture with a fixed number of cells. For each plate we have that, according to the design described above, each factor combination is assigned to a well. The response is the number of cells in the well after a specified period of time. For the statistical analysis we use as response the logarithm of the number of cells. This logarithmic transformation removes skewness present in the original data. The relevant

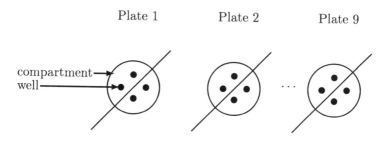

FIGURE 2.4. *The design of the cell proliferation experiment.*

issues here are the comparison of the two drugs (A and B) and the study of the effect of the presence or absence of the growth stimulating factor. The data are given in Table 2.4 and graphically presented in Figure 2.5.

A possible model can be written as

$$Y_{ijk} = \mu + \alpha_i + \beta_j + (\alpha\beta)_{ij} + p_k + c_{ik} + \varepsilon_{ijk}, \qquad (2.6)$$

where, for $k = 1, \ldots 9$, $j = 1, 2$; $i = 1, 2$,

Y_{ijk} is the logarithm of the cell count for well j in compartment i of plate k,

μ is the overall mean,

α_i is the main effect parameter for gsf i,

β_j is the main effect parameter for drug j,

$(\alpha\beta)_{ij}$ is an interaction parameter,

p_k is the random effect of plate k,

c_{ik} is the random effect of compartment i within plate k,

ε_{ijk} is the random error for well j in compartment i of plate k.

The assumptions for the random elements are

the p_k are i.i.d. $N(0, \sigma_p^2)$,

the c_{ik} are i.i.d. $N(0, \sigma_c^2)$,

the ε_{ijk} are i.i.d. $N(0, \sigma^2)$,

the p_k, c_{ik} and ε_{ijk} are independent.

A better understanding for this model can be obtained from Table 2.9 on page 43, where we explain the design structure of this experiment.

Note that gsf− corresponds to $i = 1$ and gsf+ to $i = 2$. Drug A corresponds to $j = 1$ and drug B to $j = 2$.

TABLE 2.4. *The cell proliferation data.*

plate	gsf = (growth stimulating factor)			
	no		yes	
	drug A	drug B	drug A	drug B
1	887	878	2133	2012
2	1022	1051	2313	2023
3	1271	1302	2838	2432
4	1943	1969	3423	3455
5	1804	1858	3968	4018
6	1550	1681	4185	3425
7	1802	1829	3542	4052
8	1549	2001	4196	4136
9	1781	1972	4507	5014

2.2   General Linear Mixed Models

Before we define general linear mixed models we recall the definition of general linear models. Any fixed-effects model that is linear in the parameters is called a general linear model. A formal definition is

$$Y = X\beta + \varepsilon, \tag{2.7}$$

where

Y is the vector that contains the responses,
X is a known matrix (design matrix, incidence matrix),
β is the vector that contains the overall mean and all the fixed effects (main effects and interactions) parameters,
ε is the vector that contains the random errors.

We assume that ε follows an N-variate normal distribution (N is the total number of observations) with zero-mean vector and variance-covariance matrix $\sigma^2 I_N$, i.e., $\varepsilon \sim N(0, \sigma^2 I_N)$. Note that this assumption is equivalent to the assumption that the components ε_i are i.i.d. $N(0, \sigma^2)$, $i = 1, \ldots, N$.

The SAS procedure GLM provides statistical inference for this type of models (in this chapter we restrict attention to univariate response models, PROC GLM is also suitable for models with multivariate responses). A comparison of the procedures GLM and MIXED is given in Section 3.8.

From the discussion in Section 2.1 it is clear that many practical examples do not fit into the general linear model framework. The main problem is that this model allows only one source of randomness (the random er-

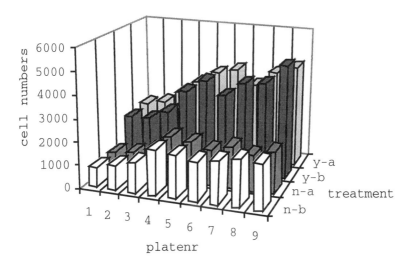

FIGURE 2.5. *The cell proliferation data.*

ror term). General linear mixed models remove this restriction. A formal definition is

$$Y = X\beta + Zb + \varepsilon, \tag{2.8}$$

with

Y, X, β, and ε as in the general linear model,
Z is a known matrix (the design or incidence matrix for the random effects),
b is the vector that contains all the random-effects variables,

and

$$\begin{pmatrix} b \\ \varepsilon \end{pmatrix} \sim N\left(\begin{pmatrix} 0 \\ 0 \end{pmatrix}, \begin{pmatrix} D & 0 \\ 0 & \Sigma \end{pmatrix} \right).$$

From this assumption it follows that the variance-covariance matrices of b and ε are given by

$$D(b) = \mathrm{Var}(b) = D,$$
$$D(\varepsilon) = \mathrm{Var}(\varepsilon) = \Sigma.$$

The assumption also implies that b and ε are independent, i.e., we assume independence between the random errors and the random effects. All examples in Section 2.1, except Model 2 in Example 2.4, have $\Sigma = \sigma^2 I_N$. In later chapters, examples with more general form for Σ will be considered. Finally note that

$$V = \mathrm{Var}(Y) = ZDZ' + \Sigma. \tag{2.9}$$

Observe that Model (2.8) collects all the measurements of all subjects into a single vector Y, whereas the models in the examples of Section 2.1, such as (2.1), (2.3), (2.4), (2.5), and (2.6) are presented for all measurements separately. A similar statement holds for the design matrices X and Z, the vector b of random effects, and the vector ε of errors. This implies that Model (2.8) can be presented without subscripts, while the earlier ones had subscripts for subjects as well as for within-subject measurements. In Section 3.4.1 an intermediate system of notation is introduced and subsequently followed. In that system, all measurements pertaining to a particular subject are grouped into a single vector indexed by i. This convention, customary in longitudinal modeling, is in contrast with the current ANOVA-type notation where the last index refers to individual replication.

The statistical analysis for general linear mixed models can be obtained from the SAS procedure MIXED. In Littell *et al* (1996) a general discussion on PROC MIXED is given, which includes a variety of applications. The further sections of this chapter will provide a short review of basic statistical tools used for general linear mixed models. We follow an example-based approach to introduce ideas on mixed models, and use Searle, Casella, and McCulloch (1992) as a basic reference for the theoretical background (especially in Sections 2.3 and 2.4).

To get a good feeling for the matrix notation in general linear mixed modeling we will revisit three examples from Section 2.1. For these examples we will specify (by enumeration *and* by using compact matrix notation) the incidence matrices X and Z, the vector $\boldsymbol{\beta}$ containing the fixed effects, the vector b containing the random effects, the vector of observations (Y) and the vector of random errors (ε). We will also provide information on the specific form of V.

EXAMPLE 2.6: BATCHES OF ANTIBIOTIC AND QUALITY CONTROL

We first revisit Example 2.1. In this example we introduced, for batches randomly selected from a population of batches, the random-effects model (2.1) and, for a specific set of batches, we proposed the fixed-effects model (2.2). The fixed-effects model is of form $Y = X\boldsymbol{\beta} + \varepsilon$ with $\boldsymbol{\beta} = (\mu, \beta_1, \ldots, \beta_8)'$. A matrix representation for this model is given in Table 2.5. Note that the first column of the design matrix X can be obtained by summing all the other columns. From this remark it is immediate that X is not of full rank. The intrinsic reason for this fact is that, by introducing the overall mean μ and the eights main effects $\beta_1, \ldots, \beta_8$, we overparameterized the model. The natural number of parameters equals the number of cell means and therefore is eight. Thinking in terms of cell means $\mu_i = E(Y_{ij})$, $i = 1, \ldots, 8$, we can consider the cell means model for which the matrix representation

TABLE 2.5. Matrix representations for the (overparameterized) fixed-effects Model (2.2).

$$
\begin{pmatrix}
Y_{11} \\ Y_{12} \\ Y_{21} \\ Y_{22} \\ Y_{31} \\ Y_{32} \\ Y_{41} \\ Y_{42} \\ Y_{51} \\ Y_{52} \\ Y_{61} \\ Y_{62} \\ Y_{71} \\ Y_{72} \\ Y_{81} \\ Y_{82}
\end{pmatrix}
=
\begin{pmatrix}
1 & 1 & 0 & 0 & 0 & 0 & 0 & 0 & 0 \\
1 & 1 & 0 & 0 & 0 & 0 & 0 & 0 & 0 \\
1 & 0 & 1 & 0 & 0 & 0 & 0 & 0 & 0 \\
1 & 0 & 1 & 0 & 0 & 0 & 0 & 0 & 0 \\
1 & 0 & 0 & 1 & 0 & 0 & 0 & 0 & 0 \\
1 & 0 & 0 & 1 & 0 & 0 & 0 & 0 & 0 \\
1 & 0 & 0 & 0 & 1 & 0 & 0 & 0 & 0 \\
1 & 0 & 0 & 0 & 1 & 0 & 0 & 0 & 0 \\
1 & 0 & 0 & 0 & 0 & 1 & 0 & 0 & 0 \\
1 & 0 & 0 & 0 & 0 & 1 & 0 & 0 & 0 \\
1 & 0 & 0 & 0 & 0 & 0 & 1 & 0 & 0 \\
1 & 0 & 0 & 0 & 0 & 0 & 1 & 0 & 0 \\
1 & 0 & 0 & 0 & 0 & 0 & 0 & 1 & 0 \\
1 & 0 & 0 & 0 & 0 & 0 & 0 & 1 & 0 \\
1 & 0 & 0 & 0 & 0 & 0 & 0 & 0 & 1 \\
1 & 0 & 0 & 0 & 0 & 0 & 0 & 0 & 1
\end{pmatrix}
\begin{pmatrix}
\mu \\ \beta_1 \\ \beta_2 \\ \beta_3 \\ \beta_4 \\ \beta_5 \\ \beta_6 \\ \beta_7 \\ \beta_8
\end{pmatrix}
+
\begin{pmatrix}
\varepsilon_{11} \\ \varepsilon_{12} \\ \varepsilon_{21} \\ \varepsilon_{22} \\ \varepsilon_{31} \\ \varepsilon_{32} \\ \varepsilon_{41} \\ \varepsilon_{42} \\ \varepsilon_{51} \\ \varepsilon_{52} \\ \varepsilon_{61} \\ \varepsilon_{62} \\ \varepsilon_{71} \\ \varepsilon_{72} \\ \varepsilon_{81} \\ \varepsilon_{82}
\end{pmatrix}
$$

TABLE 2.6. Matrix representation for the fixed-effects Model (2.2), rewritten in terms of the cell means.

$$
\begin{pmatrix}
Y_{11} \\ Y_{12} \\ Y_{21} \\ Y_{22} \\ Y_{31} \\ Y_{32} \\ Y_{41} \\ Y_{42} \\ Y_{51} \\ Y_{52} \\ Y_{61} \\ Y_{62} \\ Y_{71} \\ Y_{72} \\ Y_{81} \\ Y_{82}
\end{pmatrix}
=
\begin{pmatrix}
1 & 0 & 0 & 0 & 0 & 0 & 0 & 0 \\
1 & 0 & 0 & 0 & 0 & 0 & 0 & 0 \\
0 & 1 & 0 & 0 & 0 & 0 & 0 & 0 \\
0 & 1 & 0 & 0 & 0 & 0 & 0 & 0 \\
0 & 0 & 1 & 0 & 0 & 0 & 0 & 0 \\
0 & 0 & 1 & 0 & 0 & 0 & 0 & 0 \\
0 & 0 & 0 & 1 & 0 & 0 & 0 & 0 \\
0 & 0 & 0 & 1 & 0 & 0 & 0 & 0 \\
0 & 0 & 0 & 0 & 1 & 0 & 0 & 0 \\
0 & 0 & 0 & 0 & 1 & 0 & 0 & 0 \\
0 & 0 & 0 & 0 & 0 & 1 & 0 & 0 \\
0 & 0 & 0 & 0 & 0 & 1 & 0 & 0 \\
0 & 0 & 0 & 0 & 0 & 0 & 1 & 0 \\
0 & 0 & 0 & 0 & 0 & 0 & 1 & 0 \\
0 & 0 & 0 & 0 & 0 & 0 & 0 & 1 \\
0 & 0 & 0 & 0 & 0 & 0 & 0 & 1
\end{pmatrix}
\begin{pmatrix}
\mu_1 \\ \mu_2 \\ \mu_3 \\ \mu_4 \\ \mu_5 \\ \mu_6 \\ \mu_7 \\ \mu_8
\end{pmatrix}
+
\begin{pmatrix}
\varepsilon_{11} \\ \varepsilon_{12} \\ \varepsilon_{21} \\ \varepsilon_{22} \\ \varepsilon_{31} \\ \varepsilon_{32} \\ \varepsilon_{41} \\ \varepsilon_{42} \\ \varepsilon_{51} \\ \varepsilon_{52} \\ \varepsilon_{61} \\ \varepsilon_{62} \\ \varepsilon_{71} \\ \varepsilon_{72} \\ \varepsilon_{81} \\ \varepsilon_{82}
\end{pmatrix}
$$

TABLE 2.7. Matrix representation for the random-effects Model (2.1).

$$
\begin{pmatrix} Y_{11} \\ Y_{12} \\ Y_{21} \\ Y_{22} \\ Y_{31} \\ Y_{32} \\ Y_{41} \\ Y_{42} \\ Y_{51} \\ Y_{52} \\ Y_{61} \\ Y_{62} \\ Y_{71} \\ Y_{72} \\ Y_{81} \\ Y_{82} \end{pmatrix}
=
\begin{pmatrix} 1 \\ 1 \\ 1 \\ 1 \\ 1 \\ 1 \\ 1 \\ 1 \\ 1 \\ 1 \\ 1 \\ 1 \\ 1 \\ 1 \\ 1 \\ 1 \end{pmatrix}
\mu +
\begin{pmatrix}
1 & 0 & 0 & 0 & 0 & 0 & 0 & 0 \\
1 & 0 & 0 & 0 & 0 & 0 & 0 & 0 \\
0 & 1 & 0 & 0 & 0 & 0 & 0 & 0 \\
0 & 1 & 0 & 0 & 0 & 0 & 0 & 0 \\
0 & 0 & 1 & 0 & 0 & 0 & 0 & 0 \\
0 & 0 & 1 & 0 & 0 & 0 & 0 & 0 \\
0 & 0 & 0 & 1 & 0 & 0 & 0 & 0 \\
0 & 0 & 0 & 1 & 0 & 0 & 0 & 0 \\
0 & 0 & 0 & 0 & 1 & 0 & 0 & 0 \\
0 & 0 & 0 & 0 & 1 & 0 & 0 & 0 \\
0 & 0 & 0 & 0 & 0 & 1 & 0 & 0 \\
0 & 0 & 0 & 0 & 0 & 1 & 0 & 0 \\
0 & 0 & 0 & 0 & 0 & 0 & 1 & 0 \\
0 & 0 & 0 & 0 & 0 & 0 & 1 & 0 \\
0 & 0 & 0 & 0 & 0 & 0 & 0 & 1 \\
0 & 0 & 0 & 0 & 0 & 0 & 0 & 1
\end{pmatrix}
\begin{pmatrix} b_1 \\ b_2 \\ b_3 \\ b_4 \\ b_5 \\ b_6 \\ b_7 \\ b_8 \end{pmatrix}
+
\begin{pmatrix} \varepsilon_{11} \\ \varepsilon_{12} \\ \varepsilon_{21} \\ \varepsilon_{22} \\ \varepsilon_{31} \\ \varepsilon_{32} \\ \varepsilon_{41} \\ \varepsilon_{42} \\ \varepsilon_{51} \\ \varepsilon_{52} \\ \varepsilon_{61} \\ \varepsilon_{62} \\ \varepsilon_{71} \\ \varepsilon_{72} \\ \varepsilon_{81} \\ \varepsilon_{82} \end{pmatrix}
$$

is given in Table 2.6.

This representation is also of form $Y = X\beta + \varepsilon$ with $\beta = (\mu_1, \ldots, \mu_8)'$. Note that the design matrix for the cell means model has full rank ($\text{rank}(X) = 8$).

The random-effects model is of form (2.8) since it can be rewritten, in matrix notation, as in Table 2.7. Note that for the random-effects model the X matrix is the vector $\mathbf{1}_{16}$ ($\mathbf{1}_n$ denotes the $(n \times 1)$ vector with all entries equal to one) and the variance-covariance matrix V can be written as

$$
\begin{aligned}
V &= ZDZ' + \Sigma \\
&= \sigma_b^2(I_8 \otimes J_2) + \sigma^2 I_{16} \\
&= I_8 \otimes (\sigma_b^2 J_2 + \sigma^2 I_2)
\end{aligned}
$$

where J_2 is a (2×2) matrix having all entries 1 and $\otimes$ denotes the direct product.

The *direct product* of an $(r \times c)$ matrix A and an $(s \times d)$ matrix B is the $(rs \times cd)$ matrix

$$
A \otimes B = \begin{pmatrix}
a_{11}B & a_{12}B & \ldots & a_{1c}B \\
a_{21}B & a_{22}B & \ldots & a_{2c}B \\
\vdots & & & \\
a_{r1}B & a_{r2}B & \ldots & a_{rc}B
\end{pmatrix}
$$

Readers interested in a nice introduction on matrix algebra and its use in linear models can read Chapter 5 in Neter *et al* (1996). At the advanced level there is Searle (1982) and an appendix in Searle *et al* (1992).

An elegant structural property of V is that it can be written as a linear combination of two known matrices $(I_8 \otimes J_2)$ and I_{16} with the variance components σ_b^2 and σ^2 as coefficients, i.e., with $V_1 = I_8 \otimes J_2$, $V_2 = I_{16}$, $\phi_1 = \sigma_b^2$ and $\phi_2 = \sigma^2$ we have that

$$V = \phi_1 V_1 + \phi_2 V_2$$

with ϕ_1 and ϕ_2 the unknown variance components.

EXAMPLE 2.7: GROWTH DATA

We refer to Chapter 2 in Searle (1982) for the notion of partitioned matrices. We can write the first model in Example 2.4 as $Y = X\beta + Zb + \varepsilon$ with

$$Y' = (Y'_{11}, \ldots, Y'_{1n_1}, Y'_{21}, \ldots, Y'_{2n_2}),$$

where $Y'_{ik} = (Y_{i1k}, Y_{i2k}, Y_{i3k}, Y_{i4k})$;

$$X' = (X'_{11} | \ldots | X'_{1n_1} | X'_{21} | \ldots | X'_{2n_2}),$$

where, for $k = 1, \ldots, n_1 = 16$,

$$X_{1k} = \begin{pmatrix} 1 & 0 & 8 & 0 \\ 1 & 0 & 10 & 0 \\ 1 & 0 & 12 & 0 \\ 1 & 0 & 14 & 0 \end{pmatrix}$$

and, for $k = 1, \ldots, n_2 = 11$,

$$X_{2k} = \begin{pmatrix} 0 & 1 & 0 & 8 \\ 0 & 1 & 0 & 10 \\ 0 & 1 & 0 & 12 \\ 0 & 1 & 0 & 14 \end{pmatrix};$$

$$\beta = (\beta_{10}, \beta_{20}, \beta_{11}, \beta_{21})';$$
$$Z = I_{27} \otimes \mathbf{1}_4;$$

and

$$b = (c_1, \ldots c_{16}, c_{17}, \ldots, c_{27})',$$

with $c_1, \ldots, c_{16}$ the random effects associated with the boys $(n_1 = 16)$ and $c_{17}, \ldots, c_{27}$ the random effects associated with the girls $(n_2 = 11)$, and

$$\varepsilon' = (\varepsilon_{111}, \varepsilon_{121}, \varepsilon_{131}, \varepsilon_{141}, \ldots, \varepsilon_{21n_2}, \varepsilon_{22n_2}, \varepsilon_{23n_2}, \varepsilon_{24n_2}).$$

From the independence assumptions we easily obtain

$$D(\boldsymbol{b}) = \sigma_c^2 I_{27},$$

$$D(\varepsilon) = \sigma^2 I_{108} = \sigma^2 (I_{27} \otimes I_4),$$

$$\begin{aligned} D(\boldsymbol{Y}) &= ZD(\boldsymbol{b})Z' + D(\varepsilon) \\ &= \sigma_c^2 (I_{27} \otimes J_4) + \sigma^2 (I_{27} \otimes I_4) \\ &= I_{27} \otimes (\sigma_c^2 J_4 + \sigma^2 I_4). \end{aligned}$$

For the second representation in Example 2.4 we have $\boldsymbol{Y} = X\boldsymbol{\beta} + \varepsilon$ with $\boldsymbol{Y}$, X, and $\boldsymbol{\beta}$ as in the first representation and

$$\varepsilon' = (\varepsilon'_{11}, \ldots, \varepsilon'_{1n_1}, \varepsilon'_{21}, \ldots, \varepsilon'_{2n_2}),$$

where

$$\varepsilon'_{ik} = (\varepsilon_{i1k}, \varepsilon_{i2k}, \varepsilon_{i3k}, \varepsilon_{i4k}).$$

We assume independence of the vectors ε_{ik} and

$$\varepsilon_{ik} \sim N(\boldsymbol{0}, \sigma^2 I_4 + \sigma_c^2 J_4).$$

EXAMPLE 2.8: CELL PROLIFERATION

We revisit Example 2.5 on cell proliferation. The data set has 36 observations. The vector $\boldsymbol{\beta}$ has 9 components (one overall mean, two main effects for 'gsf', two main effect for 'drug' and four 'gsf $*$ drug' interaction parameters).

Therefore the incidence matrix X is a (36×9) matrix. The random-effects part of this mixed model has a $\boldsymbol{b}$ vector with 27 components (9 components for the plates and 18 components to describe the compartments), the corresponding Z matrix is a (36×27) matrix. The first 9 columns correspond to the incidence of the plate effects, the last 18 columns correspond to the incidence of the compartment effects. It is important to note that the matrix for the compartment effects can be obtained as the interaction between 'plate' and 'gsf'.

Using direct products it is easy to see that the explicit form is $\boldsymbol{Y} = X\boldsymbol{\beta} + Z\boldsymbol{b} + \varepsilon$ with

$$\begin{aligned} X &= (\boldsymbol{1}_{36} \mid \boldsymbol{1}_9 \otimes I_2 \otimes \boldsymbol{1}_2 \mid \boldsymbol{1}_9 \otimes \boldsymbol{1}_2 \otimes I_2 \mid \boldsymbol{1}_9 \otimes I_2 \otimes I_2) \\ &= (\boldsymbol{1}_{36} \mid X_{\text{gsf}} \mid X_{\text{drug}} \mid X_{\text{gsf}*\text{drug}}), \end{aligned}$$

$$\begin{aligned} Z &= (I_9 \otimes \boldsymbol{1}_2 \otimes \boldsymbol{1}_2 \mid I_9 \otimes I_2 \otimes \boldsymbol{1}_2) \\ &= (Z_{\text{plate}} \mid Z_{\text{plate}*\text{gsf}}), \end{aligned}$$

$$\beta' = (\mu, \alpha_1, \alpha_2, \beta_1, \beta_2, (\alpha\beta)_{11}, (\alpha\beta)_{12}, (\alpha\beta)_{21}, (\alpha\beta)_{22}),$$
$$b' = (p_1, \ldots, p_9, c_{11}, c_{21}, \ldots, c_{19}, c_{29}),$$
$$Y' = (Y_{111}, Y_{121}, Y_{211}, Y_{221}, \ldots, Y_{219}, Y_{229}),$$
$$\varepsilon' = (\varepsilon_{111}, \varepsilon_{121}, \varepsilon_{211}, \varepsilon_{221}, \ldots, \varepsilon_{219}, \varepsilon_{229}).$$

Readers less familiar with this matrix notation can consult the explicit form of the vectors and matrices in $Y = X\beta + Zb + \varepsilon$ in Appendix D.

The variance-covariance matrix V can then be written as

$$
\begin{aligned}
V &= ZDZ' + \Sigma \\
&= \sigma^2_{\text{plate}} Z_{\text{plate}} Z'_{\text{plate}} + \sigma^2_{\text{plate}*\text{gsf}} Z_{\text{plate}*\text{gsf}} Z'_{\text{plate}*\text{gsf}} + \Sigma \\
&= \sigma^2_{\text{plate}}(I_9 \otimes \mathbf{1}_4)(I_9 \otimes \mathbf{1}'_4) + \sigma^2_{\text{plate}*\text{gsf}}(I_{18} \otimes \mathbf{1}_2)(I_{18} \otimes \mathbf{1}'_2) + \sigma^2 I_{36} \\
&= \sigma^2_{\text{plate}}(I_9 \otimes J_4) + \sigma^2_{\text{plate}*\text{gsf}}(I_{18} \otimes J_2) + \sigma^2 I_{36}.
\end{aligned}
$$

Note that, similar to the previous example, we have that V has structure

$$V = \phi_1 V_1 + \phi_2 V_2 + \phi_3 V_3,$$

with $\phi_1 = \sigma^2_{\text{plate}}$, $\phi_2 = \sigma^2_{\text{plate}*\text{gsf}}$ and $\phi_3 = \sigma^2$.

In all three examples the dispersion matrix of Y takes the form

$$V = \sum_{i=1}^{L} \phi_i V_i$$

with ϕ_i, $i = 1, \ldots, L$, a finite number of variance and covariance parameters and V_i known matrices. In these examples we introduce covariance parameters in V via random effects that are independent of the random errors (except for Model 2 in Example 2.4).

A consequence is that we model covariance parameters in terms of variance components of random effects. This way of modeling is somewhat restrictive, since it results in a variance-covariance matrix with covariance entries that are non-negative ($\phi_j \geq 0$, $j = 1, \ldots, L$). The form also excludes more complex correlation structures such as serial correlation. However, for the remainder of this chapter it is not really restrictive to work with a matrix V that is a linear combination of known matrices V_i and variance components ϕ_i as weights, $i = 1, \ldots, L$. A general way to think about V is to see the dispersion matrix as a function of the variance and covariance parameters $\phi_1, \ldots, \phi_L$, i.e., $V \equiv V(\phi_1, \ldots, \phi_L)$. This is consistent with Nelder's (1954) views who observed that negative variance components do exist and are a natural concept if particular observations are negatively correlated with each other. The assumption of non-negative variance components is used as the default for the estimation procedures in PROC MIXED. If necessary the default can be changed by specifying 'nobound' as option in the PARMS statement (see Littell *et al* 1996 for details).

2.3   Variance Components Estimation and Best Linear Unbiased Prediction

2.3.1   Variance Components Estimation

Different methods have been developed to estimate the parameters $\phi_1, \ldots, \phi_L$ in $V(\phi_1, \ldots, \phi_L)$. The Henderson (1953) method, using the expected mean squares approach, and minimum norm quadratic unbiased estimation (MINQUE, Rao 1971a, 1971b) have become very popular.

Nowadays mainly likelihood based methods are used. The default method used in the SAS procedure MIXED is based on a likelihood criterion, vid., restricted maximum likelihood (REML) estimation, which corrects for the well-known downward bias in the classical maximum likelihood estimators of variance components. This extends the concept of classical least squares regression situations where an unbiased estimator of the residual variance is obtained from dividing the error sum of squares by an appropriate number of degrees of freedom.

For example, in the case of a sample $Y_1, \ldots, Y_N$ from a univariate normal distribution with mean μ and variance σ^2, the ML estimator for σ^2 equals

$$\frac{1}{N} \sum_{i=1}^{N} (Y_i - \overline{Y})^2, \tag{2.10}$$

where $\overline{Y}$ is the sample mean. This estimator is biased downward. Indeed, it is well-known that an unbiased estimator is given by the sample variance

$$S^2 = \frac{1}{N-1} \sum_{i=1}^{N} (Y_i - \overline{Y})^2. \tag{2.11}$$

The factor $N-1$ accounts for the loss of one degree of freedom in estimating μ by $\overline{Y}$, which the factor N does not. In Example 2.9 we discuss this simple situation in detail.

A similar phenomenon is seen in standard one-way ANOVA models. To illustrate this, consider Model (2.2) in Example 2.1 where we have $a =$

8 groups with $n = 2$ observations per group. The ML estimator for the residual variance σ^2 equals

$$\frac{\sum\limits_{i=1}^{a} \sum\limits_{j=1}^{n} (Y_{ij} - \overline{Y}_{i.})^2}{N},$$

where $\overline{Y}_{i.}$ is the sample mean in group i and $N = na$ is the total number of observations. In contrast, an unbiased estimator equals

$$\frac{\sum\limits_{i=1}^{a} \sum\limits_{j=1}^{n} (Y_{ij} - \overline{Y}_{i.})^2}{N - a}, \tag{2.12}$$

where we correct for the loss of $a = 8$ degrees of freedom due to the estimation of the within-group means. This case is discussed further in Example 2.10.

EXAMPLE 2.9

Take the situation considered above where $Y_1, \ldots, Y_N$ is a sample from a $N(\mu, \sigma^2)$ distribution. Then, in terms of Model (2.8), $\mathbf{Y} = (Y_1, \ldots, Y_N)'$, $V = \sigma^2 I_N$, $X = \mathbf{1}_N$ (rank$(X) = 1$) and $\boldsymbol{\beta} = \mu$.

In the discussion of residual variance formulae (2.10) and (2.11), it was indicated that the former is biased because it fails to account for one degree of freedom spent in estimating the population mean. On the other hand, if the population mean is known, then the maximum likelihood estimator $\sum_{i=1}^{N}(Y_i - \mu)^2/N$ is unbiased. Hence, the bias in (2.10) is caused by the fact that the mean has to be estimated.

This suggests that the procedure can be made unbiased by ensuring that mean and variance estimation are based on statistically independent information. To this end, note that the sample mean $\overline{Y}$ can be written as

$$\overline{Y} = \left(\frac{1}{N} \ \frac{1}{N} \ \cdots \ \frac{1}{N} \right) \mathbf{Y} = \frac{1}{N} \mathbf{1}_N' \mathbf{Y} = \frac{1}{N} X' \mathbf{Y}. \tag{2.13}$$

Let us now choose $N-1$ additional linear combinations $\mathbf{k}_i' \mathbf{Y}$ ($i = 1, \ldots, N-1$), and group their coefficient vectors $\mathbf{k}_i$ into a $(N \times (N-1))$ matrix K. We impose the requirements that the vectors $\mathbf{k}_i$ are linearly independent (to ensure that no information of the original sample is lost) and that $X'\mathbf{Y}$ and $K'\mathbf{Y}$ are statistically independent (to ensure that mean and variance estimation can be based on independent information). The latter requirement is equivalent with Cov$(K'\mathbf{Y}, X'\mathbf{Y}) = 0$ or $K'X = 0$.

In the current example, $X = \mathbf{1}_N$ and thus the condition is that the vectors $\mathbf{k}_i$ are linearly independent and that the elements of each $\mathbf{k}_i$ have zero sum. One such choice is

$$K' = \begin{pmatrix} 1 - \dfrac{1}{N} & -\dfrac{1}{N} & \cdots & -\dfrac{1}{N} & -\dfrac{1}{N} \\[2mm] -\dfrac{1}{N} & 1 - \dfrac{1}{N} & \cdots & -\dfrac{1}{N} & -\dfrac{1}{N} \\[2mm] \vdots & \vdots & \ddots & \vdots & \vdots \\[2mm] -\dfrac{1}{N} & -\dfrac{1}{N} & \cdots & 1 - \dfrac{1}{N} & -\dfrac{1}{N} \end{pmatrix}$$

$$= \left(I_{N-1} - \dfrac{J_{N-1}}{N} \; \vdots \; -\dfrac{\mathbf{1}_{N-1}}{N} \right).$$

This yields

$$K'\mathbf{Y} = \begin{pmatrix} Y_1 - \overline{Y} \\ Y_2 - \overline{Y} \\ \vdots \\ Y_{N-2} - \overline{Y} \\ Y_{N-1} - \overline{Y} \end{pmatrix}.$$

Another choice is given by so-called pairwise contrasts:

$$K' = \begin{pmatrix} 1 & -1 & 0 & \cdots & 0 & 0 \\ 0 & 1 & -1 & \cdots & 0 & 0 \\ \vdots & \vdots & \vdots & \ddots & \vdots & \vdots \\ 0 & 0 & 0 & \cdots & 1 & -1 \end{pmatrix}$$

yielding

$$K'\mathbf{Y} = \begin{pmatrix} Y_1 - Y_2 \\ Y_2 - Y_3 \\ \vdots \\ Y_{N-2} - Y_{N-1} \\ Y_{N-1} - Y_N \end{pmatrix}.$$

The resulting vector $K'\mathbf{Y}$ of *error contrasts* (Harville 1977) then follows a $N(0, \sigma^2 K'K)$ distribution.

The corresponding log-likelihood function (called restricted log-likelihood) equals

$$\ell_{\text{REML}}(\sigma^2)$$

$$= -\frac{N-1}{2}\log 2\pi - \frac{1}{2}\log|\sigma^2 K'K| - \frac{1}{2}Y'K(\sigma^2 K'K)^{-1}K'Y$$

$$= -\frac{N-1}{2}\log 2\pi - \frac{1}{2}\log|K'K| - \frac{N-1}{2}\log\sigma^2$$

$$-\frac{1}{2}Y'K(\sigma^2 K'K)^{-1}K'Y. \tag{2.14}$$

The likelihood equation is

$$\frac{d\ell_{\mathrm{REML}}(\sigma^2)}{d\sigma^2} \equiv -\frac{1}{2}\left(\frac{N-1}{\sigma^2} - \frac{Y'K(K'K)^{-1}K'Y}{\sigma^4}\right) = 0.$$

The solution of this equation, which is the REML estimator for σ^2, is given by

$$\widehat{\sigma}^2 = \frac{Y'K(K'K)^{-1}K'Y}{N-1}. \tag{2.15}$$

Even though this estimator apparently depends on the non-unique contrast matrix K', one can show that

$$K(K'K)^{-1}K' = I_N - X(X'X)^{-1}X'$$

(see Searle *et al* 1992, p. 452 for details), which in this specific example reduces to

$$I_N - X(X'X)^{-1}X' = I_N - \frac{J_N}{N}$$

and therefore (2.15) can be rewritten as

$$\widehat{\sigma}^2 = \frac{Y'(I_N - \frac{J_N}{N})Y}{N-1} = \frac{\sum_{i=1}^{N}(Y_i - \overline{Y})^2}{N-1}$$

which is equal to (2.11) and hence independent of K.

EXAMPLE 2.10

For Example 2.1, we rewrite (2.2) as a cell means model

$$Y = X\beta + \varepsilon,$$

where the only variance component is the residual (error) variance σ^2. Here, $X = I_a \otimes 1_n$ ($\mathrm{rank}(X) = a$), $\beta = (\mu_1, \ldots, \mu_a)'$, $N = an$ and $V = \sigma^2 I_N$.

One possible choice for an $((N-a) \times N)$ matrix K' satisfying $K'X = 0$ is

$$K' = I_a \otimes \left(I_{n-1} - \frac{J_{n-1}}{n} \; \middle| \; -\frac{1_{n-1}}{n}\right).$$

It immediately follows from the complete similarity with the choice of K' in Example 2.9 that $K'X = 0$. Further,

$$K'Y \sim N(0, \sigma^2 K'K)$$

and the corresponding log-likelihood equals (2.14) in which the factor $N-1$ is replaced by $N - a$. Therefore, the corresponding REML estimator is readily seen to be

$$\widehat{\sigma}^2 = \frac{Y'(I_N - X(X'X)^{-1}X')Y}{N - a}. \tag{2.16}$$

In this case,

$$I_N - X(X'X)^{-1}X' = I_N - I_a \otimes \frac{J_n}{n} = I_a \otimes \left(I_n - \frac{J_n}{n}\right)$$

such that (2.16) reduces to (2.12).

The same ideas can be applied to obtain REML estimates for the variance components in any multivariate normal model

$$Y \sim N(X\beta, V),$$

and hence also for the general linear mixed model. We refer to Section 3.4.3 for more details. However, it should be emphasized that only in particular cases, e.g., the fixed-effects models considered in Examples 2.9 and 2.10, closed form solutions for the REML estimators of the variance components can be obtained. In most cases the restricted log-likelihood must be maximized in an iterative way. SAS uses the ridge-stabilized Newton-Raphson algorithm (see Littell et al 1996, p. 498). For more details on computational aspects we refer to our Section 3.4.5 and Chapter 8 in Searle et al (1992).

2.3.2   Best Linear Unbiased Prediction (BLUP)

In Section 2.3.1 we focused attention on estimation of the variance components associated with the random effects and the error term. In a number of situations interest is also in predicting the components of the b vector. We will not discuss prediction in great detail but we sketch the main ideas for the simple random-effects model (2.1)

$$Y_{ij} = \mu + b_i + \varepsilon_{ij} \qquad j = 1, \ldots, n; i = 1, \ldots, a,$$

introduced in Example 2.1 and further discussed in Example 2.6. The scale parameters in this model are σ_b^2 and σ^2. The single location parameter is μ.

Since $b_i = (\overline{Y}_{i.} - \mu) - \bar{\varepsilon}_{i.}$, we expect b_i to be positive (negative) if $\overline{Y}_{i.}$ is considerably larger (smaller) than μ (the unknown overall mean). This is a heuristic argument in favor of using information provided by $\overline{Y}_{i.}$ to predict b_i.

We therefore propose as predictor the conditional mean of b_i given $\overline{Y}_{i.}$, i.e.,

$$\widehat{b}_i = E(b_i \mid \overline{Y}_{i.}).$$

Using

$$\begin{pmatrix} b_i \\ \overline{Y}_{i.} \end{pmatrix} \sim N \left(\begin{pmatrix} 0 \\ \mu \end{pmatrix}, \begin{pmatrix} \sigma_b^2 & \sigma_b^2 \\ \sigma_b^2 & \sigma_b^2 + \dfrac{\sigma^2}{n} \end{pmatrix} \right)$$

it can be shown that

$$\begin{aligned} \widehat{b}_i &= E(b_i|\overline{Y}_{i.}) \\ &= E(b_i) + \frac{\mathrm{Cov}(b_i, \overline{Y}_{i.})}{\mathrm{Var}(\overline{Y}_{i.})}(\overline{Y}_{i.} - E(\overline{Y}_{i.})) \\ &= \frac{\sigma_b^2}{\sigma_b^2 + \dfrac{\sigma^2}{n}}(\overline{Y}_{i.} - \mu) = \frac{n\sigma_b^2}{n\sigma_b^2 + \sigma^2}(\overline{Y}_{i.} - \mu). \end{aligned}$$

Our prediction for b_i is therefore a contraction of the difference $\overline{Y}_{i.} - \mu$, i.e., $\widehat{b}_i$ is a shrinkage estimator as it 'shrinks' $(\overline{Y}_{i.} - \mu)$ towards the expected value of b_i, which is 0. If the variance component for 'batch' is high compared to the variance component for samples within the batch $(\sigma_b^2 \gg \sigma^2)$, the best linear unbiased predictor will be very close to $(\overline{Y}_{i.} - \mu)$. It means that the information from the other batches is not very useful to make predictions on the i-th batch. If however $\sigma_b^2 \ll \sigma^2$, the estimator will shrink towards the expected value 0. Furthermore, the higher the number of observations per batch, the more the observed value $(\overline{Y}_{i.} - \mu)$ will be taken into account in the prediction.

Note that our predictor still contains a number of nuisance parameters that need to be estimated. It is easy to show that, conditional on V, the solution of the ML equation for μ is

$$\widehat{\mu}_{\mathrm{ML}} = \frac{\displaystyle\sum_{i=1}^{a} \frac{\overline{Y}_{i.}}{\mathrm{Var}\overline{Y}_{i.}}}{\displaystyle\sum_{i=1}^{a} \frac{1}{\mathrm{Var}\overline{Y}_{i.}}} = \frac{\displaystyle\sum_{i=1}^{a} \frac{Y_{i.}}{\sigma^2 + n\sigma_b^2}}{\displaystyle\sum_{i=1}^{a} \frac{n}{\sigma^2 + n\sigma_b^2}}.$$

See Section 3.3 in Searle *et al* (1992) for a derivation of this result.

To obtain a workable expression for $\widehat{b}_i$ one typically replaces μ by $\widehat{\mu}_{\mathrm{ML}}$ and the variance components by their REML estimators. As notation we use $\hat{b}_{i,\text{BLUP}}$. One can show that this estimator fits into the theory on best linear unbiased predictors. A deeper discussion is beyond the scope of this chapter. A more rigorous way to define predictors for b_i is based on Bayesian methods. This approach is considered in some detail in Section 3.11. See also Chapter 7 of Searle *et al* (1992) for more details.

EXAMPLE 2.11

The actual value of the BLUP for b_i in Example 2.1 is

$$\hat{b}_{i,BLUP} = \frac{\hat{\sigma}_b^2}{\hat{\sigma}_b^2 + \hat{\sigma}^2/2}(\overline{y}_{i.} - \overline{y}_{..})$$

For the first batch we obtain (cf. the SAS output Section 2.3.3).

$$\hat{b}_{1,BLUP} = \frac{120}{120 + 4.06/2}(41 - 44.94) = -3.87.$$

This result is in accordance with the SAS output given in Section 2.3.3.

2.3.3   Examples and the SAS Procedure MIXED

Two models are fitted to the data of Example 2.1. In the first model we consider 'batch' as a fixed effect. We show how ML and REML estimates can be obtained from PROC MIXED. In the second model we consider 'batch' as a random effect. Both the batch and the residual variance component are estimated by the REML procedure. We also show how the best linear unbiased predictions for the random batch effects can be obtained.

For the first model the ML and REML estimates of the residual variance can be obtained from the following SAS program

```
proc mixed data = quality method = ml covtest;
class batch;
model eff = batch;
run;

proc mixed data = quality method = reml covtest;
class batch;
model eff = batch;
run;
```

The PROC MIXED statement calls the mixed procedure. One of the possible options in the PROC MIXED statement is the choice of the estimation method for the variance components. Since REML estimation is the default, specifying 'method=reml' in the second part of the program is superfluous. All the classification variables that appear in the model statement or in the random statement (see the second program) must be declared as classification variables in the CLASS statement.

In the MODEL statement the response variable (eff = efficiency or concentration) is placed left of the equality sign and one puts the fixed effect 'batch' on the right hand side. The only variance component in this model is the residual variance, which does not have to be specified explicitly in the mixed model procedure. The 'covtest' option in the PROC MIXED statement requests the printing of standard errors and test statistics for the variance and covariance parameters. As can be learnt from the discussion in Appendix B these test results have to be used with care.

For the second model the REML estimates of the two variance components (σ_b^2 and σ^2) and the best linear unbiased predictions for the batch effects are obtained from the following SAS program

```
proc mixed data = quality method = reml covtest;
class batch;
model eff = ;
random batch / s;
run;
```

Now the MODEL statement only contains 'eff' on the left hand side of the equality sign. The only location parameter in the model is the overall mean, its presence is implicitly assumed in the MIXED procedure. The 'batch' effect is now a random effect. This is specified in the RANDOM statement. The option 's' (or 'solution'), added to the RANDOM statement, gives the best linear unbiased predictions for the random batch effects.

For the first model (fixed effects), the ML and REML estimates of the residual variance are given by 2.03 and 4.06 respectively. This clearly underlines the difference between ML and REML as illustrated in Example 2.10. In fact, $N = na = 16$ and $N - a = 16 - 8 = 8$, explaining why the ML variance estimate is twice the REML estimate. The corresponding standard deviations are estimated to be 1.43 and 2.02, for ML and REML respectively.

For the second model (random effects), the two variance components can be obtained from the table 'Covariance Parameter Estimates (REML)'. The REML estimate for the residual variance equals 4.06. The best linear unbiased predictions can be read from the table 'Solution for Random Effects'. The prediction for 'batch 1' is -3.87, as calculated in Example 2.11.

TABLE 2.8. *REML estimates for the covariance parameters and the random effects for Model (2.1) fitted to the antibiotic data of Example 2.1.*

Effect	Parameter	Estimate (s.e.)
Variance of b_i (batch):		
$\quad$ var(b_i)	σ_b^2	120.00 (65.24)
Residual variance:		
$\quad$ var(ε_{ij})	σ^2	4.06 (2.03)
Random effects:		
$\quad$ Batch 1	b_1	-3.87 (4.09)
$\quad$ Batch 2	b_2	-11.25 (4.09)
$\quad$ Batch 3	b_3	1.54 (4.09)
$\quad$ Batch 4	b_4	8.42 (4.09)
$\quad$ Batch 5	b_5	15.80 (4.09)
$\quad$ Batch 6	b_6	-8.30 (4.09)
$\quad$ Batch 7	b_7	10.88 (4.09)
$\quad$ Batch 8	b_8	-13.21 (4.09)

```
              Covariance Parameter Estimates (REML)

    Cov Parm        Estimate      Std Error      Z    Pr > |Z|

    BATCH        120.00000000    65.23635316    1.84    0.0658
    Residual       4.06250000     2.03125000    2.00    0.0455


                   Solution for Random Effects

Parameter        Estimate         SE Pred    DDF        T   Pr > |T|

BATCH 1       -3.87195903      4.09240263      8    -0.95    0.3718
BATCH 2      -11.24711908      4.09240263      8    -2.75    0.0251
BATCH 3        1.53649168      4.09240263      8     0.38    0.7171
BATCH 4        8.41997439      4.09240263      8     2.06    0.0736
BATCH 5       15.79513444      4.09240263      8     3.86    0.0048
BATCH 6       -8.29705506      4.09240263      8    -2.03    0.0772
BATCH 7       10.87836108      4.09240263      8     2.66    0.0289
BATCH 8      -13.21382843      4.09240263      8    -3.23    0.0121
```

These results are summarized in Table 2.8. In the remainder of this book, we will generally prefer to present selected results in tabulated form rather than as raw SAS output.

2.4 Fixed Effects: Estimation and Hypotheses Testing

In this section we present an overview of inferential techniques for fixed effects. Illustrations are provided based on the examples of Section 2.1. For a more detailed treatment of these topics the reader is referred to Appendix A.

2.4.1 General Considerations

As shown in Appendix A.1, the maximum likelihood estimator for β in Model (2.8) equals the generalized least squares estimator

$$\widehat{\beta}_{\text{GLS}} = (X'V^{-1}X)^{-1}X'V^{-1}\boldsymbol{Y}. \tag{2.17}$$

In case the model is overparameterized, $X'V^{-1}X$ is not of full rank such that its inverse does not exist and should be replaced with a generalized inverse. For general matrices A it can be shown that there exist matrices A^-, termed generalized inverses, satisfying $AA^-A = A$. For non-singular square matrices, the generalized inverse is unique and coincides with the inverse of A, i.e., $A^- = A^{-1}$. The consequences for parameter interpretation are discussed in Appendix A, where it will be shown that only certain parameter combinations can be uniquely estimated (estimable parameters).

The variance-covariance matrix of $\widehat{\beta}_{\text{GLS}}$ can be shown to be

$$D(\widehat{\beta}_{\text{GLS}}) = (X'V^{-1}X)^-. \tag{2.18}$$

In the derivation leading to (2.17) it has been implicitly assumed that the covariance matrix V defined in (2.9) is known. The simplest solution is to assume $V = \sigma^2 I_N$, which completely ignores the correlation structure in the data. This leads to the well-known ordinary least squares (OLS) estimator

$$\widehat{\beta}_{\text{OLS}} = (X'X)^- X'\boldsymbol{Y}. \tag{2.19}$$

One can show that GLS estimators perform better than OLS estimators. Here, better performance means that one can prove that, compared to OLS estimators, GLS estimators generally have smaller variance, i.e., they are more efficient.

Another approach consists of replacing V by an estimator $\hat{V}$, yielding

$$\widehat{\beta} = (X'\hat{V}^{-1}X)^- X'\hat{V}^{-1}\boldsymbol{Y}. \tag{2.20}$$

The estimator $(X'\widehat{V}^{-1}X)^-$ for (2.18) is biased downwards since the variability introduced by working with estimated variance components in V, rather than with the known variance components, is not taken into account in our approximation for $(X'V^{-1}X)^-$. Alternatives were proposed by Kackar and Harville (1984) and Nabugoomu and Allen (1994). Since these ideas are not followed up in the current implementation of PROC MIXED, they will not be discussed further.

When interest is in the estimation of a linear combination $h'\beta$ of the fixed-effects parameters β, one uses $h'\widehat{\beta}$ of which the variance $\mathrm{Var}(h'\widehat{\beta})$ is estimated by $h'(X'\widehat{V}^{-1}X)^-h$. In addition, McLean and Sanders (1988) have shown that the distribution of

$$\frac{h'\widehat{\beta} - h'\beta}{\sqrt{h'(X'\widehat{V}^{-1}X)^-h}} \tag{2.21}$$

can be well approximated by a t-distribution with ν degrees of freedom (df).

As always in linear models, the degrees of freedom of the t-statistic are found from the degrees of freedom available to estimate the variance $h'(X'V^{-1}X)^-h$. In some situations this variance is the expected mean square that corresponds to one of the random effects or to the random error (see the first question in Example 2.12 on page 41 and Tables 2.9 and 2.10 on pages 43 and 44 respectively for a specific example). In such case the degrees of freedom equal the degrees of freedom associated with the mean square used to estimate the expected mean square under consideration. More often, especially in unbalanced designs, no such correspondence exists and the degrees of freedom need to be approximated. One possible choice are the degrees of freedom of the chi-squared distribution which best approximates the distribution of $h'(X'\widehat{V}^{-1}X)^-h$. This procedure, which is due to Satterthwaite (1941), is described in some detail in Appendix A.4.

Compared to the fixed-effects Model (2.7), testing hypotheses for fixed effects in a mixed model by an appropriate F-test (the default in PROC MIXED) is much more complex. The intuitive reason is clear: the fixed-effects model has only one variance component (the residual or error variance) and all fixed effects are tested against the error variance; a mixed model however contains different variance components and a particular fixed-effects hypothesis must be tested against the appropriate background variability, which can be expressed in terms of the variance components present in the model.

If the data are balanced and if the hypothesis states that all levels of a specific fixed-effects factor are the same, the background variability that serves as denominator in the F-test can be selected by looking at the expected mean squares in the ANOVA table associated with the problem under consideration (use e.g., PROC GLM to obtain expected mean squares). If more complex linear hypotheses of the form

$$H_0 : H'\beta = 0 \qquad \text{versus} \qquad H_1 : H'\beta \neq 0$$

are tested and/or if the data are unbalanced, more complicated expressions show up as background variability used as denominator in the appropriate F-test. The derivation of such approximate F-tests is sketched in Appendix A.2. Further, approximate degrees of freedom need to be determined. An overview of several methods available to this end in the MIXED procedure is presented in Appendix A.3. In the remainder of this chapter emphasis will be put on the Satterthwaite procedure, which is discussed in detail in Appendix A.4.

EXAMPLE 2.12

Assume that, for Example 2.5, the following two questions need to be answered:
(1) Is the mean response (= logarithm of the cell count) for drug A and drug B the same or different ?
(2) What is the mean response for drug A ?

The parameter behind **Question 1** is

$$\mu_{.1} - \mu_{.2} = \beta_1 + \frac{1}{2}\left((\alpha\beta)_{11} + (\alpha\beta)_{21}\right) - \beta_2 - \frac{1}{2}\left((\alpha\beta)_{12} + (\alpha\beta)_{22}\right).$$

Note that $\mu_{.1} - \mu_{.2}$ is of form $h_1'\beta$ with

$$\beta' = (\mu, \alpha_1, \alpha_2, \beta_1, \beta_2, (\alpha\beta)_{11}, (\alpha\beta)_{12}, (\alpha\beta)_{21}, (\alpha\beta)_{22})$$

and

$$h_1' = (0, 0, 0, 1, -1, 0.5, -0.5, 0.5, -0.5).$$

For this balanced design example we have

$$h_1'\widehat{\beta} = \overline{Y}_{.1.} - \overline{Y}_{.2.}$$

and

$$\text{Var}(\overline{Y}_{.1.} - \overline{Y}_{.2.})$$

$$= \left(\frac{1}{18}\right)^2 \text{Var}(Y_{.1.} - Y_{.2.})$$

$$= \left(\frac{1}{18}\right)^2 \text{Var}\left(\sum_{i=1}^{2}\sum_{k=1}^{9}(\mu + \alpha_i + \beta_1 + (\alpha\beta)_{i1} + p_k + c_{ik} + \varepsilon_{i1k}\right)$$

$$\left. - \mu - \alpha_i - \beta_2 - (\alpha\beta)_{i2} - p_k - c_{ik} - \varepsilon_{i2k}\right)$$

$$= \frac{1}{18}\mathrm{Var}(\varepsilon_{111} - \varepsilon_{121}) = \frac{\sigma^2}{9}.$$

The REML estimates of the variance components are

$$\widehat{\sigma}_p^2 = 0.0803, \qquad \widehat{\sigma}_c^2 = 0.00345, \qquad \widehat{\sigma}^2 = 0.00495. \tag{2.22}$$

Therefore the actual value of the estimator of $\mathrm{Var}(\overline{Y}_{.1.} - \overline{Y}_{.2.})$ is given by

$$\boldsymbol{h}_1'(X'\widehat{V}^{-1}X)^-\boldsymbol{h}_1 = \frac{\widehat{\sigma}^2}{9} = 0.00055.$$

The parameter behind **Question 2** is

$$\mu_{.1} = \mu + \frac{1}{2}(\alpha_1 + \alpha_2) + \beta_1 + \frac{1}{2}\left((\alpha\beta)_{11} + (\alpha\beta)_{21}\right).$$

Note that $\mu_{.1}$ is of form $\boldsymbol{h}_2'\boldsymbol{\beta}$ with $\boldsymbol{\beta}$ as in Question 1 and

$$\boldsymbol{h}_2' = (1, 0.5, 0.5, 1, 0, 0.5, 0, 0.5, 0).$$

We have $\boldsymbol{h}_2'\widehat{\boldsymbol{\beta}} = \overline{Y}_{.1.}$ and

$$\mathrm{Var}(\overline{Y}_{.1.})$$

$$= \left(\frac{1}{18}\right)^2 \mathrm{Var}\left(\sum_{i=1}^{2}\sum_{k=1}^{9}(\mu + \alpha_i + \beta_1 + (\alpha\beta)_{i1} + p_k + c_{ik} + \varepsilon_{i1k})\right)$$

$$= \left(\frac{1}{18}\right)^2 (36\sigma_p^2 + 18\sigma_c^2 + 18\sigma^2) = \frac{1}{18}(2\sigma_p^2 + \sigma_c^2 + \sigma^2).$$

Therefore the actual value of $\mathrm{Var}(\overline{Y}_{.1.})$ is given by

$$\boldsymbol{h}_2'(X'\widehat{V}^{-1}X)^-\boldsymbol{h}_2 = \frac{1}{18}(2\widehat{\sigma}_p^2 + \widehat{\sigma}_c^2 + \widehat{\sigma}^2) = 0.00939.$$

We now want to construct approximate $(1 - \alpha)100\%$ confidence limits for $\mu_{.1} - \mu_{.2}$, respectively $\mu_{.1}$. Since the test statistic (2.21) is approximately t-distributed, the confidence limits assume the following form ($\ell = 1, 2$):

$$\boldsymbol{h}_\ell'\widehat{\boldsymbol{\beta}} \pm t_{\nu_\ell}\left(1 - \frac{\alpha}{2}\right)\sqrt{\boldsymbol{h}_\ell'(X'\widehat{V}^{-1}X)^-\boldsymbol{h}_\ell}.$$

We now discuss how to obtain ν_ℓ ($\ell = 1, 2$). The degrees of freedom that correspond with the mean squares of the fixed-effects and random-effects

TABLE 2.9. *Design structure.*

SOURCE		df
BLOCK (plate)		8
residual (σ_p^2)	8	
WHOLE PLOT (compartment)		9
gsf	1	
residual (σ_c^2)	8	
SPLIT PLOT (random error)		18
drug	1	
gsf $*$ drug	1	
residual (σ^2)	16	

factors can easily be obtained from the specific design structure of this experiment, given in Table 2.9. In Table 2.10 we give the expected mean squares. In Appendix C we show how the expected mean squares can be obtained. In the table $\phi(\cdot)$ denotes a fixed effects contribution to the expected mean square under consideration (we do not include the specific form of $\phi(\cdot)$).

From Table 2.9 it is immediate that $\nu_1 = 16$, since $\mathrm{Var}(\overline{Y}_{.1.} - \overline{Y}_{.2.}) = \sigma^2/9$. Therefore the 95% approximate confidence limits for $\mu_{.1} - \mu_{.2}$ are given by

$$(\overline{y}_{.1.} - \overline{y}_{.2.}) \pm t(0.975; 16)\sqrt{0.00055}$$

$$= \quad -0.0133 \pm 2.12 \times 0.02345 = -0.0133 \pm 0.0497.$$

While the determination of ν_1 was based on classical ANOVA results, the determination of ν_2 is less straightforward. However, an intuitively appealing approximation exists in this case, since $h'(X'\widehat{V}^{-1}X)^- h$ can be expressed as a linear combination of mean squares, i.e., $a_1\mathrm{MS}_1 + \ldots + a_s\mathrm{MS}_s$. Here, $a_1, \ldots, a_s$ are constants and $\mathrm{MS}_1, \ldots, \mathrm{MS}_s$ refer to the mean squares corresponding to the various sources of variability (s is the total number of sources). It is indicated in Appendix A.4 that in this case Satterthwaite's approximate degrees of freedom ν_2 can be written as

$$\nu_2 = \frac{(a_1\mathrm{MS}_1 + \ldots + a_s\mathrm{MS}_s)^2}{\dfrac{(a_1\mathrm{MS}_1)^2}{\mathrm{df}_1} + \ldots + \dfrac{(a_s\mathrm{MS}_s)^2}{\mathrm{df}_s}},$$

with df_t the degrees of freedom for MS_t, $t = 1, \ldots, s$.

TABLE 2.10. *Expected Mean Squares.*

Factor	df	Expected Mean Squares
plate	8	$\sigma^2 + 2\sigma_c^2 + 4\sigma_p^2$
gsf	1	$\sigma^2 + 2\sigma_c^2 + \phi(\text{gsf})$
compartment (plate * gsf)	8	$\sigma^2 + 2\sigma_c^2$
drug	1	$\sigma^2 + \phi(\text{drug})$
gsf * drug	1	$\sigma^2 + \phi(\text{gsf} * \text{drug})$
residual	16	σ^2

In our particular example, it follows from Table 2.10 that

$$E(\text{MS(plate)}) = \sigma^2 + 2\sigma_c^2 + 4\sigma_p^2, \tag{2.23}$$
$$E(\text{MS(residual)}) = \sigma^2, \tag{2.24}$$

where MS(plate) is the notation for 'plate mean square' and MS(residual) refers to 'residual mean square'.

The actual values for MS(plate) and MS(residual) are obtained by plugging the REML estimates (2.22) for the variance components into (2.23) and (2.24). This yields

MS	actual value
plate	0.3329
residual	0.00495

and therefore

$$\nu_2 = \frac{\left(\frac{1}{2}0.3329 + \frac{1}{2}0.00495\right)^2}{\dfrac{\left(\dfrac{0.3329}{2}\right)^2}{8} + \dfrac{\left(\dfrac{0.00495}{2}\right)^2}{16}} = 8.24 \approx 8.$$

Hence, the 95% approximate confidence limits for $\mu_{.1}$ are given by

$$\overline{y}_{.1.} \pm t(0.975; 8)\sqrt{0.00938} = 7.7 \pm 2.306 \times 0.0968 = 7.7 \pm 0.223.$$

Next, assume that we want to test the null hypothesis of no difference between drug A and drug B against the alternative that there is a difference between the drugs, i.e.,

$$H_0 : \mu_{.1} - \mu_{.2} = 0 \qquad \text{versus} \qquad H_1 : \mu_{.1} - \mu_{.2} \neq 0.$$

With h_1 and β as above we have $\mu_{.1} - \mu_{.2} = H'\beta$, with $H = h_1$. Further, we know that the variance of $H'\widehat{\beta}$ is $\sigma^2/9$ and σ^2 can be estimated based on 16 degrees of freedom. The actual values for $H'\widehat{\beta}$ and $\widehat{\sigma}^2/9$ are -0.0133 and 0.00055, and rank$(H) = 1$. As discussed in Appendix A.2 these elements can now be used to construct the following Wald-type test statistic F with realized value F^*:

$$F = \frac{(H'\widehat{\beta})'(H'(X'\widehat{V}^{-1}X)^-H)(H'\widehat{\beta})}{\text{rank}(H)}$$

$$F^* = (-0.0133)(0.00055)^{-1}(-0.0133)$$
$$= 0.32.$$

Under H_0, F approximately follows an F-distribution.

Denoting a random variable that follows an F-distribution with ν_1 and ν_2 degrees of freedom by F_{ν_1,ν_2} and F^* for its realized value, the p-value corresponding to the above test is given by

$$p = \text{Prob}(F_{\nu_1,\nu_2} \geq F^*) = \text{Prob}(F_{1,16} \geq 0.32) = 0.58.$$

We conclude that there is no significant difference between drug A and drug B.

Next, assume that interest is in the more complex null hypothesis of no difference between the four treatments, i.e.,

$$H_0 : \mu_{11} = \mu_{12} = \mu_{21} = \mu_{22}$$

versus the alternative of at least one difference. The null hypothesis can be written as $H'\beta$ with β as above and

$$H' = \begin{pmatrix} 0 & 1 & -1 & 0 & 0 & 1 & 0 & -1 & 0 \\ 0 & 1 & -1 & 0 & 0 & 0 & 1 & 0 & -1 \\ 0 & 0 & 0 & 1 & -1 & 1 & -1 & 0 & 0 \end{pmatrix}.$$

It can be shown that the actual value of the F-statistic is 155.8 and that the denominator degrees of freedom are 11.7. Finally note that rank$(H) = 3$ and that $\text{Prob}(F_{3,11} \geq 155.8) < 0.0001$, hence the null hypothesis is clearly rejected.

EXAMPLE 2.13: EFFICIENCY IN ESTIMATING FIXED EFFECTS

In Example 2.3 we want to compare drug A and drug B. To keep the discussion simple, we consider the following simplified version of Model (2.4):

$$Y_{ij} = \mu + \tau_i + p_j + \varepsilon_{ij}, \tag{2.25}$$

where, for $j = 1, \ldots, 19$ and $i = 1, 2$,

Y_{ij} is the dbp of patient j assigned to drug i,

μ is the overall mean,

τ_i is the main effect parameter of treatment i,

p_j is the random effect of patient j,

ε_{ij} is the random error of patient j assigned to drug i.

A first estimator of the drug effect is based on the within patients information. Patients #4 and #16 cannot be used since they contribute a single measurement only (for drugs B and A respectively). The estimator for drug effect, based on within patient information, is

$$(\widehat{\tau_2 - \tau_1})_w = \frac{1}{17} \sum_{j \neq 4,16} (Y_{2j} - Y_{1j}),$$

where the summation is over all 19 patients except Patients #4 and #16. Note that for each $j = 1, \ldots, 19$, $E(Y_{2j} - Y_{1j}) = \tau_2 - \tau_1$. Therefore $(\widehat{\tau_2 - \tau_1})_w$ is an unbiased estimator for $\tau_2 - \tau_1$. The variance of this estimator is

$$\mathrm{Var}_w = \mathrm{Var}((\widehat{\tau_2 - \tau_1})_w) = \left(\frac{1}{17}\right)^2 \sum_{j \neq 4,16} \mathrm{Var}(\varepsilon_{2j} - \varepsilon_{1j}) = \frac{2\sigma^2}{17}.$$

So the variance only contains the variance component σ^2. The actual value of $(\widehat{\tau_2 - \tau_1})_w$ is 9.412.

It will now be illustrated how the information in the two incompletely measured individuals #4 and #16 can be incorporated into the estimator. We have $E(Y_{2,16} - Y_{1,4}) = \tau_2 - \tau_1$. Therefore the actual value of $Y_{2,16} - Y_{1,4}$, which is 4, also provides information on $\tau_2 - \tau_1$. We call $Y_{2,16} - Y_{1,4}$ an estimator based on between patients information. In general we write $(\widehat{\tau_2 - \tau_1})_B$ for the between patients estimator for $\tau_2 - \tau_1$ (which in this simple example reduces to $Y_{2,16} - Y_{1,4}$). The variance of this estimator is

$$\mathrm{Var}_B = \mathrm{Var}((\widehat{\tau_2 - \tau_1})_B) = \mathrm{Var}(Y_{2,16} - Y_{1,4}) = 2(\sigma_p^2 + \sigma^2).$$

From the REML estimates $\hat{\sigma}_p^2 = 85.04$ and $\hat{\sigma}^2 = 56.87$ we obtain as estimates for Var_w and Var_B, $2\hat{\sigma}^2/17 = 6.69$ and $2(\hat{\sigma}_p^2 + \hat{\sigma}^2) = 283.82$.

It can be shown that the GLS procedure, described in the general discussion preceding the examples, is the linear combination of $(\widehat{\tau_2 - \tau_1})_w$ and $(\widehat{\tau_2 - \tau_1})_B$ that has minimal variance. The combined estimator is given by

$$(\widehat{\tau_2 - \tau_1})_c = K \left\{ \frac{(\widehat{\tau_2 - \tau_1})_B}{\mathrm{Var}_B} + \frac{(\widehat{\tau_2 - \tau_1})_w}{\mathrm{Var}_w} \right\},$$

with $K = \dfrac{\text{Var}_B \text{Var}_W}{\text{Var}_B + \text{Var}_W}$. The variance of $(\widehat{\tau_2 - \tau_1})_c$ is

$$\text{Var}((\widehat{\tau_2 - \tau_1})_c) = K^2 \left(\frac{1}{\text{Var}_B} + \frac{1}{\text{Var}_W} \right) = K.$$

Estimators are obtained by replacing σ^2 and σ_p^2 by the REML estimators. The actual values for $(\widehat{\tau_2 - \tau_1})_c$ and the estimate of the variance are 9.287 and 6.536. The actual value 6.536 is slightly smaller than 6.69, the estimated value for $\text{Var}((\widehat{\tau_2 - \tau_1})_w)$. The reason is of course that additional (between patients) information has been used to obtain this estimate. In this specific example not much precision is gained because only two observations are missing and moreover the estimate for the between patients variability is very large.

The variance of $(\widehat{\tau_2 - \tau_1})_c$, the combined estimator, is a non-linear function of the variance components. We therefore have to use the general Satterthwaite procedure described in Appendix A.4 rather than its simplified version used in Example 2.12 (page 43).

Let us sketch the procedure for this particular example. The degrees of freedom are approximated by

$$\nu \approx \frac{2(h'(X'\widehat{V}^{-1}X)^- h)^2}{\text{Var}(h'(X'\widehat{V}^{-1}X)^- h)}.$$

The denominator is in turn approximated by (p indicates 'patient' and e 'residual'):

$$\text{Var}(h'(X'\widehat{V}^{-1}X)^- h) \approx \text{Var}(\widehat{\sigma}_p^2)M_p^2 + \text{Var}(\widehat{\sigma}^2)M_e + \text{Cov}\,(\widehat{\sigma}_p^2, \widehat{\sigma}^2)M_p M_e,$$

where the variances and covariances are replaced by their REML estimates:

parameter	estimate
$\text{Var}(\widehat{\sigma}_p^2)$	1530
$\text{Var}(\widehat{\sigma}^2)$	388.6
$\text{Cov}(\widehat{\sigma}_p^2, \widehat{\sigma}^2)$	-183.6

Expressions for M_p and M_e are found in Appendix A.4. Here they take the values $M_p = 0.00106$ and $M_e = 0.11335$.

Finally note that $E(h'(X'\widehat{V}^{-1}X)^- h)$ is estimated by 6.536, the estimate for K. This yields

$$\nu \approx \frac{2 \times (6.536)^2}{1530(0.00106)^2 + 388.6(0.1135)^2 - 183.6(0.00106)(0.1135)} = 17.3.$$

The 95% approximate confidence limits for $\tau_2 - \tau_1$ are given by

$$9.287 \pm t(0.975; 17)\sqrt{6.536} = 9.287 \pm 2.11\sqrt{6.536} = 9.287 \pm 5.4.$$

2.4.2   Examples and the SAS Procedure MIXED

Mixed models are fitted to both the cell proliferation data (Example 2.5) and the data of the cross-over trial (Example 2.3). We show how results on estimation and testing, discussed in Examples 2.12–2.13 can be obtained from PROC MIXED.

THE SAS PROGRAM

For the cell proliferation data, the estimates for $\mu_{.1} - \mu_{.2}$ and $\mu_{.1}$ and the p-values for the two null hypotheses $H_0 : \mu_{.1} - \mu_{.2} = 0$ and $H_0 : \mu_{11} = \mu_{21} = \mu_{12} = \mu_{22}$ can be obtained from the following SAS program

```
proc mixed data = cellprol covtest;
class plate gsf drug;
model y = gsf drug gsf*drug / ddfm = satterth;
random plate plate*gsf;
lsmeans drug;
estimate 'mean of drug A'
     INT 1 GSF 0.5 0.5 DRUG 1 0 GSF*DRUG 0.5 0 0.5 0;
estimate 'drug A versus drug B'
     DRUG 1 -1 GSF*DRUG 0.5 -0.5 0.5 -0.5;
contrast 'drug A versus drug B'
     DRUG 1 -1 GSF*DRUG 0.5 -0.5 0.5 -0.5;
contrast 'diff in 4 pop means'
     GSF 1 -1 DRUG 0 0 GSF*DRUG 1 0 -1 0,
     GSF 1 -1 DRUG 0 0 GSF*DRUG 0 1 0 -1,
     GSF 0 0 DRUG 1 -1 GSF*DRUG 1 -1 0 0;
run;
```

Since 'plate', 'drug', and 'gsf' are classification variables, they all appear in the CLASS statement. In the MODEL statement we put the response variable (y) left of the equality sign, while the fixed effect factors 'gsf', 'drug' and their interaction 'gsf*drug' are placed right of the equality sign. The random effects are specified in the RANDOM statement. To obtain the denominator degrees of freedom of the F-tests and the degrees of freedom of the t-statistics we specify as an option in the MODEL statement that the Satterthwaite procedure is needed. We therefore add the option 'ddfm=satterth'. Note that the default method for the determination of the degrees of freedom is the containment method, which will be discussed in Section 3.5.2 (page 84) and in Appendix A.3. The estimate for $\mu_{.1}$ with its standard error and degrees of freedom can be obtained by two equivalent statements, the LSMEANS statement and the ESTIMATE statement. In the latter statement, the elements of h_2' of the linear combination of interest $\mu_{.1} = h_2'\beta$ must be specified. To estimate $\mu_{.1} - \mu_{.2} = h_1'\beta$ we also use an ESTIMATE statement.

Specific hypotheses can be tested using the CONTRAST statement. For the first hypothesis $H_0 : \mu_{.1} - \mu_{.2} = 0$ the matrix H' is a row vector. For the second hypothesis $H_0 : \mu_{11} = \mu_{21} = \mu_{12} = \mu_{22}$, the three rows of the H' matrix have to be described, separated by a colon.

For the cross-over experiment, an estimate of the difference between drug B and A, can be obtained from the following program

```
proc mixed data = crossover covtest;
class patient drug;
model dbp = drug / ddfm = satterth;
random patient;
estimate 'drug B versus drug A' drug -1 1;
run;
```

Both patient and drug are classification variables, specified in the CLASS statement. The Satterthwaite procedure is chosen again to determine the degrees of freedom. 'Drug' is the fixed effect, specified in the MODEL statement, and 'patient' is the random effect, specified in the RANDOM statement. An estimate of the difference of means of drug B and A is obtained from the ESTIMATE statement.

THE RESULTS

The results of the first program are summarized in Table 2.11. The estimated mean of drug A is 7.7034 with an estimated standard error equal to 0.097 $(= \sqrt{0.00939})$ and 8.24 degrees of freedom; the difference between the means of drug A and B is estimated to be -0.0133 with standard error 0.023 $(= \sqrt{0.00055})$ and 16 degrees of freedom. These results are of course in correspondence with Example 2.12.

The F-value for testing $H_0 : \mu_{.1} - \mu_{.2} = 0$ (drug A versus drug B), is 0.32. The numerator and denominator degrees of freedom of the F-statistic are given by 1 and 16, and the p-value is 0.577. The F-value for $H_0 : \mu_{11} =

TABLE 2.11. *Results from fitting the SAS program on page 49 to the cell prolif-eration data.*

Effect	Estimate (s.e.)		ddf	p-value
ESTIMATE Statement Results:				
Mean of drug A	7.703(0.097)		8.24	<0.0001
Drug A versus drug B	-0.013(0.023)		16	0.5776
Least Squares Means:				
Drug a	7.703(0.097)		8.24	<0.0001
Drug b	7.717(0.097)		8.24	<0.0001
Effect	F-statistic	ndf	ddf	p-value
CONTRAST Statement Results:				
Drug A versus drug B	0.32	1	16	0.5776
Difference in 4 pop. means	155.80	3	11.7	0.0001

$\mu_{21} = \mu_{12} = \mu_{22}$ (difference in 4 population means) is 155.8. The numerator and denominator degrees of freedom of the F-statistic are given by 3 and 11.7, and the p-value for this null hypothesis is smaller than 0.0001.

Finally, the least squares means results provide exactly the same informa-tion for the mean of drug A as obtained from the ESTIMATE statement. These findings are in correspondence with Example 2.12.

For the second program the estimate of the difference of the least squares means of drug B and A, obtained from the ESTIMATE statement, is given by 9.287(2.557), with 17.3 denominator degrees of freedom ($p = 0.0020$). The results are in correspondence with Example 2.13. Note that the stan-dard error is the square root of the estimated value of K, i.e., $\sqrt{6.536} = 2.5566$ (see page 47).

2.5   Case Studies

2.5.1   Cell Proliferation

In Example 2.12 we answered, for the cell proliferation experiment (de-scribed in Example 2.5), a few specific questions. We now give a full sta-tistical analysis of this example. Recall the notation for the fixed effects:

	drug	
gsf	A	B
$-$	μ_{11}	μ_{12}
$+$	μ_{21}	μ_{22}

Note that $\mu_{ij} = \mu + \alpha_i + \beta_j + (\alpha\beta)_{ij}$ for each cell mean. Relevant questions include:

(i) Is there interaction between the fixed effects 'gsf' and 'drug' ?

(ii) Is the mean response (= logarithm of the cell count) different for drug A and drug B ?

(iii) Is there a shift in mean response in the presence of the gsf ?

(iv) Is there a difference in the mean responses for drug A and drug B in either absence or presence of the gsf ?

To start answering these questions we run the following SAS program (which is the first part of the program given in Section 2.4.2)

```
proc mixed data = cellprol covtest;
class plate gsf drug;
model y = gsf drug gsf*drug / ddfm = satterth;
random plate plate*gsf;
run;
```

The results are displayed in Table 2.12.

Recall that the variance component for 'compartment' corresponds with 'plate*gsf' in the output (see also Table 2.10). From the output it is clear that the estimated variance component for 'plate' is high compared to the other components. For example, $\hat{\sigma}_p^2$ is 16.22 times $\hat{\sigma}^2$, showing that the variability between plates is much larger than the variability between wells within compartments.

Table 2.12 also gives the fixed effects F-tests. The significance of the interaction 'gsf*drug' is borderline. The factor 'gsf' is highly significant, the drug effect is not significant at all.

To obtain the generalized least squares estimators for the means ($\mu_{i\cdot}$, $\mu_{\cdot j}$ and μ_{ij}) with their standard errors and degrees of freedom we use the LSMEANS statement and insert the following lines in the above program.

```
lsmeans gsf;
```

TABLE 2.12. *Results from fitting the SAS program on page 51 to the cell prolif-eration data.*

Effect	Param.	Estimate (s.e.)			
Covariance Parameters:					
Plate	σ_p^2	0.0803 (0.0416)			
Plate*Gsf	σ_c^2	0.0035 (0.0031)			
Residual	σ^2	0.0050 (0.0018)			
Effect		F-statistic	ndf	ddf	p-value
Test of Fixed Effects:					
Gsf		463.14	1	8	<0.0001
Drug		0.32	1	16	0.5776
Gsf*Drug		3.93	1	16	0.0648

```
lsmeans drug;
lsmeans gsf*drug / adjust = tukey;
lsmeans gsf*drug / slice = gsf;
```

The first statement provides the estimates for $\mu_{1.}$ and $\mu_{2.}$, the overall means for gsf− and gsf+. The second statement provides the estimates for $\mu_{.1}$ and $\mu_{.2}$, the overall means for drug A and drug B. The corresponding standard errors and degrees of freedom (according to the Satterthwaite procedure) are also given. The output from this extra part of the program is displayed in Table 2.13.

From the 'Least Squares Means' panel in Table 2.13 it is easily seen that addition of the growth stimulating factor to a compartment increases the average response from 7.320 to 8.100. There is almost no difference in average response for drug A and drug B. Also note that the information obtained for drug A is (of course) in correspondence with what we discussed in Question 2 of Example 2.12.

The highest least squares mean is obtained for μ_{21} ('gsf*drug y a' in the output). The approximate 95% confidence limits for μ_{21} are

$$\bar{y}_{21.} \pm t(0.975; 9) \times 0.099 = 8.117 \pm 2.26 \times 0.099 = 8.117 \pm 0.0224.$$

The degrees of freedom, used in the previous expression, are obtained from the Satterthwaite procedure.

Information on pairwise differences of means can be obtained from 'Differences of Least Squares Means' panel in Table 2.13. The Tukey-Kramer adjustment for multiple comparisons is used (see the SAS manual 1996 on

TABLE 2.13. *Results from fitting the extra code on page 52 to the cell proliferation data.*

Effect	Estimate (s.e.)	ddf	p-value
Least Squares Means:			
Gsf n	7.320(0.098)	8.57	<0.0001
Gsf y	8.100(0.098)	8.57	<0.0001
Drug a	7.703(0.097)	8.24	<0.0001
Drug b	7.717(0.097)	8.24	<0.0001
Gsf*Drug n a	7.290(0.099)	9.06	<0.0001
Gsf*Drug n b	7.350(0.099)	9.06	<0.0001
Gsf*Drug y a	8.117(0.099)	9.06	<0.0001
Gsf*Drug y b	8.084(0.099)	9.06	<0.0001

Tests of Effect Slices					
Effect	Slice	F-statistic	ndf	ddf	p-value
Gsf*DRUG	Gsf n	3.26	1	16	0.0900
Gsf*DRUG	Gsf y	1.00	1	16	0.3320

Level 1		Level 2					
Gsf	Drug	Gsf	Drug	Diff. (s.e.)	ddf	p-value	p (adj.)
Differences of Least Squares Means:							
n	a	n	b	-0.060(0.033)	16	0.0900	0.3072
n	a	y	a	-0.827(0.043)	14.8	<0.0001	<0.0001
n	a	y	b	-0.794(0.043)	14.8	<0.0001	<0.0001
n	b	y	a	-0.768(0.043)	14.8	<0.0001	<0.0001
n	b	y	b	-0.734(0.043)	14.8	<0.0001	<0.0001
y	a	y	b	0.033(0.033)	16	0.3320	0.7513

the procedure MULTTEST and Westfall and Young 1993). The difference between two means is only significant if the levels of the gsf factor differ.

The two drugs are compared in the absence and presence of the growth stimulating factor in the panel entitled 'Test of Effect Slices' in Table 2.13. None of the two comparisons lead to a significant result at the 5% significance level, but the two drugs differ significantly at the 10% significance level if no growth stimulating factor is added.

Finally, we show how to estimate and to test a specific estimable linear combination $h'\beta$. We only need to specify h' in an ESTIMATE statement or a CONTRAST statement (see also the discussion in Section 2.4.2). As an example we consider $\mu_{11} - \mu_{22}$, i.e., the difference between the two treatment combinations 'gsf∗drug n a' and 'gsf∗drug y b'. This difference can be written as

$$\mu_{11} - \mu_{22} = (\alpha_1 - \alpha_2) + (\beta_1 - \beta_2) + ((\alpha\beta)_{11} - (\alpha\beta)_{22}).$$

To obtain confidence limits for $\mu_{11} - \mu_{22}$ and to test the null hypothesis $\mu_{11} - \mu_{22} = 0$ we insert the following lines in the SAS program on page 52.

```
estimate 'GSF-, DRUG A versus GSF+, DRUG B'
    GSF 1 -1 DRUG 1 -1  GSF*DRUG 1 0 0 -1;
contrast 'GSF-, DRUG A versus GSF+, DRUG B'
    GSF 1 -1 DRUG 1 -1  GSF*DRUG 1 0 0 -1;
```

The estimated difference between these two means is $-0.794(0.043)$. Hence, the t-statistic equals -18.38 (ddf=14.8) with associated $p < 0.0001$. The test statistic, produced by the CONTRAST statement, statistic for the null hypothesis $\mu_{11} - \mu_{22} = 0$ is approximately F-distributed with 1 and 14 (≈ 14.8) degrees of freedom. The actual value is 337.9, hence the p-value is very small and the two treatments are significantly different.

2.5.2   A Cross-Over Experiment

In Example 2.3 we wrote a simple cross-over experiment as a mixed model and in Example 2.13 we analyzed the diastolic blood pressure data given in Table 2.3, thereby ignoring the period effect. Here, we fit the data to the more complex mixed model (2.4) including the period effect.

The general model can be fitted and the generalized least squares estimates for the two drugs can be obtained by submitting the following SAS program

```
proc mixed data = crossover covtest;
class patient drug period;
model y = drug period / s ddfm = satterth;
random patient;
lsmeans drug;
run;
```

The two fixed effects 'drug' and 'period' appear in the MODEL statement. Apart from the Satterthwaite ('ddfm=satterth') option, we add the option 's' (producing the generalized least squares estimates for the fixed effects) to the model statement. The random effect 'patient' appears in the RANDOM statement. Finally, the generalized least squares means for drug A and drug B are obtained from the LSMEANS statement. The SAS output is summarized in Table 2.14.

TABLE 2.14. *Results from fitting the SAS program on page 54 to the cross-over trial.*

Effect	Param.	Estimate (s.e.)	ddf	p-value
Fixed Effects:				
Intercept	μ	113.063 (3.014)	31	<0.0001
Drug A	τ_1	-9.354 (2.623)	16.3	0.0025
Period 1	π_1	1.255 (2.625)	16.3	0.6389
Least Squares Means:				
Drug A	τ_1	104.336 (2.796)	27	<0.0001
Drug B	τ_2	113.690 (2.802)	27.1	<0.0001
Covariance Parameters:				
Patient effect	σ_p^2	83.589 (39.281)		
Residual variance	σ^2	59.696 (21.302)		

Effect	Param.	F-statistic	ndf	ddf	p-value
Tests of Fixed Effects:					
Drug	$\tau_2 - \tau_1$	12.72	1	16.3	0.0025
Period	$\pi_2 - \pi_1$	0.23	1	16.3	0.6389

As can be seen from the covariance parameters in Table 2.14 the patient variance component (σ_p^2) is larger than the residual variance component (σ^2). This is an indication that the cross-over trial design is an appropriate choice. This finding has the following consequence: if the same treatment would be given to the same patient in both periods, the variance of the difference between the two measurements on this patient will be considerably smaller than the variance of the difference between two measurements on different patients receiving the same treatment. The explanation for this finding follows from the fact that, with $j \neq j'$,

$$\text{Var}(Y_{ijk} - Y_{ij'k}) = 2\sigma^2$$

and that, with $k \neq k'$ (and $j = j'$ or $j \neq j'$)

$$\text{Var}(Y_{ijk} - Y_{ij'k'}) = 2(\sigma_p^2 + \sigma^2).$$

The estimates are $2\hat{\sigma}^2 = 119.4$ and $2(\hat{\sigma}_p^2 + \hat{\sigma}^2) = 286.6$.

The generalized least squares estimates of the overall mean (μ) and the main effects $(\tau_1, \tau_2, \pi_1$ and $\pi_2)$ are given in the fixed effects panel in Table 2.14. The main effects of drug B (τ_2) and of period two (π_2) are taken to be zero (the SAS choice to handle the overparameterization). Generalized least squares estimates of estimable linear combinations of the fixed effects parameters can be obtained from this table. As an example we have that

$\mu_{1.}$, the mean response if treated with drug A, can be written as $\mu_{1.} = \mu + \tau_1 + (\pi_1 + \pi_2)/2$ and therefore can be estimated by

$$\widehat{\mu}_{1.} = 113.062 - 9.354 + \frac{1}{2}1.255 = 104.335.$$

This estimated value (and the corresponding standard error and degrees of freedom) for the mean diastolic blood pressure after treatment with drug A is of course also obtained from the 'Least Squares Means' panel.

From the 'Tests of Fixed Effects' panel in Table 2.14 it can be seen that there is a significant difference in diastolic blood pressure for drug A and drug B (p-value is 0.0025). We further see that the period effect is not significant, such that Model (2.4) effectively reduces to the simplified Model (2.25) of Example 2.13.

The least squares means for treatments A and B are 104.33 and 113.69 and the corresponding standard errors are small, i.e., drug A is more successful than drug B in lowering the diastolic blood pressure.

2.5.3 A Multicenter Trial

In this example we give variations on Example 2.2 where we studied the efficacy of a new drug in decreasing blood pressure. In Example 2.2 the response variable is 'difference in blood pressure before and after treatment (=difbp)', a variable derived from the separate values of blood pressure before and after treatment. The original data are given in Table 2.15. In the table, x and y denote the blood pressures before and after treatment respectively. Unlike the model given in Example 2.2, we now treat y as response and x as covariate. The intuitive motivation is to allow comparison of the response with the baseline value x.

MODEL 1

This comparison will be done in a model with 'treatment' as fixed-effects factor and 'country' as random-effects factor.

$$Y_{ijk} = \mu + \tau_i + \beta x_{ijk} + c_j + \varepsilon_{ijk},$$

where, for $k = 1, \ldots, n_{ij}$; $j = 1, \ldots, 9$; $i = 1, 2$,

Y_{ijk} is the blood pressure of person k assigned to treatment i and from country j,

μ is the overall mean,

τ_i is the main effect parameter for treatment i,

TABLE 2.15. *Blood Pressure Data.*

x	y	x	y	x	y	x	y	x	y	x	y
Australia		92	55	98	55	96	72	82	73	79	35
Drug		77	77	95	95	102	60	74	36	97	55
126	82	77	44	102	58	74	34	104	55	93	43
78	73	**Canada**		102	92	72	44	Placebo		81	44
89	72	Drug		77	77	83	83	98	55	87	68
106	89	93	56	95	95	68	46	66	56	78	50
91	51	103	82	64	121	48	64	79	73	85	82
79	40	101	54	78	62	68	66	150	150	Placebo	
74	52	78	44	106	56	83	44	73	49	107	88
67	56	49	35	98	88	92	36	96	54	121	121
108	33	89	37	103	102	80	55	84	100	151	54
108	96	84	37	86	69	Placebo		77	59	98	60
Placebo		80	46	85	38	77	83	88	42	71	48
119	58	97	54	68	36	88	97	77	64	86	38
56	33	Placebo		Placebo		104	120	108	110	89	43
74	69	96	42	73	43	99	40	85	34	83	56
93	79	85	88	99	31	58	37	140	68	76	45
62	66	85	34	97	63	70	56	**South**		100	39
122	107	72	32	103	35	88	84	**Africa**		77	40
Belgium		90	53	81	53	77	61	Drug		63	64
Drug		97	32	84	75	76	44	114	47	69	53
109	57	71	61	116	49	80	59	73	40	58	50
64	87	84	36	94	94	67	50	96	96	76	55
65	39	**France**		104	86	88	34	69	32	96	102
64	63	Drug		103	51	62	42	113	67	113	45
92	42	125	91	**Great**		**Korea**		89	80	135	82
115	57	143	52	**Britain**		Drug		86	43	103	40
72	36	97	54	Drug		88	41	99	35	80	67
106	54	120	64	84	70	121	105	116	104	73	56
Placebo		Placebo		88	88	109	96	118	38	**Sweden**	
95	44	105	63	80	61	129	46	100	60	Drug	
64	66	84	57	64	70	93	36	65	34	66	42
86	54	107	70	46	33	87	37	70	35	72	41
126	51	**Germany**		77	71	127	47	58	30	Placebo	
99	34	Drug		101	37	102	39	78	30	65	63

β is the regression coefficient, i.e., the slope that describes the linear trend between response and regressor,

x_{ijk} is the baseline value for the blood pressure of person k,

c_j is the random effect for country j,

ε_{ijk} is the random error of person k assigned to treatment i and from country j.

Below we will discuss some other possible models that could be used to fit this data set.

Model 1 is fitted by the following SAS program:

```
proc mixed data = multicnt covtest;
class country treatm;
model y = x treatm / s ddfm = satterth;
random country / s;
run;
```

The option 's' has been added to the RANDOM statement to generate the best linear unbiased predictors (introduced in Section 2.3.2) for the random country effects. In the MODEL statement we specify the presence in the model of x, a continuous covariate. The model fitting results are given in Table 2.16.

The mean blood pressure after treatment with drug and placebo respectively for a patient with baseline blood pressure x can be estimated by using the generalized least squares estimates shown in the 'Fixed Effects' panel of Table 2.16. We deduce

$$\begin{aligned}
\widehat{\mu}(\text{drug}, x) &= \widehat{\mu} + \widehat{\tau}_1 + \widehat{\beta}x = 27.50 - 2.39 + 0.37x, \\
\widehat{\mu}(\text{placebo}, x) &= \widehat{\mu} + \widehat{\tau}_2 + \widehat{\beta}x = 27.50 + 0.37x.
\end{aligned}$$

Thus, the mean responses of the treatments 'drug' and 'placebo' differ (for a fixed x) with -2.386, the drug causing a somewhat lower value for blood pressure than placebo. This treatment effect however is not significant as τ_1 is not significantly different from 0 (p-value is 0.447). The same test can be found in the 'Tests of Fixed Effects' panel. The F-statistic for the treatment effect is equal to the square of the t-value of the parameter τ_1 ($F = t^2 = (-0.76)^2 = 0.58$)). The p-value is of course 0.447.

From the 'Tests of Fixed Effects' panel we see that $H_0 : \beta = 0$ is rejected (p-value is 0.0001), i.e., patients with high baseline blood pressure also have high response values. This means that such patients have high blood pressure values (after having received 'drug' or 'placebo').

Information on the best linear unbiased predictors can be read from the

TABLE 2.16. *Results from fitting the SAS program on page 58 to the multicenter trial.*

Effect	Param.	Estimate (s.e.)	ddf	p-value
Fixed Effects:				
Intercept	μ	27.497 (7.828)	138	0.0006
Baseline	β	0.370 (0.082)	172	<0.0001
Treatment Drug	τ_1	-2.386 (3.132)	173	0.4471
Covariance Parameters:				
Country effect	σ_c^2	13.982 (18.292)		
Residual variance	σ^2	438.911 (47.408)		
Random Effects:				
Australia	c_1	2.172 (3.124)	2.29	0.5508
Belgium	c_2	-1.682 (3.124)	2.29	0.6382
Canada	c_3	-3.320 (3.101)	2.34	0.3822
France	c_4	-0.541 (3.418)	1.66	0.8915
Germany	c_5	3.247 (2.957)	2.72	0.3600
Great Britain	c_6	2.071 (2.881)	2.93	0.5253
Korea	c_7	0.489 (2.971)	2.68	0.8809
South Africa	c_8	-2.240 (2.711)	3.42	0.4622
Sweden	c_9	-0.197 (3.581)	1.39	0.9629

Effect	Param.	F-statistic	ndf	ddf	p-value
Tests of Fixed Effects:					
Baseline	β	20.27	1	172	<0.0001
Treatment	$\tau_2 - \tau_1$	0.58	1	173	0.4471

'Random Effects' panel. The smallest prediction is seen for Canada, while Germany has the largest estimated random effect. However, since $\hat{\sigma}_c^2 \ll \hat{\sigma}^2$, the differences are presumably due to random fluctuation only.

Let us consider two more general forms of the mixed model discussed above. In Model 2 we include possible interaction between treatment and baseline value, i.e., the slope describing the linear trend between response and regressor is β_1 for 'drug' (treatment 1) and β_2 for 'placebo' (treatment 2), respectively. Such model takes form

TABLE 2.17. *Results from fitting the SAS program on page 60 to the multicenter trial.*

Effect	F-statistic	ndf	ddf	p-value
Tests of Fixed Effects:				
Baseline	20.27	1	171	<0.0001
Treatment	0.22	1	174	0.6419
Baseline*Treatment	0.41	1	174	0.5214

MODEL 2

$$Y_{ijk} = \mu + \tau_i + \beta_i x_{ijk} + c_j + \varepsilon_{ijk},$$

where

β_i gives the slope of the linear relation between response and covariate for treatment i ($i = 1$ is drug, $i = 2$ is placebo).

All the other quantities are as in Model 1. Note that for $\beta_1 = \beta_2 = \beta$ (i.e., regression lines parallel), Model 2 reduces to Model 1.

This model can be fitted adding the interaction term to the program

```
proc mixed data = multicnt covtest;
class country treatm;
model y = x treatm x*treatm / s ddfm = satterth;
random country / s;
run;
```

The tests of fixed effects are summarized in Table 2.17.

The interaction is not significant. So there is no reason to prefer Model 2 over Model 1, i.e., it seems all right to assume parallel regression lines for the different treatment levels.

In Model 3 we allow for different treatment effects in different countries. This can be translated by adding an interaction between treatment and country. This model takes form

MODEL 3

$$Y_{ijk} = \mu + \tau_i + \beta x_{ijk} + c_j + (\tau c)_{ij} + \varepsilon_{ijk},$$

where $(\tau c)_{ij}$ is the random interaction effect.

All other quantities are as in Model 1. This extension of Model 1 introduces an extra variance component in the model ($\sigma^2_{\tau c}$ with (τc) a shorthand notation for treatment*country). To find out whether Model 3 improves the fit compared to Model 1 we can compare the likelihood of Model 1 (without $\sigma^2_{\tau c}$) and Model 3 (with $\sigma^2_{\tau c}$).

First the log-likelihoods for the two models can be obtained by submitting the following SAS program

```
proc mixed data = multicnt covtest;
class country treatm;
model y = x treatm / s ddfm = satterth;
random country;
run;

proc mixed data = multicnt covtest;
class country treatm;
model y = x treatm / s ddfm = satterth;
random country country*treatm;
run;
```

In Model 3 the random effect country*treatment (variance component: $\sigma^2_{\tau c}$) has been added, leading to an actual value of 1610.83 for the deviance. For Model 1 the actual deviance value is 1611.89.

The difference in deviance,

$$\text{deviance (Model 1)} - \text{deviance (Model 3)} = 1.06,$$

is small, suggesting that the simpler model is probably appropriate. More formal tests for significance for variance components will be discussed in Section 3.9.1.

3

Linear Mixed Models for Longitudinal Data

Geert Verbeke

3.1 Introduction

In medical science, studies are often designed to investigate changes in a specific parameter which is measured repeatedly over time in the participating subjects. This allows one to model the process of change within individuals. Although this process occurs in every individual, the inter subject variability can be high. For example, using data of 955 men, Brant *et al* showed that the average rates of increase of systolic blood pressure (SBP) are smallest in the younger age groups, and greatest in the older age groups, that obese individuals tend to have a higher SBP than non-obese individuals, and that individuals in more recent birth cohorts have lower SBP's than those born before 1910. However, these factors are not sufficient to explain all the heterogeneity between individuals since, after correction for age, obesity and birth cohort, individuals with SBP's above (below) average at initial examination, still have slower (faster) rates of longitudinal change in SBP.

Long-term longitudinal studies are the most appropriate studies for the investigation of individual changes over time and for the study of effects of aging and other factors likely to influence change. In principle, continuous data from designed longitudinal experiments can often be analyzed with classical multivariate regression techniques. However, such methods impose model assumptions that are usually not met in observational studies, since the circumstances under which the measurements are collected cannot always fully be controlled. That is, individuals can enter the study at any time, they can also withdraw from the study at any time, for different reasons such as lost to follow up or death. Moreover, not only may individuals be observed a different number of times, at different periods of time, the intervals between observations may be different as well.

One of the frequently used alternatives is the linear mixed-effects model

(Laird and Ware 1982, and Harville 1977), in which the repeated measurements are modeled using a linear regression model, with parameters which are allowed to vary over individuals, and which are therefore called random effects or subject-specific regression coefficients. Since there is too little data on a single person to estimate its regression parameters, and to avoid theoretical obstacles, one often assumes that the random effects are independently and identically distributed random variables. Their distribution is referred to as the mixing distribution.

Since the subject-specific regression parameters reflect the natural heterogeneity in the population and because they can also be interpreted as the deviation of the evolution of a specific subject from the overall population average evolution, they are usually assumed to follow a Gaussian distribution. Their mean then reflects the average evolution in the population, and is therefore called the vector of fixed effects. The assumption of a Gaussian mixture is not only intuitive, it is also mathematically convenient because it implies that both the marginal distribution of the data and the posterior distribution of the random effects are Gaussian, which considerably simplifies the estimation procedure.

In Section 3.2, we will introduce a longitudinal data set on prostate cancer, which will be used throughout this chapter to illustrate all aspects of the linear mixed model in the context of repeated measurements. Section 3.3 shows how linear mixed models naturally arise from analyzing regression parameters obtained from fitting linear regression models to the data of each subject separately. The general linear mixed model will then be presented in Section 3.4, where also some estimation methods will be discussed. The Sections 3.5 to 3.7 show how the SAS procedure MIXED can be used to fit such models, and to test hypotheses about the parameters which describe the average evolution of the response variable over time. Another SAS procedure frequently used for the analysis of longitudinal data is PROC GLM. The two procedures will be compared in Section 3.8. The Sections 3.9 and 3.10 are devoted to the comparison of models with the same mean structure but different covariance structures. In Section 3.11, it will be shown how Bayesian methods are used to estimate the random effects in linear mixed models, and how the so-obtained empirical Bayes estimates can be interpreted. In practice, it is not always obvious how to select an appropriate model for a data set at hand. We will therefore present some general guidelines for model construction in Section 3.12. Section 3.13 generalizes some well-known diagnostic tools used in ordinary least squares regression to the framework of linear mixed models. We refer to Chapter 4 for an extensive illustration of the use of linear mixed models for the analysis of four longitudinal data sets taken from the literature.

3.2 The Study of Natural History of Prostate Disease

During the last five years, many papers have been published on the natural history of prostate disease, see for example Carter *et al* (1992a, 1992b) and Pearson *et al* (1991, 1994). According to Carter and Coffey (1990), prostate disease is one of the most common and most costly medical problems in the United States, and prostate cancer has become the second leading cause of male cancer deaths. It is therefore very important to look for markers which can detect the disease in an early stage. The prostate specific antigen (PSA) is such a marker. PSA is an enzyme produced by both normal and cancerous prostate cells, and its level is related to the volume of prostate tissue. Still, an elevated PSA level is not necessarily an indicator of prostate cancer because also patients with benign prostatic hyperplasia (BPH) have an enlarged volume of prostate tissue and therefore also an increased PSA level. This overlap of the distribution of PSA values in patients with prostate cancer and BPH has limited the usefulness of a single PSA value as a screening tool since, according to Pearson *et al* (1991), up to 60% of BPH patients may be falsely identified as potential cancer cases based on a single PSA value.

Based on clinical practice, researchers have hypothesized that the rate of change in PSA level might be a more accurate method of detecting prostate cancer in the early stages of the disease. This has been extensively investigated by Pearson *et al* (1994) who analyzed repeated PSA measures from the Baltimore Longitudinal Study of Aging (BLSA), using linear mixed models. In the following sections, we will use their data and their models to illustrate all features of linear mixed models in the context of longitudinal data.

The BLSA (Pearson *et al* 1994) is a unique resource for rapidly evaluating longitudinal hypotheses because of the availability of data from repeated clinical examinations and a bank of frozen blood samples from the same individuals over 30 years of follow-up (where new studies would require many years to conduct). Participants in the BLSA, return approximately every two years for three days of biomedical and psychological examinations. Over 1400 men with an average of almost 7 visits and 16 years of follow-up have participated in the study since its inception in 1958. BLSA participants are volunteers who are predominantly white (95 per cent), well-educated (over 75 per cent have bachelor's degrees), and financially comfortable (82 per cent).

A retrospective case-control study was undertaken that utilized frozen serum samples from 18 BLSA participants identified as prostate cancer

TABLE 3.1. *Description of study participants, by diagnostic group. The cancer cases are subdivided in local/regional (L/R) and metastatic (M) cancer cases.*

			Cancer Cases	
	Controls	BPH cases	L/R	M
Number of participants	16	20	14	4
Age at diagnosis (years)				
median	66	75.9	73.8	72.1
range	56.7-80.5	64.6-86.7	63.6-85.4	62.7-82.8
Years of follow up				
median	15.1	14.3	17.2	17.4
range	9.4-16.8	6.9-24.1	10.6-24.9	10-25.3
Time between measurements (years)				
median	2	2	1.7	1.7
range	1.1-11.7	0.9-8.3	0.9-10.8	0.9-4.8
Number of measurements per individual				
median	8	8	11	9.5
range	4-10	5-11	7-15	7-12

cases, 20 cases of BPH, and 16 controls with no clinical signs of prostate disease. In order to be eligible for the analyses, men had to meet several criteria:

1. seven or more years of follow-up prior to diagnosis of prostate cancer, simple prostatectomy for BPH, or exclusion of prostate disease by a urologist,

2. confirmation of the pathological diagnosis, and

3. no prostate surgery prior to diagnosis.

To the extent possible, age at diagnosis and years of follow-up was matched for the control, BPH and cancer groups. However, due to the high prevalence of BPH in men over age 50, it was difficult to find age-matched controls with no evidence of prostate disease. In fact, the control group remained significantly younger at first visit and at diagnosis compared to the BPH group, which makes it necessary to control for age at diagnosis in all statistical analyses.

A description of the data, differentiating between local/regional (L/R) cancer cases and metastatic cancer cases, is given in Table 3.1. The number of repeated PSA measurements per individual varies between 4 and 15, and

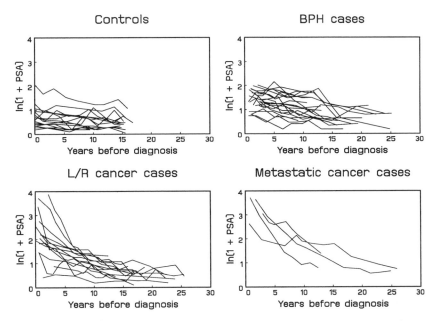

FIGURE 3.1. *Longitudinal trends in PSA in men with prostate cancer, benign prostatic hyperplasia, or no evidence of prostate disease.*

the follow-up period ranges from 6.9 to 25.3 years. Since it was anticipated that PSA values would increase exponentially in prostate cancer cases, the responses were transformed to $\ln(PSA + 1)$. These transformed individual profiles are shown in Figure 3.1.

3.3   A Two-Stage Analysis

Following Pearson *et al* (1994), we assume that every individual transformed profile (Figure 3.1) can be well approximated by a quadratic function of time, expressed in years before diagnosis. We can then fit such a function to the data of each individual separately, resulting in estimates for the subject-specific intercept and the two subject-specific slopes for each subject in the data set. Further, analysis of covariance techniques can then be used to investigate what factors (diagnostic groups, age, ...) influence a subject's evolution over time. These two steps (two stages) can be formalized as follows.

Let the random variable $Y_{ij} = \boldsymbol{Y}_i(t_{ij})$ denote the transformed PSA-level $\ln(1 + PSA)$ of the ith individual, measured at t_{ij} years before diagnosis.

We then assume that Y_{ij} satisfies

$$Y_{ij} = \beta_{1i} + \beta_{2i}t_{ij} + \beta_{3i}t_{ij}^2 + \varepsilon_{ij}, \quad j = 1, \ldots, n_i \qquad (3.1)$$

where n_i is the number of repeated measurements available for the ith individual, and where all error components ε_{ij} are assumed to be independently normally distributed with mean zero and variance σ^2. Note how (3.1) can be rewritten as

$$\boldsymbol{Y_i} = Z_i\,\boldsymbol{\beta_i} + \boldsymbol{\varepsilon_i}, \qquad (3.2)$$

where $\boldsymbol{Y_i}$ equals $(Y_{i1}, Y_{i2}, \ldots, Y_{in_i})'$, $\boldsymbol{\varepsilon_i}$ equals $(\varepsilon_{i1}, \varepsilon_{i2}, \ldots, \varepsilon_{in_i})'$, $\boldsymbol{\beta_i}$ equals $(\beta_{1i}, \beta_{2i}, \beta_{3i})'$, and where Z_i is the $(n_i \times 3)$ matrix, the columns of which contain only ones, all time points t_{ij} and all squared time points t_{ij}^2. The above model can now be seen as a linear regression model, and the vector $\boldsymbol{\beta_i}$ of unknown parameters can be estimated by replacing $\boldsymbol{Y_i}$ in the ordinary least squares estimator $\boldsymbol{\beta}_{i,\mathrm{OLS}} = (Z_i'Z_i)^{-1}Z_i'\boldsymbol{Y_i}$, by the vector $\boldsymbol{y_i}$ of observed values, leading to $\widehat{\boldsymbol{\beta}}_{i,\mathrm{OLS}}$.

In a second step, each of the components of the $\widehat{\boldsymbol{\beta}}_{i,\mathrm{OLS}}$ is further analyzed in order to investigate what factors affect these subject-specific regression coefficients. For the prostate data for example, we assume the following analysis of covariance models:

$$\begin{cases} \widehat{\beta}_{1i,\mathrm{OLS}} = \beta_1 Age_i + \beta_2 C_i + \beta_3 B_i + \beta_4 L_i + \beta_5 M_i + b_{1i} \\[2mm] \widehat{\beta}_{2i,\mathrm{OLS}} = \beta_6 Age_i + \beta_7 C_i + \beta_8 B_i + \beta_9 L_i + \beta_{10} M_i + b_{2i} \\[2mm] \widehat{\beta}_{3i,\mathrm{OLS}} = \beta_{11} Age_i + \beta_{12} C_i + \beta_{13} B_i + \beta_{14} L_i + \beta_{15} M_i + b_{3i}, \end{cases} \qquad (3.3)$$

in which Age_i equals the subject's age at diagnosis ($t = 0$), and where C_i, B_i, L_i and M_i are indicator variables defined to be one if the subject is a control, a BPH-case, a local cancer case, or a metastatic cancer case respectively, and zero otherwise. We also assume that the error components b_{1i}, b_{2i} and b_{3i} are normally distributed with mean zero. The above models describe how the individual profiles depend on age and how they differ between diagnostic groups. For example β_2, β_3, β_4 and β_5 are the average intercept for the controls, the BPH cases, the L/R cancer cases and the metastatic cancer cases, after correction for age at diagnosis. All three models in (3.3) can now be fitted separately using ordinary least squares regression, and contrasts of the parameters can be used to estimate differences between the four diagnostic groups. The results can be summarized as follows. The subject-specific regression parameters $\widehat{\boldsymbol{\beta}}_{i,\mathrm{OLS}}$ do not seem to depend on age at diagnosis (at the 5% level of significance), but we found highly significant differences between the diagnostic groups. No significant differences were found between the controls and the BPH cases, and the two groups of cancer patients only differ with respect to their intercepts.

A more efficient analysis could be performed by taking into account the dependence between the different components in $\widehat{\boldsymbol{\beta}}_{i,\text{OLS}}$. This can be done by fitting the multivariate model

$$\widehat{\boldsymbol{\beta}}_{i,\text{OLS}} = B_i \boldsymbol{\beta} + \boldsymbol{b_i}, \tag{3.4}$$

where B_i is the appropriate (3×15) matrix of covariates, and where $\boldsymbol{\beta}$ is equal to $(\beta_1, \ldots, \beta_{15})'$. We then assume that the vector $\boldsymbol{b_i} = (b_{1i}, b_{2i}, b_{3i})'$ follows a multivariate normal distribution with mean vector zero, and general covariance matrix D.

Note, that the estimated regression coefficients $\widehat{\boldsymbol{\beta}}_{i,\text{OLS}}$ can be viewed as summary statistics for the actual data. Other frequently used summary statistics are the area under each individual profile (AUC), the mean response for each individual, largest observation (peak), the half-time,... (see for example Weiner 1981 and Rang and Dale 1990). These are then analyzed in a second step, similar to our analysis of $\widehat{\boldsymbol{\beta}}_{i,\text{OLS}}$.

The reason why the above two-stage fitting procedure is frequently used is that one believes that the $\widehat{\boldsymbol{\beta}}_{i,\text{OLS}}$ are good approximations to the real subject-specific regression parameters $\boldsymbol{\beta}_i$. However, more efficient estimators for $\boldsymbol{\beta}$ can be obtained if no extra variability would be introduced due to the estimation of the $\boldsymbol{\beta}_i$. We then act as if all $\boldsymbol{\beta}_i$ were known, replacing (3.4) in the second stage by

$$\boldsymbol{\beta}_i = B_i \boldsymbol{\beta} + \boldsymbol{b_i}. \tag{3.5}$$

Replacing $\boldsymbol{\beta}_i$ in (3.2) by (3.5) then yields

$$\boldsymbol{Y_i} = X_i \boldsymbol{\beta} + Z_i \boldsymbol{b_i} + \boldsymbol{\varepsilon_i}, \tag{3.6}$$

where $X_i = Z_i B_i$ is a $(n_i \times 15)$ matrix of covariates, and where all other components are as defined before. For the prostate cancer data for example, the resulting model for Y_{ij}, $j = 1, \ldots, n_i$, equals

$$\begin{aligned} Y_{ij} &= \boldsymbol{Y_i}(t_{ij}) \\ &= \beta_1 Age_i + \beta_2 C_i + \beta_3 B_i + \beta_4 L_i + \beta_5 M_i \\ &\quad + (\beta_6 Age_i + \beta_7 C_i + \beta_8 B_i + \beta_9 L_i + \beta_{10} M_i) \times t_{ij} \\ &\quad + (\beta_{11} Age_i + \beta_{12} C_i + \beta_{13} B_i + \beta_{14} L_i + \beta_{15} M_i) \times t_{ij}^2 \\ &\quad + b_{1i} + b_{2i} \times t_{ij} + b_{3i} \times t_{ij}^2 + \varepsilon_{ij}. \end{aligned} \tag{3.7}$$

In general, model (3.6) is called a linear mixed (-effects) model with fixed effects $\boldsymbol{\beta}$ and random effects $\boldsymbol{b_i}$. The fixed effects are regression parameters which are assumed to be the same for all subjects, while the random effects are subject-specific regression coefficients. In Section 3.4, we will introduce the general linear mixed model and it will be shown how such models can be fitted without having to do a two-stage analysis explicitly.

3.4   The General Linear Mixed-Effects Model

3.4.1   The Model

In general, a linear mixed-effects model can be defined as any model which satisfies (Laird and Ware 1982)

$$
\begin{cases}
\boldsymbol{Y_i} = X_i \boldsymbol{\beta} + Z_i \boldsymbol{b_i} + \boldsymbol{\varepsilon_i} \\[2mm]
\boldsymbol{b_i} \sim N(\boldsymbol{0}, D), \\[2mm]
\boldsymbol{\varepsilon_i} \sim N(\boldsymbol{0}, \Sigma_i), \\[2mm]
\boldsymbol{b_1}, \ldots, \boldsymbol{b_N}, \boldsymbol{\varepsilon_1}, \ldots, \boldsymbol{\varepsilon_N} \text{ independent,}
\end{cases}
\tag{3.8}
$$

where $\boldsymbol{Y_i}$ is the n_i dimensional response vector for subject i, $1 \leq i \leq N$, N is the number of subjects, X_i and Z_i are $(n_i \times p)$ and $(n_i \times q)$ dimensional matrices of known covariates, $\boldsymbol{\beta}$ is the p dimensional vector containing the fixed effects, $\boldsymbol{b_i}$ is the q dimensional vector containing the random effects, and $\boldsymbol{\varepsilon_i}$ is a n_i dimensional vector of residual components. Finally, D is a general $(q \times q)$ covariance matrix with (i, j) element $d_{ij} = d_{ji}$ and Σ_i is a $(n_i \times n_i)$ covariance matrix which depends on i only through its dimension n_i, i.e. the set of unknown parameters in Σ_i will not depend upon i.

Very often, Σ_i is chosen to be equal to $\sigma^2 I_{n_i}$ where I_{n_i} denotes the identity matrix of dimension n_i. We then call model (3.8) the conditional independence model, since it implies that the n_i responses on individual i are independent, conditional on $\boldsymbol{b_i}$ and $\boldsymbol{\beta}$. In the sequel of this chapter, Σ_i will be assumed to be $\sigma^2 I_{n_i}$, unless stated otherwise.

It follows from (3.8) that, conditional on the random effect $\boldsymbol{b_i}$, $\boldsymbol{Y_i}$ is normally distributed with mean vector $X_i \boldsymbol{\beta} + Z_i \boldsymbol{b_i}$ and with covariance matrix Σ_i. Further, $\boldsymbol{b_i}$ is assumed to be normally distributed with mean vector $\boldsymbol{0}$ and covariance matrix D. Let $f(\boldsymbol{y_i}|\boldsymbol{b_i})$ and $f(\boldsymbol{b_i})$ be the corresponding density functions. We then have that the marginal density function of $\boldsymbol{Y_i}$ is calculated by

$$
f(\boldsymbol{y_i}) = \int f(\boldsymbol{y_i}|\boldsymbol{b_i}) \, f(\boldsymbol{b_i}) \, d\boldsymbol{b_i}
$$

which can easily be shown to be the density function of a n_i dimensional normal distribution with mean vector $X_i\beta$ and with covariance matrix $V_i = Z_iDZ_i'+\Sigma_i$. Unless the data are analyzed in a Bayesian framework (see e.g., Gelman *et al* 1995), inference is based on this marginal distribution for the response Y_i. This is also the approach used in the SAS procedure PROC MIXED. Note that the marginal model

$$Y_i \sim N(X_i\beta, Z_iDZ_i' + \Sigma_i) \qquad (3.9)$$

does not imply that Y_i satisfies the hierarchical model (3.8). Hence, inferences based on the marginal model do not explicitly assume the presence of random effects representing the natural heterogeneity between subjects. A simple example of the difference between marginal and hierarchical models is given in Section 3.6.

In the sequel of this section, we will discuss how the parameters in the marginal distribution (3.9) can be estimated. Later, in Section 3.11, it will be shown how the random effects can be estimated under the explicit assumption that Y_i satisfies model (3.8).

Let α denote the vector of all variance and covariance parameters (usually called variance components) found in V_i, i.e. α consists of the $q(q+1)/2$ different elements in D and of all parameters in Σ_i. Finally, let $\theta = (\beta', \alpha')'$ be the vector of all parameters in the marginal model for Y_i.

The classical approach to inference is based on estimators obtained from maximizing the marginal likelihood function

$$L_{\mathrm{ML}}(\theta) = \prod_{i=1}^{N} \left\{ (2\pi)^{-n_i/2} |V_i(\alpha)|^{-\frac{1}{2}} \right.$$
$$\left. \times \exp\left(-\frac{1}{2}(Y_i - X_i\beta)' V_i^{-1}(\alpha)(Y_i - X_i\beta) \right) \right\} \quad (3.10)$$

with respect to θ. Let us first assume α to be known. The maximum likelihood estimator (MLE) of β, obtained from maximizing (3.10), conditional on α is then given by (Laird and Ware 1982)

$$\widehat{\beta} = \left(\sum_{i=1}^{N} X_i'W_iX_i \right)^{-1} \sum_{i=1}^{N} X_i'W_iy_i \qquad (3.11)$$

and its variance-covariance matrix then equals

$$\mathrm{var}(\widehat{\beta})$$
$$= \left(\sum_{i=1}^{N} X_i'W_iX_i \right)^{-1} \left(\sum_{i=1}^{N} X_i'W_i\mathrm{var}(Y_i)W_iX_i \right) \left(\sum_{i=1}^{N} X_i'W_iX_i \right)^{-1} \quad (3.12)$$

$$= \left(\sum_{i=1}^{N} X_i' W_i X_i \right)^{-1},$$

(3.13)

where W_i equals $V_i^{-1}(\boldsymbol{\alpha})$.

Note that a sufficient condition for (3.11) to be unbiased is that the mean $E(\boldsymbol{Y_i})$ is correctly specified as $X_i \boldsymbol{\beta}$. However, the equivalence of (3.12) and (3.13) also assumes the covariance matrix to be correctly specified. Thus, an analysis based on (3.13) will not be robust with respect to model deviations in the covariance structure. Liang and Zeger (1986) therefore propose inferential procedures based on the so-called sandwich estimator for $\text{var}(\widehat{\boldsymbol{\beta}})$, obtained from replacing $\text{var}(\boldsymbol{Y_i})$ in (3.12) by $\boldsymbol{r_i r_i'}$, where $\boldsymbol{r_i} = \boldsymbol{y_i} - X_i \boldsymbol{\beta}$. The resulting estimator can then be shown to be consistent, as long as the mean is correctly specified in the model. An example of the use of standard errors obtained from the above sandwich estimator is given in Section 4.2.

When $\boldsymbol{\alpha}$ is not known, but an estimate $\widehat{\boldsymbol{\alpha}}$ is available, we can set $\widehat{V_i} = V_i(\widehat{\boldsymbol{\alpha}}) = \widehat{W_i}^{-1}$, and estimate $\boldsymbol{\beta}$ by using the expression (3.11) in which W_i is replaced by $\widehat{W_i}$. Estimates of the standard errors of $\widehat{\boldsymbol{\beta}}$ can then be obtained by replacing $\boldsymbol{\alpha}$ by $\widehat{\boldsymbol{\alpha}}$ in (3.12) and in (3.13) respectively, which are both available in the SAS procedure MIXED (1996). However, as noted by Dempster, Rubin and Tsutakawa (1981), they underestimate the variability of $\widehat{\boldsymbol{\beta}}$ because they do not take into account the variability introduced by estimating $\boldsymbol{\alpha}$. The procedure MIXED therefore accounts for this downward bias by using approximate t- and F-statistics for testing hypotheses about $\boldsymbol{\beta}$. This will be further discussed in Sections 3.5.2 and 3.7.

Two frequently used methods for estimating $\boldsymbol{\alpha}$ are maximum likelihood estimation and restricted maximum likelihood estimation which we will now briefly discuss.

3.4.2   Maximum Likelihood Estimation

The maximum likelihood estimator (MLE) of $\boldsymbol{\alpha}$ is obtained by maximizing (3.10) with respect to $\boldsymbol{\alpha}$, after $\boldsymbol{\beta}$ is replaced by (3.11). This approach arises naturally when we consider the estimation of $\boldsymbol{\beta}$ and $\boldsymbol{\alpha}$ simultaneously by maximizing the joint likelihood (3.10). The resulting estimators will be denoted by $\widehat{\boldsymbol{\beta}}_{\text{ML}}$ and $\widehat{\boldsymbol{\alpha}}_{\text{ML}}$. Standard errors could then be obtained by estimating the inverse Fisher information matrix. This approach would yield an estimator for the covariance matrix of $\widehat{\boldsymbol{\beta}}_{\text{ML}}$ which would take into account the extra variability due to the estimation of $\boldsymbol{\alpha}$. However, as discussed in Section 3.4.1, this is not the approach followed by the MIXED procedure.

3.4.3 Restricted Maximum Likelihood Estimation

In practice, linear mixed models often contain many fixed effects. For example, model (3.7) for the prostate cancer data has a fifteen-dimensional vector β of parameters in the mean structure. In such cases, it may be important to estimate the variance components, explicitly taking into account the loss of the degrees of freedom involved in estimating the fixed effects. This can be done via restricted maximum likelihood estimation (REML), which was introduced in Section 2.3.1 for the estimation of the residual variance in two univariate normal models. In order to extend these ideas to the general linear mixed model, we first combine all N subject-specific regression models (3.8) to one model

$$Y = X\beta + Zb + \varepsilon, \tag{3.14}$$

where the vectors Y, b and ε, and the matrix X are obtained from stacking the vectors Y_i, b_i and ε_i, and the matrices X_i respectively, underneath each other, and where Z is the block-diagonal matrix with blocks Z_i on the main diagonal and zeros elsewhere. The dimension of Y equals $\sum_{i=1}^{N} n_i$ and will be denoted by n.

The marginal distribution for Y is normal with mean vector $X\beta$ and with covariance matrix $V(\alpha)$ equal to the block-diagonal matrix with blocks V_i on the main diagonal and zeros elsewhere. Hence, the REML estimator for the variance components α is obtained from maximizing the likelihood function of a set of error contrasts $U = K'Y$ where K is a $(n \times (n-p))$ full-rank matrix with columns orthogonal to the columns of the X matrix. The vector U then follows a normal distribution with mean vector zero and covariance matrix $K'V(\alpha)K$, which is not depending on β anymore. Further, Harville (1974) has shown that the likelihood function of the error contrasts can be written as

$$
\begin{aligned}
L(\alpha) &= (2\pi)^{-(n-p)/2} \left| \sum_{i=1}^{N} X_i' X_i \right|^{1/2} \\
&\times \left| \sum_{i=1}^{N} X_i' V_i^{-1} X_i \right|^{-1/2} \prod_{i=1}^{N} |V_i|^{-\frac{1}{2}} \\
&\times \exp\left\{ -\frac{1}{2} \sum_{i=1}^{N} \left(Y_i - X_i\widehat{\beta} \right)' V_i^{-1} \left(Y_i - X_i\widehat{\beta} \right) \right\}, \tag{3.15}
\end{aligned}
$$

where $\widehat{\beta}$ is given by (3.11). Hence, the resulting REML estimator $\widehat{\alpha}$ does not depend on the error contrasts (i.e., the choice of K).

Note that the maximum likelihood estimator for the mean of a univariate normal population and for the vector of regression parameters in a linear regression model are independent of the residual variance σ^2. Hence, the estimates for the mean structures of the two examples in Section 2.3.1 do not change if REML estimates are used for the variance components, rather than ML estimates. However, it follows from (3.11) that this no longer holds in the general linear mixed model. Hence we have that, although REML estimation is only with respect to the variance components in the model, the 'REML' estimator for the vector of fixed effects is not identical to its ML estimator. This will be illustrated in Section 3.5.2 where model (3.7) will be fitted to the prostate cancer data.

Finally, note that the likelihood function in (3.15) equals

$$L(\boldsymbol{\alpha}) = C \left| \sum_{i=1}^{N} X_i' W_i(\boldsymbol{\alpha}) X_i \right|^{-\frac{1}{2}} L_{\mathrm{ML}}(\widehat{\boldsymbol{\beta}}(\boldsymbol{\alpha}), \boldsymbol{\alpha}) \tag{3.16}$$

where C is a constant not depending on $\boldsymbol{\alpha}$, where as before $W_i(\boldsymbol{\alpha})$ equals $V_i^{-1}(\boldsymbol{\alpha})$, and where $L_{\mathrm{ML}}(\boldsymbol{\beta}, \boldsymbol{\alpha}) = L_{\mathrm{ML}}(\boldsymbol{\theta})$ is the ML likelihood function given by (3.10). Because $\left| \sum_{i=1}^{N} X_i' W_i(\boldsymbol{\alpha}) X_i \right|$ in (3.16) does not depend on $\boldsymbol{\beta}$, it follows that the REML estimators for $\boldsymbol{\alpha}$ and for $\boldsymbol{\beta}$ can also be found by maximizing the so-called REML likelihood function

$$L_{\mathrm{REML}}(\boldsymbol{\theta}) = \left| \sum_{i=1}^{N} X_i' W_i(\boldsymbol{\alpha}) X_i \right|^{-\frac{1}{2}} L_{\mathrm{ML}}(\boldsymbol{\theta}) \tag{3.17}$$

with respect to all parameters simultaneously ($\boldsymbol{\alpha}$ and $\boldsymbol{\beta}$).

JUSTIFICATION OF REML ESTIMATION

The main justification of the REML approach has been given by Patterson and Thompson (1971) who prove that, in the absence of information on $\boldsymbol{\beta}$, no information about $\boldsymbol{\alpha}$ is lost when inference is based on $\boldsymbol{U}$ rather than on $\boldsymbol{Y}$. More precisely, $\boldsymbol{U}$ is marginally sufficient for $\boldsymbol{\alpha}$ in the sense described by Sprott (1975) (see also Harville 1977). Further, Harville (1974) has shown that, from a Bayesian point of view, using only error contrasts to make inferences on $\boldsymbol{\alpha}$ is equivalent to ignoring any prior information on $\boldsymbol{\beta}$ and using all the data to make those inferences.

3.4.4   Comparison between ML and REML Estimation

Maximum likelihood estimation and restricted maximum likelihood estimation both have the same merits of being based on the likelihood principle which leads to useful properties such as consistency, asymptotic normality, and efficiency. ML estimation also provides estimators of the fixed effects, while REML estimation, on itself, does not. On the other hand, for balanced mixed ANOVA models, the REML estimates for the variance components are identical to classical ANOVA-type estimates obtained from solving the equations which set mean squares equal to their expectations, which have optimal minimum variance properties and which do not rely on any normality assumption since only moment assumptions are involved (Harville 1977, and Searle, Casella, and McCulloch 1992).

Also with regard to the mean squared error for estimating $\boldsymbol{\alpha}$, there is no indisputable preference for either one of the two estimation procedures, since it depends on the specifics of the underlying model, and possibly on the true value of $\boldsymbol{\alpha}$. For ordinary ANOVA or regression models, the ML estimator of the residual variance σ^2 has uniformly smaller mean squared error than the REML estimator when $p = \text{rank}(X) \leq 4$ but the opposite is true when $p > 4$ and $n - p$ is sufficiently large ($n - p > 2$ suffices if $p > 12$). More details on this and related topics can be found in Harville (1977).

3.4.5 Model-Fitting Procedures

In the literature, several methods for the actual calculation of the ML or REML estimates have been described. Dempster, Laird and Rubin (1977) for example, have introduced the EM algorithm for the calculation of MLE's based on incomplete data, and have illustrated how it can be used for the estimation of variance components in mixed-model analysis of variance. Laird and Ware (1982) have shown how this EM algorithm not only can be applied to obtain MLE's, but also to calculate the REML estimates through an empirical Bayesian approach. Note that, strictly speaking, no data are missing: The EM algorithm is only used to 'estimate' the unobservable parameters, i.e., the random effects $\boldsymbol{b}_i$. The main advantage of the EM algorithm is that the general theory (Dempster *et al* 1977) assures that each iteration increases the likelihood. However, Laird and Ware (1982) report slow convergence of the estimators of the variance components, especially when the maximum likelihood is on or near the boundary of the parameter space. We refer to Section 5.9 for more details on the EM algorithm.

Therefore, one nowadays usually uses Newton-Raphson-based procedures to estimate all parameters in the model. Details about the implementation of such algorithms, together with expressions for all first and second order derivatives of L_{ML} and L_{REML} with respect to all parameters in $\boldsymbol{\theta}$ can be found in Lindstrom and Bates (1988).

3.5   Example

To illustrate the topics raised in Section 3.4, we now fit model (3.7) using the SAS procedure MIXED (SAS 1992, 1996). The program will be presented in Section 3.5.1, together with some available options. In Section 3.5.2, we will interpret all components in the SAS-output. Finally, it will be shown in Section 3.5.3 how problems of convergence of the iterative maximization program, due to small variance components, can be circumvented.

3.5.1   The SAS Program

Let the variable *group* indicate whether a subject is a control (*group* = 1), a BPH case (*group* = 2), a local cancer case (*group* = 3) or a metastatic cancer case (*group* = 4). From now on, for reasons explained further in Section 3.5.3, we express time in decades before diagnosis, rather than years before diagnosis. Further, we define the variable *timeclss* to be equal to *time*. This will enable us to consider time as a continuous covariate and as a classification variable (a factor in the ANOVA terminology) simultaneously. As before, the variable *age* measures the age of the subject at the time of diagnosis. Finally, *id* is a variable containing the subject's identification label, and *lnpsa* is the logarithmic transformation $\ln(1+x)$ of the original PSA measurements. We can then use the following program to fit model (3.7), in which all t_{ij} have been divided by 10:

```
proc mixed data = prostate method = ml covtest;
class id group timeclss;
model lnpsa = group age group*time age*time
              group*time2 age*time2 / noint solution;
random intercept time time2 / type = un subject = id g;
repeated timeclss / type = simple subject = id;
run;
```

Before presenting the results of this analysis, we shortly discuss the statements and options used in the above program.

THE PROC MIXED STATEMENT

This statement calls the procedure MIXED and specifies that the data are stored in the SAS data set 'prostate'. If no data set is specified, then the most recently created data set is used. In general, there are two ways of setting up data sets containing repeated measurements. One way is to define a variable for each variable measured, and for each time point in the data set at which at least one subject was measured. Each subject then corresponds to exactly one record (one line) in the data set. This setup is convenient when the data are highly balanced, i.e., when all measurements are taken at only a few number of time points. However, this approach leads to huge data matrices with many missing values in cases of highly unbalanced data such as the prostate data. Therefore, the MIXED procedure requires that the data set is structured such that each record corresponds to the measurements available for a subject at only one moment in time. For example, 5 repeated measurements for individual i are put into 5 different records. This has the additional advantage that time-varying covariates (such as time) can be easily incorporated into the model. An identification variable id is then needed to link measurements to subjects, and a time variable is used to order the repeated measurements within each individual. For example, our prostate cancer data set is set up in the following way:

OBS	ID	LNPSA	TIME	AGE	GROUP
1	1	0.405	1.94	72.4	2
2	1	0.336	1.44	72.4	2
3	1	0.693	1.20	72.4	2
...	..	.....	....	....	.
461	54	0.182	0.46	62.9	1
462	54	0.262	0.25	62.9	1
463	54	0.182	0.00	62.9	1

The option 'method = ' specifies the estimation method. In this book, we will always specify 'method = ML' or 'method = REML' requesting ML or REML estimation respectively. However it is also possible to use the non-iterative MIVQUE0 method (minimum variance quadratic unbiased estimation), which is used by default to compute starting values for the iterative ML and REML estimation procedures. We refer to the SAS manual (1996) for a treatment of the MIVQUE0 method. If no method is specified, then REML estimation is used by default.

Finally, in SAS version 6.12, no asymptotic standard errors for the variance components are given by default. However they can be obtained from specifying the 'covtest' option. We refer to Appendix B for a discussion on the use and the interpretation of standard errors for variance components estimators.

THE CLASS STATEMENT

This statement specifies which variables should be considered as factors. Such classification variables can be either character or numeric. Internally, each of these factors will correspond to a set of dummy variables in the way described in the SAS manual on linear models (Section 5.5, 1991).

THE MODEL STATEMENT

The MODEL statement names the response variable (one and only one) and all fixed effects, which determine the X_i matrices. Note that in order to have the same parameterization for the mean structure as model (3.7), no overall intercept (using the 'noint' option) nor overall linear or quadratic time effects should be included into the model, since otherwise the mean structure is parameterized using contrasts between the intercepts and slopes of the first three diagnostic groups and those for the last group. Although this would facilitate the testing of group differences (see also Section 3.5.2), it complicates the interpretation of the parameter estimates.

Finally, the 'solution' option is used to request the printing of the estimates for all the fixed effects in the model, together with standard errors, t-statistics and corresponding p-values for testing their significance.

THE RANDOM STATEMENT

This statement is used to define the random effects in the model, i.e., the matrices Z_i containing the covariates with subject-specific regression coefficients. Note that when random intercepts are required, this should be specified explicitly, which is in contrast to the MODEL statement where an intercept is included by default.

The 'subject = ' option is used to identify the subjects in our data set. All records with the same value for id are assumed to be from the same subject, whereas records with different values for id are assumed to contain independent data. This option also defines the block-diagonality of the matrix Z, and of the covariance matrix $\mathcal{D}$ of b in (3.14). The variable id is permitted to be continuous as well as categorical (specified in the CLASS statement). However, when id is continuous, PROC MIXED considers a record to be from a new subject whenever the value of id changes from the previous record. Hence, one then should first sort the data by the values of id. On the other hand, using a continuous id variable reduces execution times for models with a large number of subjects (manual PROC MIXED).

The 'type = ' option specifies the covariance structure D for the random

TABLE 3.2. *Overview of frequently used covariance structures which can be specified in the RANDOM and REPEATED statements of the SAS procedure MIXED. The σ-parameters are used to denote variances and covariances, while the ρ-parameters are used for correlations.*

Structure	Example
Unstructured type=UN	$\begin{pmatrix} \sigma_1^2 & \sigma_{12} & \sigma_{13} \\ \sigma_{12} & \sigma_2^2 & \sigma_{23} \\ \sigma_{13} & \sigma_{23} & \sigma_3^2 \end{pmatrix}$
Simple Variance Components type=SIMPLE type = VC	$\begin{pmatrix} \sigma^2 & 0 & 0 \\ 0 & \sigma^2 & 0 \\ 0 & 0 & \sigma^2 \end{pmatrix}^{(1)}$ or $\begin{pmatrix} \sigma_1^2 & 0 & 0 \\ 0 & \sigma_2^2 & 0 \\ 0 & 0 & \sigma_3^2 \end{pmatrix}^{(2)}$
Compound symmetry type=CS	$\begin{pmatrix} \sigma_1^2+\sigma^2 & \sigma_1^2 & \sigma_1^2 \\ \sigma_1^2 & \sigma_1^2+\sigma^2 & \sigma_1^2 \\ \sigma_1^2 & \sigma_1^2 & \sigma_1^2+\sigma^2 \end{pmatrix}$
Banded type=UN(2)	$\begin{pmatrix} \sigma_1^2 & \sigma_{12} & 0 \\ \sigma_{12} & \sigma_2^2 & \sigma_{23} \\ 0 & \sigma_{23} & \sigma_3^2 \end{pmatrix}$
First-order autoregressive type=AR(1)	$\begin{pmatrix} \sigma^2 & \rho\sigma^2 & \rho^2\sigma^2 \\ \rho\sigma^2 & \sigma^2 & \rho\sigma^2 \\ \rho^2\sigma^2 & \rho\sigma^2 & \sigma^2 \end{pmatrix}$
Toeplitz type=TOEP	$\begin{pmatrix} \sigma^2 & \sigma_{12} & \sigma_{13} \\ \sigma_{12} & \sigma^2 & \sigma_{12} \\ \sigma_{13} & \sigma_{12} & \sigma^2 \end{pmatrix}$
Toeplitz (1) type=Toep(1)	$\begin{pmatrix} \sigma^2 & 0 & 0 \\ 0 & \sigma^2 & 0 \\ 0 & 0 & \sigma^2 \end{pmatrix}$
Heterogeneous compound symmetry type=CSH	$\begin{pmatrix} \sigma_1^2 & \rho\sigma_1\sigma_2 & \rho\sigma_1\sigma_3 \\ \rho\sigma_1\sigma_2 & \sigma_2^2 & \rho\sigma_2\sigma_3 \\ \rho\sigma_1\sigma_3 & \rho\sigma_2\sigma_3 & \sigma_3^2 \end{pmatrix}$
Heterogeneous first-order autoregressive type=ARH(1)	$\begin{pmatrix} \sigma_1^2 & \rho\sigma_1\sigma_2 & \rho^2\sigma_1\sigma_3 \\ \rho\sigma_1\sigma_2 & \sigma_2^2 & \rho\sigma_2\sigma_3 \\ \rho^2\sigma_1\sigma_3 & \rho\sigma_2\sigma_3 & \sigma_3^2 \end{pmatrix}$
Heterogeneous Toeplitz type=TOEPH	$\begin{pmatrix} \sigma_1^2 & \rho_1\sigma_1\sigma_2 & \rho_2\sigma_1\sigma_3 \\ \rho_1\sigma_1\sigma_2 & \sigma_2^2 & \rho_1\sigma_2\sigma_3 \\ \rho_2\sigma_1\sigma_3 & \rho_1\sigma_2\sigma_3 & \sigma_3^2 \end{pmatrix}$

[1] Example : repeated timeclss / type = simple subject = id;
[2] Example : random intercept time time2 / type = simple subject = id;

TABLE 3.3. *Overview of frequently used (stationary) spatial covariance structures, which can be specified in the RANDOM and REPEATED statements of the SAS procedure MIXED. The correlations are positive decreasing functions of the Euclidean distances d_{ij} between the observations. The coordinates of the observations, used to calculate these distances are given by a set of variables the names of which are specified in the list 'list'. The variance is denoted by σ^2, and ρ defines how fast the correlations decrease as functions of the d_{ij}.*

Structure	Example
Power type=SP(POW)(*list*)	$\sigma^2 \begin{pmatrix} 1 & \rho^{d_{12}} & \rho^{d_{13}} \\ \rho^{d_{12}} & 1 & \rho^{d_{23}} \\ \rho^{d_{13}} & \rho^{d_{23}} & 1 \end{pmatrix}$
Exponential type=SP(EXP)(*list*)	$\sigma^2 \begin{pmatrix} 1 & \exp(-d_{12}/\rho) & \exp(-d_{13}/\rho) \\ \exp(-d_{12}/\rho) & 1 & \exp(-d_{23}/\rho) \\ \exp(-d_{13}/\rho) & \exp(-d_{23}/\rho) & 1 \end{pmatrix}$
Gaussian type=SP(GAU)(*list*)	$\sigma^2 \begin{pmatrix} 1 & \exp(-d_{12}^2/\rho^2) & \exp(-d_{13}^2/\rho^2) \\ \exp(-d_{12}^2/\rho^2) & 1 & \exp(-d_{23}^2/\rho^2) \\ \exp(-d_{13}^2/\rho^2) & \exp(-d_{23}^2/\rho^2) & 1 \end{pmatrix}$

effects b_i. In our example, we specified 'type = un' which corresponds to a general unstructured covariance matrix, i.e., a symmetric positive (semi-) definite $(q \times q)$ matrix D. Many other covariance structures can be specified, some of which are shown in Table 3.2 and Table 3.3. We further refer to the SAS manual (1996) for a complete list of possible structures. Although many structures are available, in longitudinal data analysis, one usually specifies 'type = UN' which does not assume the random-effects covariance matrix to be of any specific form.

Finally, specifying the option 'g' requests that the random-effects covariance matrix D is printed, printing blanks for all values that are zero.

THE REPEATED STATEMENT

The REPEATED statement is used to specify the Σ_i matrices in the mixed model. The repeated effects define the ordering of the repeated measurements within each subject. These effects (in the example 'timeclss') must be classification variables, which is why we needed two versions of our time variable: a continuous version 'time' needed in the MODEL statement as well as in the RANDOM statement, and a classification version 'timeclss' needed in the REPEATED statement. Usually, one will specify only one repeated effect. Its levels should then be different for each observation within a subject. If not, PROC MIXED constructs identical rows in Σ_i corresponding to the observations with the same level, yielding a singular Σ_i and an infinite likelihood. If the data are ordered similarly for each subject, and any missing data are denoted with missing values, then specifying a repeated effect is not necessary (see Section 5.7 for an example). In this case, the name 'DIAG' appears as the repeated effect in the printed output. Note that this is not the same as completely omitting the REPEATED statement which would not allow to specify parametric forms for Σ_i, other than the simple form $\sigma^2 I_{n_i}$. The options for the REPEATED statement are similar to those for the RANDOM statement.

For example, the option 'subject = ' identifies the subjects in the data set, and complete independence is assumed across subjects. It therefore defines the block-diagonality of the covariance matrix Σ of ε in (3.14). With respect to the variable *id*, the same remarks hold as the ones stated in our description of the RANDOM statement. Although this is strictly speaking not required, the RANDOM and REPEATED statement often have the same options 'subject = *id*', as was the case in our example.

Further, the 'type = ' option specifies the covariance structure Σ_i for the error components ε_i. All covariance structures described for the RANDOM statement can also be specified here. Very often, one selects 'type = simple' which corresponds to the most simple covariance structure $\Sigma_i = \sigma^2 I_{n_i}$. This assumes that all variability in the data which is not taken into account by the random effects (which model the stochastic variability between subjects) is purely measurement error. In Section 3.13.3, we will discuss how this assumption can be checked, and how appropriate alternative covariance structures for the error components ε_i can be found. We also refer to Chapter 4 in the book by Davidian and Giltinan for a discussion in the context of non-linear mixed models. Finally, if no REPEATED statement is used, PROC MIXED automatically fits a simple covariance structure for the residual components.

3.5.2   The SAS Output

PARAMETER ESTIMATES AND RELATED TOPICS

Table 3.4 shows the maximum likelihood as well as the restricted maximum likelihood estimates for all parameters in the marginal model (3.7). The standard errors for the estimates of the variance components α are calculated from inverting minus the matrix of second order partial deriva-

TABLE 3.4. *Maximum likelihood and restricted maximum likelihood estimates (MLE and REMLE) and standard errors for all fixed effects and all variance components in model (3.7), with time expressed in decades before diagnosis.*

Effect	Parameter	MLE (s.e.)	REMLE (s.e.)
Age effect	β_1	0.026 (0.013)	0.027 (0.014)
Intercepts:			
control	β_2	-1.077 (0.919)	-1.098 (0.976)
BPH	β_3	-0.493 (1.026)	-0.523 (1.090)
L/R cancer	β_4	0.314 (0.997)	0.296 (1.059)
Met. cancer	β_5	1.574 (1.022)	1.549 (1.086)
Age×time effect	β_6	-0.010 (0.020)	-0.011 (0.021)
Time effects:			
control	β_7	0.511 (1.359)	0.568 (1.473)
BPH	β_8	0.313 (1.511)	0.396 (1.638)
L/R cancer	β_9	-1.072 (1.469)	-1.036 (1.593)
Met. cancer	β_{10}	-1.657 (1.499)	-1.605 (1.626)
Age×time^2 effect	β_{11}	0.002 (0.008)	0.002 (0.009)
Time^2 effects:			
control	β_{12}	-0.106 (0.549)	-0.130 (0.610)
BPH	β_{13}	-0.119 (0.604)	-0.158 (0.672)
L/R cancer	β_{14}	0.350 (0.590)	0.342 (0.656)
Met. cancer	β_{15}	0.411 (0.598)	0.395 (0.666)
Covariance of $\boldsymbol{b}_i$:			
var(b_{1i})	d_{11}	0.398 (0.083)	0.452 (0.098)
var(b_{2i})	d_{22}	0.768 (0.187)	0.915 (0.230)
var(b_{3i})	d_{33}	0.103 (0.032)	0.131 (0.041)
cov(b_{1i}, b_{2i})	$d_{12} = d_{21}$	-0.443 (0.113)	-0.518 (0.136)
cov(b_{2i}, b_{3i})	$d_{23} = d_{32}$	-0.273 (0.076)	-0.336 (0.095)
cov(b_{3i}, b_{1i})	$d_{13} = d_{31}$	0.133 (0.043)	0.163 (0.053)
Residual variance:			
var(ε_{ij})	σ^2	0.028 (0.002)	0.028 (0.002)

tives of the log-likelihood function (ML or REML) with respect to $\boldsymbol{\alpha}$. The standard errors for the fixed-effects estimates are calculated by replacing $\boldsymbol{\alpha}$ in (3.13) by $\widehat{\boldsymbol{\alpha}}$, as discussed in Section 3.4.1.

As can be expected from the theory in Section 3.4, the ML estimates deviate most from the REML estimates for the variance components in the

Average profiles

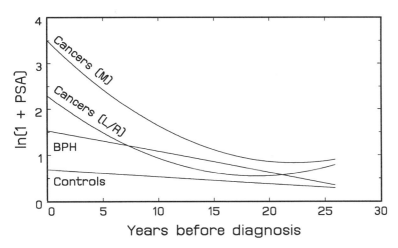

FIGURE 3.2. *Fitted average profiles for males with median ages at diagnosis, based on the model (3.7), where the parameters are replaced by their REML estimates.*

model. In fact, all REML estimates are larger in absolute value than the ML estimates. Note that the same is true for the REML estimates for the residual variance in normal populations or in linear regression models when compared with their ML estimates, as described in Section 2.3.1. Further, we have that Table 3.4 illustrates the fact that the REML estimates for the fixed effects are also different from their ML estimates. For the remainder of this Chapter, we will only consider REML estimation, unless stated otherwise. Hence all SAS output shown, and all results discussed are obtained from REML estimation. Figure 3.2 shows, for each diagnostic group separately, the fitted average profile for a male of median age at diagnosis.

Further investigating the estimates for the parameters in the mean structure shows that no significant interaction seems to be present between the age effect and the linear and quadratic time effects, suggesting that only a subject's intercept (= PSA value at time of diagnosis) is influenced by age, and not the complete evolution of PSA over time. Also, the quadratic time effects seem to be similar for the two cancer groups but also for the two non-cancer groups, although these last two groups probably do not evolve quadratically over time. This is also suggested by the average fitted profiles in Figure 3.2. Finally, it should be noted that for the control patients, there is almost no evidence that there is any change over time at all for their PSA level.

Some of the above hypotheses can easily be tested using the ratio of the parameter estimate of interest over its estimated standard error as test statistic. It then follows from the theory of maximum likelihood (see for example Serfling 1980) that this ratio, which is called a t-statistic and therefore denoted by t, is asymptotically normally distributed. In finite samples however, the distribution of t is not normal. For data satisfying certain types of balance and for some special unbalanced cases, t has an exact t-distribution. In general however, t is only approximately t-distributed, and the appropriate number of degrees of freedom needs to be estimated from the data.

The calculation PROC MIXED uses by default for random-effects models is the so-called containment method. Suppose we want to calculate the appropriate number of degrees of freedom to test the significance of the interaction of age with the quadratic time effect. We then need to proceed as follows. For each specified random effect which syntactically contains our fixed effect $age \times time2$ of interest (possibly as a component in interaction or nested effects), we compute their rank contribution to the matrix $(X|Z)$ obtained from merging the covariate matrices X and Z from the general model (3.14). The smallest of these ranks is then used as number of degrees of freedom for our t-distribution. When no random effects contain the fixed effect we want to test, then the number of degrees of freedom is taken equal to $n - \text{rank}(X|Z)$. Helms (1992) proposes to use $n - \text{rank}(X|Z)$, even when the random effects contain the fixed effect under consideration.

In our example, $age \times time2$ is not part of any of the random effects specified in our model. Hence we need to calculate $\text{rank}(X|Z)$. The matrices X and Z contain 15 and $54 \times 3 = 162$ columns respectively, resulting in 177 columns for the matrix $(X|Z)$ of which only 164 columns are linearly independent of each other. Therefore, the p-value SAS reports for testing the significance of β_{11}, is based on a t-distribution with $n - \text{rank}(X|Z) = 463 - 164 = 299$ degrees of freedom, and is equal to $p = 0.7982$. The same procedure is followed for all fixed effects specified in the model, and the results are shown in a separate table called 'Solution for fixed effects', containing the parameter estimates, their estimated standard errors, the t-statistic with appropriate number of degrees of freedom, and the corresponding p-value. However, this is only done when the option 'solution' has been specified in the MODEL statement. In our example, the containment method leads to t-distributions with 299 degrees of freedom for all fixed effects in the model.

Other methods for estimating the appropriate number of degrees of freedom are available within PROC MIXED, all leading to different results. However, in the analysis of longitudinal data, one usually has a fair number of blocks in the matrix Z (corresponding to different subjects). This results in numbers of degrees of freedom which are large enough in order to lead to very similar p-values. We refer to the manual of PROC MIXED (SAS 1996) and to Appendix A.3 for more information on the different methods for calculating the number of degrees of freedom.

With respect to the estimates of the variance components α, SAS version 6.11 also reports by default Wald statistics, defined as the ratio of the parameter estimate over its estimated standard error, as well as p-values obtained from comparing these Wald statistics to a standard normal distribution. In SAS version 6.12, these can be obtained from specifying the 'covtest' option (see Appendix B for a discussion). Note that, for the variances in α, such p-values are of limited value. Suppose for example, we are interested in testing whether or not the quadratic time effects differ between subjects, i.e., whether a quadratic time effect was necessary in the RANDOM statement. This is more then just testing whether or not the variance d_{33} of the random slopes for $time2$ equals zero. Indeed, if no third random effect would have been included, then no covariances between this random effect and the others would have been included either. So, instead of just testing $H_0 : d_{33} = 0$ we should test $H_0 : d_{13} = d_{23} = d_{33} = 0$, which will be described in Section 3.9.

Further, the p-values reported for the variance components are based on the asymptotic normality of the parameter estimators. However, this does not hold whenever the true parameter values are on the boundary of the parameter space. Now, if we would test $H_0 : d_{33} = 0$, then under the null hypothesis, d_{33} would be on the boundary, hence the standard maximum likelihood theory cannot be applied. Obviously, this argument does not hold for testing significance of the covariances, so the reported p-values can then be used, at the condition that the corresponding variances are not zero. For example, if random intercepts and slopes are needed in the model, we can use the reported p-values to test whether these intercepts and slopes are correlated. It would then follow from Table 3.4 that all correlations between random effects are strongly significant and that the only positive correlation is the one between the random intercepts and random slopes for $time^2$.

Apart from estimates for all parameters in the marginal model, estimated standard errors for these estimates and associated test statistics and p-values, much more information, which we will now describe, can be found in the SAS output.

INFORMATION ON THE ITERATION PROCEDURE

First of all, an 'Estimation Iteration History' table is given, describing the iteration history, i.e. the process of maximizing the likelihood function (or equivalently, the log-likelihood function). This table is of the following form:

REML Estimation Iteration History

Iteration	Evaluations	Objective	Criterion
0	1	-259.0577593	
1	2	-753.2423823	0.00962100
2	1	-757.9085275	0.00444385
.	.	. . . .	. . . .
6	1	-760.8988784	0.00000003
7	1	-760.8988902	0.00000000

Convergence criteria met.

The objective function is, apart from a constant which does not depend on the parameters, minus twice the log-likelihood function. In case of REML estimation, the exact relation between L_{REML} and the objective function OF_{REML} is given by

$$\ln(L_{\text{REML}}(\boldsymbol{\theta})) = -\frac{1}{2}\{(n-p)\,\ln(2\pi) + OF_{\text{REML}}(\boldsymbol{\theta})\}. \quad (3.18)$$

For ML estimation, the above equation becomes

$$\ln(L_{\text{ML}}(\boldsymbol{\theta})) = -\frac{1}{2}\{n\,\ln(2\pi) + OF_{\text{ML}}(\boldsymbol{\theta})\}.$$

Hence, our final parameter estimates are those which minimize this objective function. The reported number of evaluations is the number of times the objective function has been evaluated during each iteration. In the 'Criterion' column, a measure of convergence is given, where a value equal to zero indicates that the iterative estimation procedure has converged. In practice, the procedure is considered to have converged whenever the convergence criterion is smaller than a so-called tolerance number which is set equal to 10^{-8} by default. Unless specified otherwise, SAS uses the relative Hessian convergence criterion defined as $|g_k' H_k^{-1} g_k|/|f_k|$, where f_k is the value of the objective function at iteration k, g_k is the gradient (vector of first order derivatives) of f_k, and H_k is the Hessian (matrix of second order derivatives) of f_k. Other possible choices are the relative function convergence criterion and the relative gradient convergence criterion defined as $|f_k - f_{k-1}|/|f_k|$ and $(\max_j |g_{kj}|)/|f_k|$ respectively, where g_{kj} is the jth element in g_k.

INFORMATION ON THE MODEL FIT

The 'Model Fitting Information' table shows the following additional information:

```
Model Fitting Information for LNPSA

Description                          Value

Observations                        463.0000
Variance Estimate                     1.0000
Standard Deviation Estimate           1.0000
REML Log Likelihood                 -31.2350
Akaike's Information Criterion      -38.2350
Schwarz's Bayesian Criterion        -52.6018
-2 REML Log Likelihood               62.4700
Null Model LRT Chi-Square            501.8411
Null Model LRT DF                     6.0000
Null Model LRT P-Value                0.0000
```

In our example, $n = \sum_{i=1}^{N} n_i = 463$ observations were used to calculate the parameter estimates. In this example, all variability is ascribed to either random effects using the RANDOM statement or to the factor *timeclss* using the REPEATED statement. SAS, version 6.11, then automatically sets the 'variance estimate' equal to one. As described in Section 3.5.1, the simple covariance structure specified in the REPEATED statement is the default structure. Hence the same model can be fitted omitting the REPEATED statement, but the variability not explained by the random effects would then not be ascribed explicitly to any effect. In that case, SAS would consider this variability as residual variability, and report it as 'variance estimate' in the 'Model Fitting Information' table. In our example, this would lead to the values $\hat{\sigma}^2 = 0.0282$ and $\hat{\sigma} = 0.1679$ on the second and third line of the above table respectively. In version 6.12 of SAS, these two lines are no longer included in this output table.

The 'Model Fitting Information' table also reports the value of the REML log-likelihood function, evaluated at the REML estimates, which can also easily be calculated from expression (3.18). In our example, this becomes $-((463 - 15) \ln(2\pi) - 760.8989)/2 = -31.2350$. Based on this value, two criteria are defined which may be helpful in selecting an appropriate covariance structure. Akaike's information criterion (AIC) is defined as $\ln(L) - \#\boldsymbol{\alpha}$ where L equals the maximized ML or REML likelihood function and where $\#\boldsymbol{\alpha}$ is the number of variance components in the model, i.e., the number of parameters in $\boldsymbol{\alpha}$. Schwarz's Bayesian information criterion (SBC) equals $\ln(L) - \#\boldsymbol{\alpha} \ln(n^*)/2$ where n^* is n in case of ML estimation and $n-p$ in case of REML estimation. In our example we have AIC $= -31.2350 - 7 = -38.2350$ and SBC $= -31.2350 - 3.5 \ln(463 - 15) = -52.6018$ respectively. We refer to Akaike (1974) and to Schwarz (1978) for more information on AIC and SBC, and to Section 3.10 for an example of how these criteria are used in mixed models.

The 'Null Model LRT Chi-Square' value is -2 times the log-likelihood from the null model minus -2 times the log-likelihood from the fitted model, where the null model is the one with the same fixed effects as the actual model, but without any random effects, and with $\Sigma_i = \sigma^2 I_{n_i}$. This statistic is then compared to a χ^2 distribution with degrees of freedom equal to the number of variance components minus 1, and the reported p-value is the upper tail area from this distribution. Since the null model equals $y = X\beta + \varepsilon$ where all components in ε are independently normally distributed with mean $\mathbf{0}$ and variance σ^2, this p-value can be used to test whether or not there is any need at all for modeling the covariance structure of the data.

F-TESTS FOR FIXED EFFECTS

The table in the output entitled 'Tests of fixed effects' summarizes results of F-tests for the significance of all effects specified in the MODEL statement:

Tests of Fixed Effects

Source	NDF	DDF	Type III F	Pr > F
GROUP	4	299	15.90	0.0001
AGE	1	299	3.48	0.0631
TIME*GROUP	4	299	7.85	0.0001
AGE*TIME	1	299	0.27	0.6026
TIME2*GROUP	4	299	4.44	0.0017
AGE*TIME2	1	299	0.07	0.7982

Table 3.5 shows for each effect in the MODEL statement, what hypothesis is tested. For continuous covariates, which do not interact with any factors (no interaction term included in the MODEL statement), this is equivalent with the t-test reported in the table 'Solution for fixed effects'. For each factor specified in the CLASS statement, it is tested whether any of the parameters assigned to this factor is significantly different from zero. The same is true for interactions of factors with other effects.

Note how each of the hypotheses in Table 3.5 can be rewritten as

$$H_0 \ : \ L\,\beta \ = \ \mathbf{0}, \tag{3.19}$$

for some specific known matrix L. The F-statistics reported in the table 'Tests of Fixed Effects' are given by

$$F \ = \ \frac{\widehat{\beta}'\,L'\,\left[L\,\left(\sum_{i=1}^{N} X_i'V_i^{-1}(\widehat{\alpha})X_i\right)^{-1}\,L'\right]^{-1}\,L\,\widehat{\beta}}{\mathrm{rank}(L)}, \tag{3.20}$$

TABLE 3.5. *Overview of the hypotheses corresponding to the tests specified in the table labeled 'Tests of Fixed Effects'.*

Source	Null hypothesis
Group	$H_1 : \beta_2 = \beta_3 = \beta_4 = \beta_5 = 0$
Age	$H_2 : \beta_1 = 0$
Time*group	$H_3 : \beta_7 = \beta_8 = \beta_9 = \beta_{10} = 0$
Age*group	$H_4 : \beta_6 = 0$
Time2*group	$H_5 : \beta_{12} = \beta_{13} = \beta_{14} = \beta_{15} = 0$
Age*time2	$H_6 : \beta_{11} = 0$

and their null distribution (distribution under $H_0 : L\beta = 0$) can be well approximated by an F-distribution (Helms 1992, see also Appendix A.2). The numerator degrees of freedom equals rank(L), and the denominator degrees of freedom reported by PROC MIXED are the same as the number of degrees of freedom used in the output table 'Solution for Fixed Effects' for the t-tests for the parameters assigned to the effect which is tested now. So, for random-effects models, the containment method (see page 84) is used by default.

Note that it follows from the way we parameterized the mean structure of our model that the F-tests reported in the above table, cannot be used to test whether the different diagnostic groups have different intercepts or slopes. For example, 4 parameters are assigned to the effect '*time2 * group*', being the slopes for the quadratic time effect for each group separately. The hypothesis tested here is therefore

$$H_5 : \beta_{12} = \beta_{13} = \beta_{14} = \beta_{15} = 0$$

rather than

$$H_0 : \beta_{12} = \beta_{13} = \beta_{14} = \beta_{15}. \tag{3.21}$$

Note that hypothesis (3.21) is also of the form $H_0 : L\beta = 0$, and can thus also be tested using an F-statistic of the form (3.20), and approximating the null distribution by an F-distribution with degrees of freedom calculated as before. We will describe in Section 3.7.1 how this can be done in PROC MIXED using the CONTRAST statement.

Another possibility is to reparameterize the mean structure, including an overall intercept, and overall slopes for the linear and quadratic time effects. The MODEL statement of our program on page 76 then needs to be replaced by

```
model lnpsa = group age time group*time age*time
              time2 group*time2 age*time2 / solution;
```

We then get the following output table 'Solution for Fixed Effects' with REML estimates and t-tests for all parameters in the reparameterized mean structure:

Solution for Fixed Effects

Parameter	Estimate	Std Error	DDF	T	Pr > |T|
INTERCEPT	1.549386	1.085611	49	1.43	0.1599
GROUP 1	-2.647811	0.393111	300	-6.74	0.0001
GROUP 2	-2.072235	0.383595	300	-5.40	0.0001
GROUP 3	-1.252982	0.393223	300	-3.19	0.0016
GROUP 4	0.000000	.	.	.	.
AGE	0.026550	0.014234	300	1.87	0.0631
TIME	-1.604904	1.625757	49	-0.99	0.3284
TIME*GROUP 1	2.172966	0.583601	300	3.72	0.0002
TIME*GROUP 2	2.000526	0.567835	300	3.52	0.0005
TIME*GROUP 3	0.568994	0.579436	300	0.98	0.3269
TIME*GROUP 4	0.000000	.	.	.	.
AGE*TIME	-0.011165	0.021423	300	-0.52	0.6026
TIME2	0.395063	0.666049	50	0.59	0.5558
TIME2*GROUP 1	-0.524586	0.234146	300	-2.24	0.0258
TIME2*GROUP 2	-0.553522	0.223216	300	-2.48	0.0137
TIME2*GROUP 3	-0.053144	0.226748	300	-0.23	0.8149
TIME2*GROUP 4	0.000000	.	.	.	.
AGE*TIME2	0.002259	0.008829	300	0.26	0.7982

The slope β_{15} for time^2 in the last group is now the parameter assigned to the overall time^2 effect, and the three parameters assigned to the interaction of *group* with *time2* are the contrasts $\beta_{12} - \beta_{15}$, $\beta_{13} - \beta_{15}$ and $\beta_{14} - \beta_{15}$ respectively (see also the original estimates in Table 3.4). It is remarkable how, for example, the t-statistic corresponding to the *time2* effect is now compared with a t-distribution with only 50 degrees of freedom, rather than the 299 degrees of freedom we had before (the t-statistic remains the same). This is because our RANDOM statement now contains the effect of interest (*time2*) such that the containment method, described earlier, leads to a different number of degrees of freedom (the other effects in the above table also have a different number of degrees of freedom). However, this does not lead to different conclusions since there is very little difference between t-distributions with 299 and 50 degrees of freedom, leading to very similar p-values ($p = 0.5535$ and $p = 0.5558$ respectively).

TABLE 3.6. *Overview of the hypotheses corresponding to the tests specified in the table labeled 'Tests of Fixed Effects' for the model with reparameterized mean structure.*

Source	Null hypothesis
Group	$H_7 : \beta_2 = \beta_3 = \beta_4 = \beta_5$
Age	$H_8 : \beta_1 = 0$
Time	$H_9 : (\beta_7 + \beta_8 + \beta_9 + \beta_{10})/4 = 0$
Time*group	$H_{10} : \beta_7 = \beta_8 = \beta_9 = \beta_{10}$
Age*group	$H_{11} : \beta_6 = 0$
Time2	$H_{12} : (\beta_{12} + \beta_{13} + \beta_{14} + \beta_{15})/4 = 0$
Time2*group	$H_{13} : \beta_{12} = \beta_{13} = \beta_{14} = \beta_{15}$
Age*time2	$H_{14} : \beta_{11} = 0$

For the reparameterized model, we get the following F-tests for the effects specified in the MODEL statement:

Tests of Fixed Effects

Source	NDF	DDF	Type III F	Pr > F
GROUP	3	300	20.13	0.0001
AGE	1	300	3.48	0.0631
TIME	1	49	0.07	0.7885
TIME*GROUP	3	300	10.41	0.0001
AGE*TIME	1	300	0.27	0.6026
TIME2	1	50	0.03	0.8616
TIME2*GROUP	3	300	5.93	0.0006
AGE*TIME2	1	300	0.07	0.7982

The hypotheses tested in the above output are shown in Table 3.6. Hence, the test for hypothesis (3.21) is now reported as the F-test corresponding to the effect of *time2*group*. Note also the change in its numerator degrees of freedom due to the fact that we now test for equality of the quadratic time effect in the four diagnostic groups, rather than testing whether there is any quadratic time effect in any of the four diagnostic groups at all. Also, under this parameterization for the mean structure, the F-test reported for *time2* tests whether there is a quadratic time effect in the overall population and is therefore not equivalent to the t-test reported for *time2* in the table labeled 'Solution for Fixed Effects', which was testing for a quadratic time effect for the metastatic cancer cases only. The same remark is true for the F-test reported for *time*.

Although fitting the reparameterized model automatically yields tests for group differences with respect to average intercepts or slopes, it often complicates the interpretation of the parameter estimates since contrasts are estimated rather than the parameters of interest. All further analyses in this chapter will therefore be based on the original model (3.7), fitted with the program on page 76, and techniques which are to be described in Section 3.7 will be used to test for group differences.

3.5.3   Estimation Problems due to Small Variance Components

When we first fitted a linear mixed model to the prostate cancer data, time was expressed in decades before diagnosis, rather than years before diagnosis as in the original data set (see Section 3.5.1). This is done to avoid that the random slopes for the linear and quadratic time effects show too little variability which might lead to divergence of the numerical maximization routine. To illustrate this, we refit our mixed model but we express time as months before diagnosis. The only output we then get is the following table describing the iteration history:

REML Estimation Iteration History

Iteration	Evaluations	Objective	Criterion
..	.	....	....
45	1	-608.8969060	142120.74213
46	1	-608.8975012	142101.06725
47	1	-608.8980963	142084.01076
48	1	-608.8986914	142067.99906
49	1	-608.8992864	142052.47348
50	1	-608.8998813	142037.00154

Did not converge.

together with the estimates at last iteration for the variance components, shown in Table 3.7. Note how the reported estimate for the variance of the random slopes for the quadratic time effect equals $\widehat{d}_{33} = 0.00000000$. This suggests that, unless this variance is negative (discussions on negative variance components are given by Nelder 1954 and Thompson 1962), it is extremely small (almost zero). In the latter case, the MIXED procedure is expected to converge to a point which is very close to the boundary of the parameter space (since only nonnegative variances are allowed), if

TABLE 3.7. *Restricted maximum likelihood estimates (REMLE) at last iteration for all variance components in model (3.7), with time expressed in months before diagnosis.*

Effect	Parameter	REMLE
Covariance of b_i:		
$\mathrm{var}(b_{1i})$	d_{11}	0.36893546
$\mathrm{var}(b_{2i})$	d_{22}	0.00003846
$\mathrm{var}(b_{3i})$	d_{33}	0.00000000
$\mathrm{cov}(b_{1i}, b_{2i})$	$d_{12} = d_{21}$	-0.00244046
$\mathrm{cov}(b_{2i}, b_{3i})$	$d_{23} = d_{32}$	-0.00000011
$\mathrm{cov}(b_{3i}, b_{1i})$	$d_{13} = d_{31}$	0.00000449
Residual variance:		
$\mathrm{var}(\varepsilon_{ij})$	σ^2	0.03259207

not on the boundary of the parameter space. This can produce numerical difficulties in the maximization process. One way of circumventing this, is by artificially enlarging the true value d_{33}.

Let the model we just fitted for Y_{ij} be written as

$$Y_{ij} = X_i^{[j]}\boldsymbol{\beta} + b_{1i} + b_{2i}t_{ij} + b_{3i}t_{ij}^2 + \varepsilon_{ij},$$

where $X_i^{[j]}$ is the jth row of X_i, where t_{ij} is time expressed as months before diagnosis, and where the random effects b_{1i}, b_{2i} and b_{3i} have covariance matrix

$$\mathrm{var}(\boldsymbol{b_i}) = D = \begin{pmatrix} d_{11} & d_{12} & d_{13} \\ d_{12} & d_{22} & d_{23} \\ d_{31} & d_{32} & d_{33} \end{pmatrix}.$$

We can then reformulate the model as

$$\begin{aligned} Y_{ij} &= X_i^{[j]}\boldsymbol{\beta} + b_{1i} + 120\, b_{2i}\left(\frac{t_{ij}}{120}\right) + (120)^2\, b_{3i}\left(\frac{t_{ij}}{120}\right)^2 + \varepsilon_{ij} \\ &= X_i^{[j]}\boldsymbol{\beta} + b_{1i}^* + b_{2i}^* t_{ij}^* + b_{3i}^* t_{ij}^{*\,2} + \varepsilon_{ij}, \end{aligned}$$

which is a new linear mixed effects model, in which t_{ij}^* is now expressed in decades before diagnosis, and where the random effects $b_{1i}^* \equiv b_{1i}$, b_{2i}^* and b_{3i}^* now have covariance matrix

$$\mathrm{var}(\boldsymbol{b_i}^*) = D^* = \begin{pmatrix} (120)^0\, d_{11} & (120)^1\, d_{12} & (120)^2\, d_{13} \\ (120)^1\, d_{12} & (120)^2\, d_{22} & (120)^3\, d_{23} \\ (120)^2\, d_{31} & (120)^3\, d_{32} & (120)^4\, d_{33} \end{pmatrix}.$$

This transformation enlarges the covariance parameters substantially which implies that the log-likelihood function becomes much flatter. The normal equations, which are the equations to be solved in the maximization algorithm, now form a system which is much more stable and which can easily be solved without any convergence problems. In general, we therefore recommend to always rescale random effects with large ranges.

3.6   The RANDOM and REPEATED Statements

In Section 3.5.1, we introduced the RANDOM statement and the REPEATED statement of PROC MIXED, and both statements were used in our program on page 76 to fit model (3.7) to the prostate cancer data. However, since the covariance structure for the error components ε_i was taken equal to $\sigma^2 I_{n_i}$, which is the default in PROC MIXED, the same model can be fitted omitting the REPEATED statement. In practice, it is often sufficient to use only a RANDOM statement or only a REPEATED statement. In the first case, a hierarchical model is assumed, in which random effects are used to describe the covariance structure in the data while all remaining variability is assumed to be purely measurement error (the components in ε_i are assumed to be independently, identically distributed). The covariance structure is then assumed to be of the form $V_i = Z_i D Z_i' + \sigma^2 I_{n_i}$. In the other case, no random effects are included indicating that no part of the observed variability in the data can be ascribed to between-subject variability. The covariance structure for the data is then completely determined by the covariance structure Σ_i for the error components ε_i, which is specified in the REPEATED statement.

It should be noted however that, although both procedures have different interpretations, they can result in identical marginal models. We hereby also refer to our discussion in Section 3.4.1 on hierarchical and marginal models. As an example, we take the so-called 'random intercepts' or 'compound symmetry' model, which assumes a covariance structure of the form

$$\text{var}(\boldsymbol{y_i}) = V_i = \begin{pmatrix} \sigma^2 + \sigma_c^2 & \sigma_c^2 & \cdots & \sigma_c^2 \\ \sigma_c^2 & \sigma^2 + \sigma_c^2 & \cdots & \sigma_c^2 \\ \vdots & \vdots & \ddots & \vdots \\ \sigma_c^2 & \sigma_c^2 & \cdots & \sigma^2 + \sigma_c^2 \end{pmatrix}, \qquad (3.22)$$

for some nonnegative value σ_c^2. Although such an assumption is often not realistic in a longitudinal-data setting (constant variance and all correlations equal), it is frequently used in practice since it immediately follows from random factor ANOVA models (see for example Neter, Wasserman, and Kutner 1990, Section 17.6 or Searle 1987, Chapter 13).

Since the covariance matrix in (3.22) can be rewritten as

$$
V_i = \begin{pmatrix} 1 \\ 1 \\ \vdots \\ 1 \end{pmatrix} \sigma_c^2 \begin{pmatrix} 1 & 1 & \cdots & 1 \end{pmatrix} + \sigma^2 \begin{pmatrix} 1 & 0 & \cdots & 0 \\ 0 & 1 & \cdots & 0 \\ \vdots & \vdots & \ddots & \vdots \\ 0 & 0 & \cdots & 1 \end{pmatrix}
$$

$$
= Z_i \mathrm{var}(b_i) Z_i' + \sigma^2 I_{n_i},
$$

it can be interpreted as the covariance structure of a linear mixed model containing only random intercepts with variance σ_c^2, which can be fitted with PROC MIXED by specifying random intercepts in the RANDOM statement and omitting the REPEATED statement. Note also that in this case no 'type = ' option is needed in the RANDOM statement since for univariate random effects b_i all types result in the same covariance structure. Further, since the option 'type = CS' in the REPEATED statement results in a covariance structure for ε_i of the same form as (3.22), the same model can be fitted without the RANDOM statement. This shows that there are sometimes several ways for specifying a given model. In such a case, it is recommended to specify the model using the REPEATED statement rather then the RANDOM statement because this can reduce the computing time considerably.

This also implies that one should not conclude that the REPEATED statement is used whenever the data are of the repeated measures type. Some repeated measures models are best expressed using the RANDOM statement (see e.g., the prostate cancer data), while there are also random effects models which do not fall into the repeated measures class but where the REPEATED statement is the simplest tool for expressing them in PROC MIXED syntax. For example, suppose 100 exams were randomly assigned for correction to 10 randomly selected teachers. If Y_{ij} then denotes the grade assigned to the jth exam by the ith observer, the following random-factor ANOVA model can be used to analyze the data:

$$
Y_{ij} = \mu + \alpha_i + \varepsilon_{ij}. \tag{3.23}
$$

The parameter μ represents the overall mean, the parameters α_i are the random observer effects, and the ε_{ij} are components of measurement error. It is hereby assumed that all α_i and ε_{ij} are independent of each other, and that they are normally distributed with mean zero and constant variances σ_c^2 and σ^2 respectively. Model (3.23) can then be fitted using the following program:

```
proc mixed;
class observer;
model Y = / solution;
```

```
repeated / type = cs subject = observer;
run;
```

In this case, no effects need to be specified in the REPEATED statement since the ordering of observations for each of the observers is of no importance for the estimation of the mean structure (just an intercept) nor for the estimation of the covariance structure (constant variance and equal correlations).

Finally, note that PROC MIXED allows the specification of a wide range of specific structures for the random-effects covariance matrix D as well as for the covariance matrix Σ_i of the residual components. A selected set of possibilities is shown in Tables 3.2 and 3.3. Therefore, combining a RANDOM statement with a REPEATED statement allows the user to fit a large variety of covariance structures, as will be illustrated for the prostate cancer data in Section 3.12.3.

3.7   Testing and Estimating Contrasts of Fixed Effects

In practice, the fit of a statistical model to the data set at hand is only the first step in a statistical analysis. One is usually primarily interested in drawing inferences on specific aspects of the fitted model. In Section 3.7.1 it will be discussed how F-tests can be constructed in SAS to simultaneously test for the significance of sets of linear combinations of the fixed effects in the model. Afterwards, we will use these techniques in Section 3.7.2 to further investigate our model for the prostate cancer data, trying to reduce the number of fixed effects in the model as much as possible. This will result in a more parsimonious mean structure which simplifies the interpretation of the final results of our analysis. Finally, it will be explained in Section 3.7.3 how linear combinations of parameters in β can be estimated with PROC MIXED, and how confidence intervals based on approximate t-tests can be calculated.

3.7.1   The CONTRAST Statement

As an example, suppose we are interested in testing whether the local cancer cases evolve differently from the metastatic cancer cases. With respect to model (3.7), this means that the null hypothesis which is to be tested is given by

$$H_0 : \begin{cases} \beta_4 = \beta_5 \\ \beta_9 = \beta_{10} \\ \beta_{14} = \beta_{15}, \end{cases}$$

which is equivalent with testing

$$H_0 : \begin{pmatrix} 0\ 0\ 0\ 1\ -1\ 0\ 0\ 0\ 0 & 0\ 0\ 0\ 0\ 0 & 0 \\ 0\ 0\ 0\ 0 & 0\ 0\ 0\ 1\ -1\ 0\ 0\ 0 & 0 \\ 0\ 0\ 0\ 0 & 0\ 0\ 0\ 0\ 0 & 0\ 0\ 0\ 1\ -1 \end{pmatrix} \boldsymbol{\beta} = 0, \quad (3.24)$$

and is therefore also of the general form (3.19) for some known matrix L. The set of linear combinations $L\boldsymbol{\beta}$ is sometimes called a contrast (or a set of contrasts) of the fixed effects $\boldsymbol{\beta}$.

Using PROC MIXED, the above contrast can be tested adding the following CONTRAST statement to our initial program on page 76:

```
contrast 'L/R can = Met can' group 0 0 1 -1,
                             group*time 0 0 1 -1,
                             group*time2 0  0 1 -1;
```

Since it is allowed to test several contrasts at once (specifying several CON-TRAST statements), a label is needed for each contrast in order to identify them in the output. This label can be up to 20 characters long and must be enclosed in single quotes. In the above example, the label was 'L/R can = Met can'. Following the label, one needs to specify the linear combinations in the contrast, i.e., the rows in the matrix L, separated by commas. Each row in L is represented by a list of the effects, specified in the MODEL statement, followed by the appropriate elements in the corresponding row of the matrix L. Effects for which the corresponding parameters only get zero weight in the linear combination may be omitted. For example, the first row in (3.24) only gives non-zero weights to parameters in $\boldsymbol{\beta}$ assigned to the *group* effect. The first two parameters assigned to this effect (β_2 and β_3) get zero weight and the other two parameters (β_4 and β_5) get weights 1 and -1 respectively. This is represented in the first row of the above CONTRAST statement. A similar argument leads to the second and third row.

The result of the above CONTRAST statement is given in an extra output table labeled 'CONTRAST Statement Results':

CONTRAST Statement Results

Source	NDF	DDF	F	Pr > F
L/R can = Met can	3	299	5.86	0.0007

The F-statistic is calculated as in expression (3.20), and the null distribution is again approximated by an F-distribution with rank$(L) = 3$ numerator degrees of freedom. The denominator degrees of freedom is taken equal to the denominator degrees of freedom of the final effect listed in the CONTRAST statement. Note that this implies that different orderings of the effects in the CONTRAST statement may yield different numbers of denominator degrees of freedom for the corresponding F-test (the F-statistic will remain the same). However, this usually does not lead to different conclusions, provided there are sufficient blocks of independent information in the data. We hereby refer to our discussion in Section 3.5.2 on the degrees of freedom reported in the tables 'Solution for Fixed Effects' and 'Tests of Fixed Effects'.

For our example, we know from the output table on page 88 that all effects specified in the MODEL statement have 299 denominator degrees of freedom leading to 299 denominator degrees of freedom for testing contrast (3.24), independent of the order of the effects in the CONTRAST statement. Since the contrast is highly significant ($p = 0.0007$), we conclude that there are some very substantial differences among the two cancer groups, with respect to the average evolution of PSA as a function of time before diagnosis. These differences, amongst others, will be further explored in Section 3.7.2.

Since, all F-tests discussed in Section 3.5.2 and reported in the table 'Tests of Fixed effects' in the SAS output are tests for hypotheses of the general form (3.19), they can also be obtained using CONTRAST statements. Table 3.8 shows which contrasts need to be specified for testing the hypotheses in Table 3.5, which are the hypotheses tested by default if the original program on page 76 is run. The results of these CONTRAST statements are given in the following table 'CONTRAST Statement Results':

CONTRAST Statement Results

Source	NDF	DDF	F	Pr > F
H1	4	299	15.90	0.0001
H2	1	299	3.48	0.0631
H3	4	299	7.85	0.0001
H4	1	299	0.27	0.6026

TABLE 3.8. *CONTRAST statements needed to test all hypotheses in Table 3.5.*

Null hypothesis	Contrast statement
$H_1 : \beta_2 = \beta_3 = \beta_4 = \beta_5 = 0$	contrast 'H1' group 1 0 0 0, group 0 1 0 0, group 0 0 1 0, group 0 0 0 1;
$H_2 : \beta_1 = 0$	contrast 'H2' age 1;
$H_3 : \beta_7 = \beta_8 = \beta_9 = \beta_{10} = 0$	contrast 'H3' group*time 1 0 0 0, group*time 0 1 0 0, group*time 0 0 1 0, group*time 0 0 0 1;
$H_4 : \beta_6 = 0$	contrast 'H4' age*time 1;
$H_5 : \beta_{12} = \beta_{13} = \beta_{14} = \beta_{15} = 0$	contrast 'H5' group*time2 1 0 0 0, group*time2 0 1 0 0, group*time2 0 0 1 0, group*time2 0 0 0 1;
$H_6 : \beta_{11} = 0$	contrast 'H6' age*time2 1;

H5	4	299	4.44	0.0017
H6	1	299	0.07	0.7982

Note that the results are exactly the same as the ones reported in the table 'Tests of Fixed Effects' on page 88.

Adding a few CONTRAST statements to our program on page 76, we can now also obtain F-tests for the hypotheses given in Table 3.6, without first having to reparameterize the mean structure of our model. The required contrasts are shown in Table 3.9, and the results are reported as follows in the SAS output:

```
                CONTRAST Statement Results

     Source      NDF    DDF        F   Pr > F

      H7          3     299     20.13   0.0001
      H8          1     299      3.48   0.0631
      H9          1     299      0.07   0.7876
      H10         3     299     10.41   0.0001
      H11         1     299      0.27   0.6026
      H12         1     299      0.03   0.8610
      H13         3     299      5.93   0.0006
      H14         1     299      0.07   0.7982
```

TABLE 3.9. *CONTRAST statements needed to test all hypotheses in Table 3.6.*

Null hypothesis	Contrast statement
$H_7 : \beta_2 = \beta_3 = \beta_4 = \beta_5$	contrast 'H7' group 1 -1 0 0, group 1 0 -1 0, group 1 0 0 -1;
$H_8 : \beta_1 = 0$	contrast 'H8' agediag 1;
$H_9 : \beta_7 + \beta_8 + \beta_9 + \beta_{10} = 0$	contrast 'H9' group*time 1 1 1 1;
$H_{10} : \beta_7 = \beta_8 = \beta_9 = \beta_{10}$	contrast 'H10' group*time 1 -1 0 0, group*time 1 0 -1 0, group*time 1 0 0 -1;
$H_{11} : \beta_6 = 0$	contrast 'H11' agediag*time 1;
$H_{12} : \beta_{12} + \beta_{13} + \beta_{14} + \beta_{15} = 0$	contrast 'H12' group*time2 1 1 1 1;
$H_{13} : \beta_{12} = \beta_{13} = \beta_{14} = \beta_{15}$	contrast 'H13' group*time2 1 -1 0 0, group*time2 1 0 -1 0, group*time2 1 0 0 -1;
$H_{14} : \beta_{11} = 0$	contrast 'H14' agediag*time2 1;

The F-statistics are still the same as the ones reported previously on page 91, but note again the differences in denominator degrees of freedom, which is a direct consequence of the way SAS calculates the degrees of freedom for the F-approximation of the null distribution of the test statistic. However, as discussed before, this does not result in different conclusions.

3.7.2 Model Reduction

In this section, we will further investigate our model for the prostate cancer data. Testing contrasts of fixed effects, we will reduce the mean structure which simplifies the interpretation of the results of our analysis. This will be done in a hierarchical way, starting with the highest-order interaction terms, deleting non-significant terms and combining parameters which do not differ significantly. All tests are performed on the 5% level of significance, and each new hypothesis is tested, conditionally on the results of the previous tests of hypotheses, i.e., non-significant parameters are deleted before new hypotheses are tested. Finally, an overall F-test will be performed, comparing our final model to the original model (3.7). All contrasts tested are shown in Table 3.10.

First of all, since the interaction of age at diagnosis with *time2* was not significant (H_6, $p = 0.7982$) it has been removed from the model. Refitting the model showed that also the linear time effect does not depend significantly on the age at diagnosis (H_4, $p = 0.3665$) such that, from now on,

TABLE 3.10. *The different steps performed in reducing the mean structure of our original linear mixed model (3.7). For each step, the null hypothesis tested and the p-value resulting from the appropriate CONTRAST statement are shown. All tests are performed conditionally on the results of the previous tests.*

Null hypothesis	p-value
$H_6 : \beta_{11} = 0$	0.7982
$H_4 : \beta_6 = 0$	0.3665
$H_{15} : \beta_{12} - \beta_{13} = \beta_{14} - \beta_{15} = 0$	0.9716
$H_{16} : \beta_{12} = \beta_{13} = 0$	0.7726
$H_{10} : \beta_7 = \beta_8 = \beta_9 = \beta_{10}$	< 0.0001
$H_{17} : \beta_7 = 0$	0.1234
$H_{18} : \beta_8 = 0$	< 0.0001
$H_{19} : A : \beta_8 = \beta_9$	< 0.0001
$B : \beta_9 = \beta_{10}$	0.0063
$C : \beta_8 = \beta_{10}$	< 0.0001
$H_7 : \beta_2 = \beta_3 = \beta_4 = \beta_5$	< 0.0001
$H_{20} : A : \beta_2 = \beta_3$	< 0.0001
$B : \beta_2 = \beta_4$	< 0.0001
$C : \beta_2 = \beta_5$	< 0.0001
$D : \beta_3 = \beta_4$	< 0.0001
$E : \beta_3 = \beta_5$	< 0.0001
$F : \beta_4 = \beta_5$	< 0.0001
$H_{21} : \beta_2 = 0$	0.1889

we will consider models with only a main age effect in the mean structure.

We already know from the F-tests for the fixed effects in the model, reported in Section 3.5.2 that not all quadratic time effects are zero, but also that they differ between groups. Further, it follows from Table 3.4 that estimates of the quadratic time effects are similar for both non-cancer groups (controls and BPH-cases) but also for both cancer groups (L/R cancer and Metastatic cancer). Because H_{15} is not rejected ($p = 0.9716$), we can reduce our model, allowing one slope for the quadratic time effect for the cancer cases, and one slope for the quadratic time effect for the non-cancer cases. After the model is refitted, it follows from the t-tests in the table with the solutions for the fixed effects (not shown here) that this last slope is not significantly different from zero (H_{16}, $p = 0.7726$) from which we may conclude that only the cancer cases show a quadratic trend for $\ln(PSA)$ as a function of time before diagnosis.

Now that the mean structure with respect to the quadratic effect of time cannot be simplified further, we consider the linear time effects. First, there are some very substantial differences among the 4 diagnostic groups (H_{10}, p < 0.0001). Further, it follows from the t-tests for the fixed effects that there is no significant time effect for the control patients (H_{17}, $p = 0.1234$) indicating that the average profile for controls does not depend on time at all. Taking this into account, the test for the significance of the linear time effect of the BPH cases (H_{18}, p < 0.0001) and the tests for pairwise differences amongst the diagnostic groups of patients with prostate disease (H_{19A}, H_{19B} and H_{19C}, with all p-values ≤ 0.0063) suggest that no further simplification with respect to the linear trend in time is possible.

Further, the intercepts differ substantially among the diagnostic groups (H_7, p < 0.0001) and all pairwise differences of intercepts are significant (H_{20A} to H_{20F} with all p-values < 0.0001). Finally, although the average PSA level for the control patients is not significantly different from zero (H_{21}, $p = 0.1889$), we will not remove the corresponding effect from the model because a point estimate for the average PSA level in the control group may be of interest.

To conclude, the above analyses suggest that only a main age-effect is needed in the model, that the ln(PSA) level does not change over time, changes linearly over time, or changes quadratically over time for the controls, the BPH cases and the cancer cases respectively. Note that, since all hypotheses in Table 3.10 were performed conditionally on the results of the previous tests, we should confirm that this reduced model is still acceptable, when compared to the complete original model (3.7). This can be done by adding the following CONTRAST statement to the program on page 76:

```
contrast 'Final model' age*time2   1,
                        age*time    1,
                        group*time2 1 -1  0  0,
                        group*time2 0  0  1 -1,
                        group*time2 1  0  0  0,
                        group*time2 0  1  0  0,
                        group*time  1  0  0  0;
```

This results in the following table in the output:

```
          CONTRAST Statement Results

Source                  NDF   DDF       F  Pr > F

Final model               6   299    0.56  0.7583
```

TABLE 3.11. *Results from fitting the final model (3.25) to the prostate cancer data, using restricted maximum likelihood estimation.*

Effect	Parameter	Estimate (s.e.)
Age effect	β_1	0.016 (0.006)
Intercepts:		
control	β_2	-0.564 (0.428)
BPH	β_3	0.275 (0.488)
L/R cancer	β_4	1.099 (0.486)
Met. cancer	β_5	2.284 (0.531)
Time effects:		
BPH	β_8	-0.410 (0.068)
L/R cancer	β_9	-1.870 (0.233)
Met. cancer	β_{10}	-2.303 (0.262)
Time^2 effects:		
cancer	$\beta_{14} = \beta_{15}$	0.510 (0.088)
Covariance of b_i:		
var(b_{1i})	d_{11}	0.443 (0.093)
var(b_{2i})	d_{22}	0.842 (0.203)
var(b_{3i})	d_{33}	0.114 (0.035)
cov(b_{1i}, b_{2i})	$d_{12} = d_{21}$	-0.490 (0.124)
cov(b_{2i}, b_{3i})	$d_{23} = d_{32}$	-0.300 (0.082)
cov(b_{3i}, b_{1i})	$d_{13} = d_{31}$	0.148 (0.047)
Residual variance:		
var(ε_{ij})	σ^2	0.028 (0.002)
Observations		463
REML log-likelihood		-20.165
-2 REML log-likelihood		40.330
Akaike's Information Criterion		-27.165
Schwarz's Bayesian Criterion		-41.579

suggesting that no important terms have been left out of the model. Note that, although the L matrix which corresponds to the above CONTRAST statement has 7 rows, there are only 6 numerator degrees of freedom for the resulting F-test. Indeed, we have that rank(L) is only 6 since the third row equals the fifth row minus the sixth row.

From now on, all further inferences will be based on the reduced final model which can be written as:

$$
\begin{aligned}
Y_{ij} &= \mathbf{Y}_i(t_{ij}) \\
&= \beta_1 Age_i + \beta_2 C_i + \beta_3 B_i + \beta_4 L_i + \beta_5 M_i \\
&\quad + (\beta_8 B_i + \beta_9 L_i + \beta_{10} M_i) \times t_{ij} \\
&\quad + \beta_{14}(L_i + M_i) \times t_{ij}^2 \\
&\quad + b_{1i} + b_{2i} \times t_{ij} + b_{3i} \times t_{ij}^2 + \varepsilon_{ij}, \quad\quad (3.25)
\end{aligned}
$$

and which can be fitted in SAS replacing the program on page 76 by

```
proc mixed data = test noclprint method = reml covtest;
class id group timeclss;
model lnpsa = group age bph*time loccanc*time
              metcanc*time cancer*time2 / noint solution;
random intercept time time2 / type = un subject = id g;
repeated timeclss / type = simple subject = id r;
run;
```

The SAS variables *cancer*, *BPH*, *loccanc* and *metcanc* are dummy variables defined to be equal to one if the patient has prostate cancer, benign prostatic hyperplasia, local prostate cancer or metastatic prostate cancer respectively, and zero otherwise. The other variables *id*, *group*, *time* and *timeclss* are as defined in Section 3.5.1. The option 'noclprint' has been added to the PROC MIXED statement to prevent printing of all levels of the variables specified in the CLASS statement.

Table 3.11 contains the parameter estimates and estimated standard errors for all fixed effects and variance components in model (3.25), together with some extra information on the fit of the model, which will be useful in the sequel. Figure 3.3 shows the average fitted profiles based on this final model, for a man of median age at diagnosis, for each of the diagnostic groups separately. Note how little difference there is with the average fitted profiles in Figure 3.2, based on the full model (3.7).

3.7.3 The ESTIMATE Statement

To illustrate the fact that cancer patients can be better discriminated from BPH cases using the rate of increase of PSA (which can only be estimated when repeated PSA-measurements are available) rather than just one single measurement of PSA (see also Section 3.2), we estimate the average difference in $\ln(1 + PSA)$ between these two groups, as well as the average difference in the rate of increase of $\ln(PSA)$ between the two groups,

Average profiles

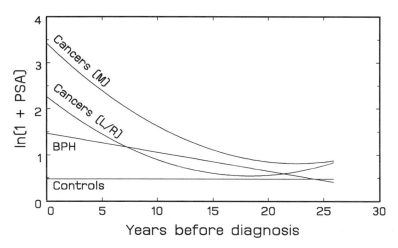

FIGURE 3.3. *Fitted average profiles for males with median ages at diagnosis, based on the final model (3.25), where the parameters are estimated using restricted maximum likelihood estimation.*

5 years prior to diagnosis. If we ignore the metastatic cancer cases, this is equivalent with estimating

$$
\begin{aligned}
\text{DIFF}(t = 5 \text{ years}) \ &= \ \left(\beta_1 \ age + \beta_4 + \beta_9 \ t + \beta_{14} \ t^2 \right)\big|_{t=0.5} \\
&\quad - \left(\beta_1 \ age + \beta_3 + \beta_8 \ t \right)\big|_{t=0.5} \\
&= \ -\beta_3 + \beta_4 - 0.5 \ \beta_8 + 0.5 \ \beta_9 + 0.25 \ \beta_{14}
\end{aligned}
$$

and

$$
\begin{aligned}
\text{DIFFRATE}(t = 5 \text{ years}) \ &= \ \frac{\partial}{\partial t} \left(\beta_1 \ age + \beta_4 + \beta_9 \ t + \beta_{14} \ t^2 \right)\bigg|_{t=0.5} \\
&\quad - \frac{\partial}{\partial t} \left(\beta_1 \ age + \beta_3 + \beta_8 \ t \right)\bigg|_{t=0.5} \\
&= \ -\beta_8 + \beta_9 + \beta_{14}
\end{aligned}
$$

which are of the form $L\beta$, for specific (1×15) matrices L. PROC MIXED allows us to estimate such linear combinations, and to construct confidence intervals based on approximate t-tests. This is done by adding the following ESTIMATE statements to our program on page 104:

```
estimate 'DIFF, t = 5yrs' group 0 -1 1 0
                         bph*time -0.5
                         loccanc*time 0.5
                         cancer*time2 0.25
```

```
                              / cl alpha = 0.05;

estimate 'DIFFRATE, t = 5yrs' bph*time -1
                              loccanc*time 1
                              cancer*time2 1
                              / cl alpha = 0.05;
```

Note that the matrices L are specified in exactly the same way as in the CONTRAST statement (see Section 3.7.1). The only difference is that now only matrices with one row are allowed, i.e., L is required to be a row-vector. The option 'cl alpha=0.05' is used to request that an approximate t-type 95% confidence interval is calculated for the linear combination specified. The output of the above additional statements is given in a new table which is labeled 'ESTIMATE Statement Results':

ESTIMATE Statement Results

Parameter	Estimate	Std Error	DDF	T
DIFF, t = 5yrs	0.22081242	0.14573103	301	1.52
DIFFRATE, t = 5yrs	-0.95067653	0.16587627	301	-5.73

Pr > |T|	Alpha	Lower	Upper
0.1308	0.05	-0.0660	0.5076
0.0001	0.05	-1.2771	-0.6243

The reported t-tests are equivalent with the F-tests we would obtain from specifying the same linear combinations in two CONTRAST statements. However, we now also get a point estimate for $L\beta$, together with its estimated standard error and a confidence interval based on the t-approximation for the t-statistic. The above table shows that, on average, five years prior to diagnosis, there is no significant difference in ln(PSA) between the local cancer cases and the BPH cases, while the rate of increase of PSA differed highly significantly. This illustrates why repeated measures of PSA are needed to discriminate between the different prostate diseases.

3.8   PROC MIXED versus PROC GLM

For balanced longitudinal data (i.e., longitudinal data where all subjects have the same number of repeated measures, taken at time points which are also the same for all subjects), one often analyses the data using the SAS procedure PROC GLM, fitting general multivariate regression models (Seber 1984, Chapters 8 and 9) to the data. Such models can also be fitted with PROC MIXED by omitting the RANDOM statement and including a REPEATED statement with option 'type=UN'. One then fits a linear model with a general unstructured covariance matrix $\Sigma = \Sigma_i$. However, the two procedures do not necessarily yield the same results: PROC GLM only takes into account the data of the completers, i.e., only the data of the subjects with all measurements available are used in the calculations. PROC MIXED on the other hand, uses all available data. Hence, patients for which not all measurements were recorded will still be taken into account in the analysis. We refer to Section 5.7 for an illustration.

The multivariate approach used in the GLM procedure produces multivariate tests for the fixed effects based on Wilk's Lambda likelihood ratio test statistic (see e.g., Rao 1973, Chapter 8 and SAS 1989, Chapter 1). The resulting F-tests are based on a better approximation to the actual distribution of the test statistic than that for the F-tests given by the MIXED procedure (see Roger and Kenward 1993). Further, apart from the multivariate tests, PROC GLM also provides a univariate analysis for the response at each time point separately. This can also be obtained with PROC MIXED, by specifying a WHERE statement. For example, an analysis of the responses at time $t = 2$ is requested by adding the following line to the main program:

```
where time = 2;
```

Note that this again may yield different results than PROC GLM due to the fact that now all second measurements are analyzed rather than only the measurements from the patients with measurements taken at all time points. Finally, the 'split unit' type of analysis provided by the GLM procedure can be obtained using PROC MIXED from fitting a compound symmetry model (see Section 3.6). However, Greenhouse-Geiser and Huynh-Feldt corrections to the F-tests are not available in the MIXED procedure, but they are not really required as it is very simple to fit and test models with more complex covariance structures.

PROC MIXED models the data of each individual separately (remember how we constructed the model for the prostate cancer data in Section 3.3). This implies that it is not assumed that an equal number of repeated observations are taken from each individual or that all individuals should be measured on the same time points. Hence, the measurements can be viewed as being taken at a continuous rather than discrete time scale. Also, the use of random effects allows us to model covariances as continuous functions of time. Another main advantage in using the MIXED procedure is the fact that all available data (not only the 'complete cases') are used in the analysis. Finally, PROC MIXED also allows us to include time-varying covariates in the mean structure, which is not possible in PROC GLM. This was illustrated in the prostate cancer example where linear as well as quadratic time effects have been included to model the mean response.

For a more elaborate discussion on the comparison between the procedures MIXED and GLM, we refer to Roger and Kenward (1993) and Roger (1993).

3.9   Tests for the Need of Random Effects

In Section 3.5.3, it was shown how variance components which are almost zero can cause convergence problems, and how one can try to solve them. On the other hand, such numerical problems might indicate that the true value of the variance component is exactly zero. For example, in the prostate cancer example, $d_{33} = 0$ would mean that no random slopes for the quadratic effect of time would be needed, i.e. that, within each diagnostic group, all individuals have the same quadratic time effect.

Also, in the Sections 3.5.2, 3.7.1 and 3.7.3 it has been explained how to construct statistical tests concerning the fixed effects included in the model, but all of this was conditional on the random effects in the model. For example, in the analysis of the prostate cancer data, we assumed random intercepts, random slopes for time, and random slopes for time^2. This was suggested by the plots of individual profiles in Figure 3.1.

Although the covariance structure may not be of primary interest, adequate covariance modeling is useful for the interpretation of the random variation in the data and it is essential to obtain valid inferences for the parameters in the mean structure of the model, which usually is of primary interest. Overparameterization of the covariance structure leads to inefficient estimation and potentially poor assessment of standard errors for estimates of the mean response profiles (fixed effects), whereas a too restrictive specification invalidates inferences about the mean response profile when the assumed covariance structure does not hold (Altham 1984).

For all these reasons, it is necessary to construct statistical tests for the significance of the random effects in the model. It has been shown in Section 3.5.2 that, due to boundary problems, the reported p-values for the variance components cannot be used for testing the need for including random effects into the model. In Section 3.9.1, we will discuss how correct tests can be obtained using likelihood ratio tests based on either the maximum likelihood or restricted maximum likelihood function. Afterwards, in Section 3.9.2, these results will be applied to the prostate cancer data.

3.9.1   The Likelihood Ratio Test

As discussed before, testing for the significance of random effects is a non-standard problem since the null hypothesis (one or more random effects have zero variance) is on the boundary of the parameter space of the alternative hypothesis. Therefore, since the usual regularity conditions in classical likelihood theory (Cox and Hinkley 1990, Chapter 9) are not satisfied, the well-known asymptotic results, such as the asymptotic normality for the estimators and the asymptotic chi-squared null distribution for the likelihood ratio test statistic, are not necessarily valid any longer.

Still, Roger and Kenward (1993) use the likelihood ratio test, based on REML likelihoods, and they apply the classical likelihood theory, ignoring the boundary problem. They also mention that ratios of maximized REML likelihoods cannot be used to test parameters in the fixed-effects part of the model. This is because different error contrasts $U = K'Y$ (see Section 3.4.3) are then used in the maximization procedures such that likelihoods would be compared, based on different observations.

Later, Stram and Lee (1994) used results for nonstandard testing situations by Self and Liang (1987) to show that the asymptotic null distribution for the likelihood ratio test statistic for testing the significance of random effects in a linear mixed-effects model is often a mixture of chi-squared distributions rather than one single chi-squared distribution. For ANOVA models with independent random effects, this was already briefly discussed by Miller (1977). Let L_{ML} denote again the likelihood function (3.10) and let $-2 \ln \lambda_N$ be the likelihood ratio test statistic defined as

$$-2 \ln \lambda_N \quad = \quad -2 \ln \left[\frac{L_{\mathrm{ML}}(\widehat{\boldsymbol{\theta}}_{\mathrm{ML},0})}{L_{\mathrm{ML}}(\widehat{\boldsymbol{\theta}}_{\mathrm{ML},1})} \right],$$

where $\widehat{\boldsymbol{\theta}}_{\mathrm{ML},0}$ and $\widehat{\boldsymbol{\theta}}_{\mathrm{ML},1}$ are the maximum likelihood estimates under the null-hypothesis and under the alternative hypothesis respectively. Stram and Lee (1994, 1995) then discuss several specific testing situations, the results of which will be presented in the following sections. Although these results were derived for the case of maximum likelihood estimation, the same results apply for restricted maximum likelihood estimation (personal communication with Daniel O. Stram). However, as mentioned before, one can then only compare models with the same mean structure since otherwise the error contrasts (see Section 3.4.3) would not be the same for the two models such that likelihoods for different data would be compared.

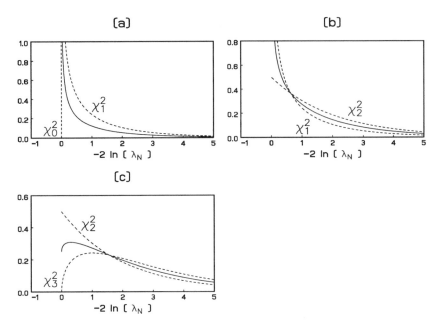

FIGURE 3.4. *Graphical representation of the asymptotic null distribution of the likelihood ratio statistic for testing the significance of random effects in a linear mixed model, for three different types of hypotheses. For each case, the distribution (solid line) is a mixture of two chi-squared distributions (dashed lines), with both weights equal to 0.5:*
(a) Case 1: no random effects versus one random effect.
(b) Case 2: one random effect versus two random effects.
(c) Case 3: two random effects versus three random effects.

CASE 1: NO RANDOM EFFECTS VERSUS ONE RANDOM EFFECT

For testing $H_0 : D = 0$ versus $H_1 : D = d_{11}$, where d_{11} is a non-negative scalar, we have that the asymptotic null distribution of $-2 \ln \lambda_N$ is a mixture of χ_1^2 and χ_0^2 with equal weights 0.5. The χ_0^2 distribution is the distribution which gives probability mass one to the value 0. The mixture is shown in panel (a) of Figure 3.4. Note that if the classical null distribution would be used, all p-values would be overestimated. Therefore, the null hypothesis would be accepted too often, resulting in incorrectly simplifying the covariance structure of the model, which may seriously invalidate inferences, as shown by Altham (1984).

CASE 2: ONE VERSUS TWO RANDOM EFFECTS

In the case one wishes to test

$$H_0 : D = \begin{pmatrix} d_{11} & 0 \\ 0 & 0 \end{pmatrix},$$

for some strictly positive d_{11}, versus H_1 that D is a (2×2) positive semi-definite matrix, we have that the asymptotic null distribution of $-2 \ln \lambda_N$ is a mixture with equal weights 0.5 for χ_2^2 and χ_1^2, shown in Figure 3.4(b). Similar to case 1, we have that ignoring the boundary problems may result in too parsimonious covariance structures.

CASE 3: q VERSUS $q + 1$ RANDOM EFFECTS

For testing the hypothesis

$$H_0 : D = \begin{pmatrix} D_{11} & \mathbf{0} \\ \mathbf{0}' & 0 \end{pmatrix}, \tag{3.26}$$

in which D_{11} is a $(q \times q)$ positive definite matrix, versus H_1 that D is a general $((q + 1) \times (q + 1))$ positive semi-definite matrix, the large-sample behavior of the null distribution of $-2 \ln \lambda_N$ is a mixture of χ_{q+1}^2 and χ_q^2, again with equal weights 0.5. A graphical representation for the case of testing two random effects $(q = 2)$ versus three random effects is given in the third panel of Figure 3.4. Again, we have that the correction due to the boundary problems reduces the p-values in order to protect against the use of oversimplified covariance structures.

CASE 4: q VERSUS $q + k$ RANDOM EFFECTS

The null distribution of $-2 \ln \lambda_N$ for testing (3.26) versus

$$H_1 : D = \begin{pmatrix} D_{11} & D_{12} \\ D_{12}' & D_{22} \end{pmatrix},$$

which is a general $((q + k) \times (q + k))$ positive semi-definite matrix, is a mixture of χ^2 random variables as well as other types of random variables formed by the lengths of projections of multivariate normal random variables upon curved as well as flat surfaces. Apart from very special cases, current statistical knowledge calls for simulation methods to estimate the appropriate null distribution.

REMARKS WITH RESPECT TO PROC MIXED

Strictly speaking, the marginal distribution corresponding to model (3.8) does not require positive definiteness of the matrix D, as long as all marginal covariance matrices $V_i = Z_i D Z_i' + \sigma^2 I_{n_i}$ are positive definite, but the model can then no longer be interpreted as a random-effects model (as was explicitly done in our formulation of model (3.8)). Further, note that the results in the above cases 1 to 4 assume that the likelihood function can be maximized over the space Ω of positive *semi*-definite matrices D, and that the estimating procedure is able to convergence for example to values of D which are positive semi-definite but not positive definite.

According to Stram and Lee (1994), this assumption did not hold for PROC MIXED when their paper was written, and they therefore discuss how the above results should be corrected if PROC MIXED is used. Since the procedure only allowed maximization of the likelihood over a subspace of Ω, the likelihood ratio statistics were typically too small. For the above third case for example, the asymptotic null distribution became a mixture of χ^2_{q+1} and χ^2_0 with equal weight 0.5.

Since release 6.10 of PROC MIXED, the only constraint on the estimate of an unstructured (option 'type = UN' in the RANDOM statement) covariance matrix D is that its diagonal elements (the variances of the random effects) are nonnegative. In some cases this can even lead to estimates of D which are not nonnegative definite. Because any symmetric matrix with at least one negative diagonal element is not positive semi-definite, we have that Ω is a subspace of the set of all symmetric matrices with nonnegative diagonal elements. Hence, we may conclude that it now has become possible to maximize the likelihood over Ω, and therefore that the original results, as described in the cases 1 to 4, are valid even when PROC MIXED is used. However, since the likelihood is now maximized over a parameter space which is larger than Ω one should check the resulting estimate $\widehat{D}$ for positive semi-definiteness.

3.9.2   Applied to the Prostate Data

For the prostate data, the hypothesis of most interest is that only random intercepts and random slopes for the linear time effect are needed, and hence that the random slopes for the quadratic time effect may be omitted (case 3). However, for illustrative purposes, we tested all hypothesis of deleting one random effect from the model, in a hierarchical way starting from the highest order time effect. Likelihood ratio tests were used, based on maximum likelihood as well as on restricted maximum likelihood esti-

TABLE 3.12. *Several random-effects models with the associated value for the log likelihood value evaluated at the parameter estimates, for maximum as well as restricted maximum likelihood estimation.*

	$\ln \left| L(\widehat{\boldsymbol{\theta}}) \right|$	
Random effects	ML	REML
Model 1: Intercepts, time, time^2	-3.575	-20.165
Model 2: Intercepts, time	-50.710	-66.563
Model 3: Intercepts	-131.218	-149.430
Model 4: _____	-251.275	-272.367

mation. The models and the associated maximized log-likelihood values are shown in Table 3.12. Further, Table 3.13 shows the likelihood ratio statistics for dropping one random effect at a time starting from the quadratic time effect. The correct asymptotic null distributions directly follow from the results described in the cases 1 to 3. We hereby denote a mixture of two chi-squared distributions with k_1 and k_2 degrees of freedom, with equal weights 0.5, by $\chi^2_{k_1:k_2}$. The naive asymptotic null distribution is the one which follows from applying the classical likelihood theory, ignoring the boundary problem for the null hypothesis, i.e., a chi-squared distribution with degrees of freedom equal to the number of free parameters which vanish under the null hypothesis. All values for $-2\ln(\lambda_N)$ are larger than 90 yielding p-values smaller than 0.0001. We conclude that the covariance structure should not be simplified deleting random effects from the model. We refer to Section 4.3 for an example where the naive and the corrected p-value differ much more.

3.10 Comparing Non-Nested Covariance Structures

So far, we have only discussed the comparison of nested covariance structures, for which the likelihood ratio test can be used. In order to extend this to the case where one wants to discriminate between models with non-nested covariance structures, we take a closer look at the previous likelihood ratio tests. Let ℓ_A and ℓ_o denote the ML (REML) log-likelihood function evaluated at the ML (REML) estimates obtained under the alternative hypothesis and the null hypothesis respectively. Further, let $\#\alpha_o$ and $\#\alpha_A$ denote the number of variance components under the null hypothesis and under the alternative hypothesis respectively. The test then rejects the null hypothesis if $\ell_A - \ell_o$ is large in comparison to the difference in degrees of

TABLE 3.13. *Likelihood ratio statistics with the correct as well as naive asymptotic null distribution for comparing random-effects models, for maximum as well as restricted maximum likelihood estimation. A mixture of two chi-squared distributions with k_1 and k_2 degrees of freedom and with equal weight for both distributions, is denoted by $\chi^2_{k_1:k_2}$.*

		Maximum likelihood	
		Asymptotic null distribution	
Hypothesis	$-2\ln(\lambda_N)$	Correct	Naive
Model 2 versus Model 1	94.270	$\chi^2_{2:3}$	χ^2_3
Model 3 versus Model 2	161.016	$\chi^2_{1:2}$	χ^2_2
Model 4 versus Model 3	240.114	$\chi^2_{0:1}$	χ^2_1
		Restricted maximum likelihood	
		Asymptotic null distribution	
Hypothesis	$-2\ln(\lambda_N)$	Correct	Naive
Model 2 versus Model 1	92.796	$\chi^2_{2:3}$	χ^2_3
Model 3 versus Model 2	165.734	$\chi^2_{1:2}$	χ^2_2
Model 4 versus Model 3	245.874	$\chi^2_{0:1}$	χ^2_1

freedom between the two models which are to be compared, or equivalently if

$$\ell_A - \mathcal{F}(\#\boldsymbol{\alpha}_A) \; > \; \ell_0 - \mathcal{F}(\#\boldsymbol{\alpha}_0)$$

for an appropriate function $\mathcal{F}(\cdot)$. For example, when tests are performed at the 5% level of significance, for hypotheses of the same form as those described in the third case in Section 3.9.1, $\mathcal{F}$ was such that

$$2\left[\mathcal{F}(\#\boldsymbol{\alpha}_A) - \mathcal{F}(\#\boldsymbol{\alpha}_0)\right] \;=\; \chi^2_{(\#\boldsymbol{\alpha}_A-\#\boldsymbol{\alpha}_0-1):(\#\boldsymbol{\alpha}_A-\#\boldsymbol{\alpha}_0),0.95}$$

where $\chi^2_{k_1:k_2,0.95}$ denotes the 95% percentile of the $\chi^2_{k_1:k_2}$ distribution. This procedure can be interpreted as a formal test of significance only if the model under the null hypothesis is nested within the model under the alternative hypothesis. However, if this is not the case, there is no reason why the above procedure could not be used as a rule of thumb, or why no other functions $\mathcal{F}(\cdot)$ could be used to construct empirical rules for discriminating between covariance structures. Other frequently used functions are shown in Table 3.14 all leading to different discriminating rules, called information criteria. Note that the AIC and SBC were already discussed in Section 3.5.2 since SAS reports these criteria by default in the 'Model Fitting Information' table. The other criteria can be requested by adding the option 'ic' to the PROC MIXED statement of the program.

TABLE 3.14. *Overview of the information criteria for comparing covariance models, which are available in PROC MIXED. We hereby define n^* equal to the total number $n = \sum_{i=1}^{N} n_i$ of observations or equal to $n - p$, depending on whether ML or REML estimation was used in the calculations.*

Criterion	Definition of $\mathcal{F}(\cdot)$
Akaike (AIC)	$\mathcal{F}(\#\boldsymbol{\alpha}) = \#\boldsymbol{\alpha}$
Schwarz (SBC)	$\mathcal{F}(\#\boldsymbol{\alpha}) = (\#\boldsymbol{\alpha} \ \ln n^*)/2$
Hannan and Quinn (HQIC)	$\mathcal{F}(\#\boldsymbol{\alpha}) = \#\boldsymbol{\alpha} \ \ln(\ln n^*)$
Bozdogan (CAIC)	$\mathcal{F}(\#\boldsymbol{\alpha}) = \#\boldsymbol{\alpha} \ (\ln n^* + 1)/2$

The model with the largest AIC, SBC, HQIC or CAIC is deemed best. We refer to the analyses of the first three case studies in Chapter 4 for some examples on the use of these criteria. Note, that these procedures only yield rules of thumb to discriminate between models with the same fixed effects, but with different covariance structures. They should not be used or interpreted as formal statistical tests of significance. In specific examples, different criteria can even lead to different models, as will be shown in Section 4.2.

3.11   Estimating the Random Effects

Although in practice one is usually primarily interested in estimating the parameters in the marginal linear mixed-effects model (the fixed effects $\boldsymbol{\beta}$ and the variance components D and σ^2), it is often useful to calculate estimates for the random effects $\boldsymbol{b}_i$ as well, since they reflect how much the subject-specific profiles deviate from the overall average profile. Such estimates can then be interpreted as residuals which may be helpful for detecting special profiles (i.e., outlying individuals) or groups of individuals evolving differently in time.

As indicated in Section 3.4.1, it is then no longer sufficient to assume that the marginal distribution of the responses $\boldsymbol{Y}_i$ is given by model (3.9), because it does not imply that the variability in the data can be explained by random effects. In this section, we will therefore explicitly assume that the hierarchical model (3.8) is appropriate. Since random effects represent natural heterogeneity between the subjects, this assumption will often be justified for data where the between-subjects variability is large in comparison to the within-subject variability. Note that this is the case for our prostate cancer data set (Figure 3.1).

Since the random effects in model (3.8) are assumed to be random variables, it is most natural to estimate them using Bayesian techniques (see for example Box and Tiao 1992, or Gelman *et al* 1995). As discussed in Section 3.4.1, the distribution of the vector Y_i of responses for the ith individual, conditional on that individual's specific regression coefficients b_i, is multivariate normal with mean vector $X_i\beta + Z_ib_i$ and with covariance matrix Σ_i, and the marginal distribution of b_i is multivariate normal with mean vector $\mathbf{0}$ and covariance matrix D. In the Bayesian literature, this last distribution is usually called the prior distribution of the parameters b_i since it does not depend on the data Y_i. Once observed values y_i for Y_i have been collected, the so-called posterior distribution of b_i, defined as the distribution of b_i, conditional on $Y_i = y_i$, can be calculated. If we denote the density function of Y_i conditional on b_i, and the prior density function of b_i by $f(y_i|b_i)$ and $f(b_i)$ respectively, we have that the posterior density function of b_i given $Y_i = y_i$ is given by

$$f(b_i|y_i) \equiv f(b_i|Y_i = y_i) = \frac{f(y_i|b_i)\,f(b_i)}{\int f(y_i|b_i)\,f(b_i)\,db_i}. \qquad (3.27)$$

For the sake of notational convenience, we hereby suppressed the dependence of all above density functions on certain components of θ.

Using the theory on general Bayesian linear models (Smith 1973 and Lindley and Smith 1972) it can be shown that (3.27) is the density of a multivariate normal distribution. Very often, b_i is estimated by the mean of this posterior distribution, called the posterior mean of b_i. This estimate is given by

$$\begin{aligned}
\widehat{b}_i(\theta) &= E\left[b_i \,|Y_i = y_i\right] \\
&= \int b_i\,f(b_i|y_i)\,db_i \\
&= DZ_i'W_i(\alpha)(y_i - X_i\beta), \qquad (3.28)
\end{aligned}$$

and the covariance matrix of the corresponding estimator equals

$$\mathrm{var}(\widehat{b}_i) = DZ_i'\left\{W_i - W_iX_i\left(\sum_{i=1}^{N}X_i'W_iX_i\right)^{-1}X_i'W_i\right\}Z_iD, \qquad (3.29)$$

where, as before, W_i equals V_i^{-1} (Laird and Ware 1982). Note that (3.29) underestimates the variability in $\widehat{b}_i - b_i$ since it ignores the variation of b_i. Therefore, one usually uses

$$\mathrm{var}(\widehat{b}_i - b_i) = D - \mathrm{var}(\widehat{b}_i) \qquad (3.30)$$

to assess the variation in $\widehat{b}_i - b_i$ (Laird and Ware 1982).

In a final step, the unknown parameters β and α in (3.28), (3.29) and (3.30) are replaced by their maximum or restricted maximum likelihood estimates. The resulting estimates for the random effects are called 'Empirical Bayes' (EB) estimates and will also be denoted by $\widehat{\boldsymbol{b}}_i$.

In PROC MIXED, the EB estimates for the random effects, as well as the estimates (3.30) needed for the calculation of approximate confidence intervals, can be obtained adding the option 'solution' to the RANDOM statement. If, for example, scatter plots or histograms of components of the $\widehat{\boldsymbol{b}}_i$ are to be made, then the estimates should also be converted to a SAS data set. This is done in the MAKE statement. The program on page 104 should then be completed as follows:

```
random intercept time time2
        / type = un subject = id g solution;
make 'solutionR' out=randeff noprint;
```

In general, the MAKE statement can be used to convert any table produced by PROC MIXED to a data set. Therefore, each table is given a label which can be found in the SAS manual (1996). The table containing the random-effects EB estimates for example, is labeled 'solutionR'. The option 'out=randeff' specifies the name of the SAS data set which will contain the requested information. Finally, the option 'noprint' avoids printing of the table in the SAS output. This option is particularly useful for large tables such as the one containing the EB estimates.

As an illustration, we calculated the EB estimates for the random effects in our final model (3.25). Frequency histograms and scatter plots of these estimates can be found in Figure 3.5. Note how the scatter plots clearly show strong negative correlations between the intercepts and slopes for time, and between the slopes for time and the slopes for time^2. On the other hand, the intercepts are positively correlated with the slopes for the quadratic time effect. This is in agreement with the estimates for the covariance parameters in D (see Table 3.11).

In practice, one often uses histograms and scatter plots of components of $\widehat{\boldsymbol{b}}_i$ for diagnostic purposes, such as the detection of outliers which are subjects who seem to evolve differently from the other subjects in the data set. For example, Morrell and Brant (1991) use scattergrams of the EB estimates to pinpoint outlying observations, DeGruttola, Lange, and Dafni (1991) report histograms of the EB estimates, and use a normal quantile plot of standardized estimated random intercepts to check their normality, and Waternaux, Laird, and Ware (1989) use several techniques based on the EB estimates to look for unusual individuals and departures from the model assumptions. The histograms in Figure 3.5 suggest the presence of

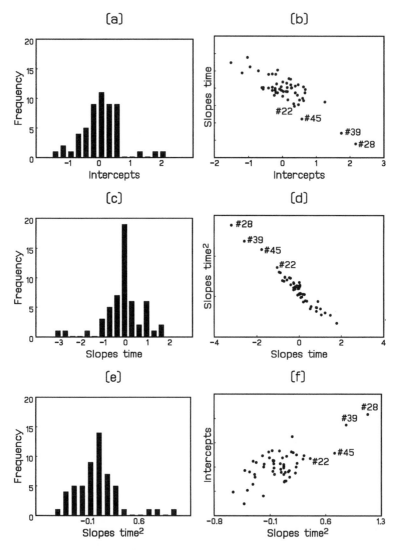

FIGURE 3.5. *Histograms (panels a, c and e) and scatter plots (panels b, d and f) of the empirical Bayes estimates for the random intercepts and slopes in the final model (3.25).*

such outliers. Furthermore, we highlighted the subjects #22, #28, #39 and #45 which are the individuals with the highest four slopes for time^2 and the smallest four slopes for time. Hence, these are the subjects with the strongest (quadratic) growth of $\ln(1 + \text{PSA})$ over time. Pearson *et al* (1994) noticed that the local/regional cancer cases #22, #28 and #39 were probably misclassified by the original methods of clinical staging and should have been included in the group of metastatic cancer cases instead.

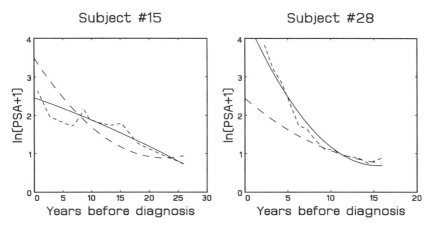

FIGURE 3.6. *Observed profiles (short dashes), population-average predicted profiles (long dashes), and subject-specific predicted profiles (solid line) for the subjects #15 and #28 of the prostate data set.*

Further, subject #45 is the metastatic cancer case with the highest rate of increase of $\ln(1 + \text{PSA})$ over time (see also Figure 3.1).

To illustrate the interpretation of the EB estimates, consider the prediction $\widehat{Y_i}$ of the ith profile. It follows from (3.28) that

$$
\begin{aligned}
\widehat{Y_i} &\equiv X_i\widehat{\beta} + Z_i\widehat{b_i} \\
&= X_i\widehat{\beta} + Z_i D Z_i' V_i^{-1}(y_i - X_i\widehat{\beta}) \\
&= \left(I_{n_i} - Z_i D Z_i' V_i^{-1}\right) X_i\widehat{\beta} + Z_i D Z_i' V_i^{-1} y_i \\
&= \Sigma_i V_i^{-1} X_i\widehat{\beta} + \left(I_{n_i} - \Sigma_i V_i^{-1}\right) y_i, \qquad (3.31)
\end{aligned}
$$

and therefore can be interpreted as a weighted mean of the population-averaged profile $X_i\widehat{\beta}$ and the observed data y_i, with weights $\Sigma_i V_i^{-1}$ and $I_{n_i} - \Sigma_i V_i^{-1}$ respectively. Note that the 'numerator' of $\Sigma_i V_i^{-1}$ is the residual covariance matrix Σ_i and the 'denominator' is the overall covariance matrix V_i. Hence, much weight will be given to the overall average profile if the residual variability is large in comparison to the between-subject variability (modeled by the random effects), while much weight will be given to the observed data if the opposite is true. As an illustration, we calculated $\widehat{Y_i}$ and $X_i\widehat{\beta}$ for the subjects #15 and #28 in the prostate data set. The resulting predicted profiles, and the observed profiles are shown in Figure 3.6. The EB estimates clearly correct the population-average profile towards the observed profile.

In the Bayesian literature, one usually refers to phenomena like those exhibited in expression (3.31), as to shrinkage (Carlin and Louis 1996, Strenio, Weisberg, and Bryk 1983). The observed data are shrunk towards the prior

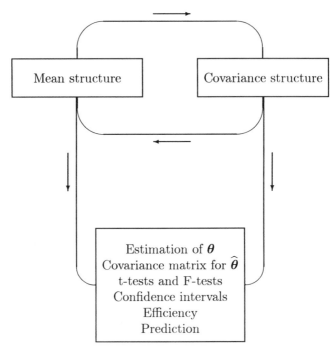

FIGURE 3.7. *Graphical representation of how the mean structure and the covariance structure of a linear mixed model influence each other, and how they affect the inference results.*

average profile which is $X_i\boldsymbol{\beta}$ since the prior mean of the random effects was zero. This is also illustrated in (3.30) which implies that for any linear combination $\boldsymbol{\lambda}$ of the random effects,

$$\text{var}(\boldsymbol{\lambda}'\widehat{\boldsymbol{b}_i}) \leq \text{var}(\boldsymbol{\lambda}'\boldsymbol{b}_i).$$

For example, the sample covariance matrix of the EB estimates $\widehat{\boldsymbol{b}_i}$ is

$$\widehat{\text{var}}(\widehat{\boldsymbol{b}_i}) = \begin{pmatrix} 0.4033 & -0.4398 & 0.1311 \\ -0.4398 & 0.7287 & -0.2532 \\ 0.1311 & -0.2532 & 0.0922 \end{pmatrix},$$

which clearly underestimates the variability in the random-effects population (compare to the elements of $\widehat{D}$ in Table 3.11).

3.12   General Guidelines for Model Construction

Under the linear mixed model (3.8), the data vector $\boldsymbol{Y}_i$ for the ith subject is assumed to be normally distributed with mean vector $X_i\boldsymbol{\beta}$ and covariance matrix $V_i = Z_i D Z_i' + \Sigma_i$. Hence, fitting linear mixed models implies that an appropriate mean structure as well as covariance structure needs to be specified. As shown in Figure 3.7, they are not independent of each other. Adequate covariance modeling is not only useful for the interpretation of the random variation in the data, it is essential to obtain valid inferences for the parameters in the mean structure, which is usually of primary interest. Too restrictive specifications invalidate inferences when the assumed structure does not hold, while overparameterization of the covariance structure leads to inefficient estimation and poor assessment of standard errors (Altham 1984). An incorrect covariance structure also affects predictions, as shown by Chi and Reinsel (1989). On the other hand, since the covariance structure models all variability in the data which is not explained by systematic trends, it highly depends on the specified mean structure.

For data sets where most variability in the measurements is due to between-subject variability, one can very often use the two-stage approach to construct an appropriate linear mixed model. This was illustrated for the prostate cancer data in Section 3.3. On the other hand, if the inter-subject variability is small in comparison to the intra-subject variability, this suggests that the covariance structure cannot be modeled using random effects but that an appropriate covariance matrix Σ_i for ε_i should be found.

In this section, some general guidelines will be discussed which can help the data analyst to select an appropriate linear mixed model for some specific data set at hand. All steps in this process will be illustrated with the prostate cancer data set.

3.12.1 Selection of a Preliminary Mean Structure

Since the covariance structure models all variability in the data which cannot be explained by the fixed effects, we start by first removing all systematic trends. As proposed by Diggle (1988) and by Diggle, Liang, and Zeger (1994) (Sections 4.4 and 5.3), we here fore use an over-elaborated model for the mean response profile. When the data are from a designed experiment in which the only relevant explanatory variables are the treatment labels, it is a sensible strategy to use a 'saturated model' for the mean structure. This incorporates a separate parameter for the mean response at each time point within each treatment group. For example, when 2 treatment groups had measurements at 4 fixed time points, we would use $p = 4 \times 2 = 8$

parameters to model $E(\mathbf{Y}_i)$. The X_i matrices would then equal

$$X_i = \begin{pmatrix} 1 & 0 & 0 & 0 & 0 & 0 & 0 & 0 \\ 0 & 1 & 0 & 0 & 0 & 0 & 0 & 0 \\ 0 & 0 & 1 & 0 & 0 & 0 & 0 & 0 \\ 0 & 0 & 0 & 1 & 0 & 0 & 0 & 0 \end{pmatrix} \quad \text{or} \quad X_i = \begin{pmatrix} 0 & 0 & 0 & 0 & 1 & 0 & 0 & 0 \\ 0 & 0 & 0 & 0 & 0 & 1 & 0 & 0 \\ 0 & 0 & 0 & 0 & 0 & 0 & 1 & 0 \\ 0 & 0 & 0 & 0 & 0 & 0 & 0 & 1 \end{pmatrix},$$

depending on whether the ith individual belongs to the first or second treatment group respectively.

For data in which the times of measurement are not common to all individuals, or when there are continuous covariates which are believed to affect the mean response, the concept of a saturated model breaks down and the choice of our most elaborate model becomes less obvious. In such cases, a plot of individual profiles often helps to select a candidate mean structure. For the prostate cancer data, the profiles (Figure 3.1) suggest to model $\ln(1 + PSA)$ as a quadratic function over time. This results in an intercept and a linear as well as quadratic time effect within each diagnostic group. Further, it has been anticipated that age is also an important prognostic covariate. We therefore also include age at diagnosis along with its interactions with time and time^2. Our preliminary mean structure therefore contains $4 \times 3 + 3 = 15$ fixed effects, represented by the vector $\boldsymbol{\beta}$. Note that this is the mean structure which was used in our initial model (3.7), and that at this stage, we deliberately favor over-parameterized models for $E(\mathbf{Y}_i)$ in order to get consistent estimators of the covariance structure in the following steps.

Once an appropriate mean structure $X_i\boldsymbol{\beta}$ for $E(\mathbf{Y}_i)$ has been selected, we use the ordinary least squares (OLS) method to estimate $\boldsymbol{\beta}$, and we hereby ignore that not all measurements are independent. It follows from the theory of generalized estimating equations (GEE), that this OLS estimator is consistent for $\boldsymbol{\beta}$ (Liang and Zeger 1986). This justifies the use of the OLS residuals $\boldsymbol{r}_i = \boldsymbol{y}_i - X_i\widehat{\boldsymbol{\beta}}_{\text{OLS}}$ for studying the dependence among the repeated measures.

3.12.2 Selection of Random-Effects

In a second step, we will select a set of random effects to be included in the covariance model. Note that random effects for time-independent covariates can be interpreted as subject-specific corrections to the overall mean structure. This makes them hard to distinguish from random intercepts. Therefore, one often includes random intercepts and random effects only for time-varying covariates. However, it will be shown in Section 4.3 that, in some applications, random effects for time-independent indicators may

OLS residual profiles

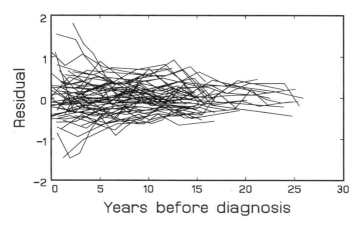

FIGURE 3.8. *Ordinary least squares (OLS) residual profiles for the prostate cancer data set.*

be useful to model differences in variability between subgroups of subjects or measurements. A helpful tool for deciding which time-varying covariates should be included in the model is a plot of the OLS residual profiles versus time. For the prostate data, this was done in Figure 3.8. When this plot shows constant variability over time, we assume stationarity (i.e., constant variance over time) and we do not include other random effects than intercepts. In cases where the variability varies over time and where there is still some remaining systematic structure in the residual profiles (i.e., where the between-subject variability is large in comparison to the overall variation), the following guidelines can be used to select one or more random effects additional to the random intercepts.

- Try to find a regression model for each residual profile in the above plot. Such models contain subject-specific parameters, and are therefore perfect candidates as random effects in our general linear mixed model. For example, if the residual profiles can be approximated by straight lines, then only random intercepts and random slopes for time would be included.

- Since our model always assumes the random effects $\boldsymbol{b}_i$ to have mean zero, we only consider covariates Z_i which have already been included as covariate in the fixed part (i.e., in X_i), or which are linear combinations of columns of X_i. Note that this condition was satisfied in the model (3.7) we used to analyze the prostate cancer data. For example, the second column of Z_i, which represents the linear random effect for time, equals the sum of the columns 7 up to 10 in X_i, which are the columns containing the linear time effects for the controls, the benign prostatic hyperplasia patients, the local cancer cases and for the metastatic cancer cases respectively.

- Morrell, Pearson, and Brant (1997) have shown that Z_i should not include a polynomial effect if not all hierarchically inferior terms are also included, and similarly for interaction terms. This generalizes the well-known results from linear regression (see e.g., Peixoto 1987, 1990) to random-effects models. It ensures the model to be invariant to coding transformations and avoids unanticipated covariance structures. This means that if, for example, we want to include quadratic random time effects, then also linear random time effects and random intercepts should be included.

- The choice of a set of random effects for the model automatically implies that the covariance matrix for Y_i is assumed to be of the general form $V_i = Z_i D Z_i' + \Sigma_i$. In the presence of random effects other than intercepts, it is often assumed (see e.g., Diggle, Liang, and Zeger 1994) that the diagonal elements in Σ_i are all equal such that the variance of $Y_i(t)$ depends on time, only through the component $Z_i(t) D Z_i'(t)$ where it is now explicitly indicated that the covariates Z_i depend on time. As an informal check for the appropriateness of the selected random effects, one can compare the fitted variance function based on a mixed-effects model with $\Sigma_i = \sigma^2 I_{n_i}$ to the sample variances of the residuals r_{ij} after grouping them into time-intervals.

In the example on prostate cancer, it was decided to include random intercepts and linear as well as quadratic random slopes for time. Note that, similar as in Section 3.12.1, we favor to include too many random effects rather than omitting some. This ensures that the remaining variability is not due to any missing random effects. However, it also should be emphasized that including high-dimensional random effects b_i with unconstrained covariance matrix D leads to complicated covariance structures, and may result in divergence of the maximization procedure.

As an informal check we subdivided the time axis in the intervals $[0, 3)$, $[3, 6)$, $[6, 9)$, $[9, 12)$, $[12, 15)$, $[15, 18)$, $[18, 21)$ and $[21, +\infty)$. Figure 3.9 compares the sample variances of the OLS residuals r_{ij} in each of the above intervals to the fitted variances obtained from calculating

$$\left(\begin{array}{ccc} 1 & t & t^2 \end{array} \right) \widehat{D} \left(\begin{array}{c} 1 \\ t \\ t^2 \end{array} \right) + \widehat{\sigma}^2$$

where $\widehat{D}$ and $\widehat{\sigma}^2$ are the REML estimates reported in Table 3.4. For each interval, the number of residuals r_{ij} used in the calculation of the sample

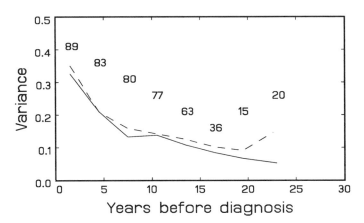

FIGURE 3.9. *Comparison of sample variances (solid line) to fitted variances (dashed line) obtained using the REML estimates in Table 3.4 for the variance components in model (3.7), at specific points in time. The numbers indicate the number of residuals r_{ij} used for the calculation of the corresponding sample variance.*

variances is indicated above the corresponding interval. In general both variance functions are quite similar, except in the last interval, which was the widest interval of all, and in which relatively few residuals were available to estimate the residual variability.

3.12.3 Selection of Residual Covariance Structure

Conditional on our selected set of random effects, we now need to specify the covariance matrix Σ_i for the error components ε_i. Many possible covariance structures are available at this stage, some of which have been described in Section 3.5.1. Unfortunately, apart from the information criteria discussed in Section 3.10, there are no general simple techniques available to compare all these models. For highly unbalanced data with many repeated measurements per subject, one usually assumes that random effects can account for most of the variation in the data and that the remaining error components ε_i have a very simple covariance structure, leading to parsimonious models for V_i.

One frequently used class of covariance structures for ε_i has been proposed by Diggle, Liang, and Zeger (1994). They assume that ε_i has constant variance and can be decomposed as $\varepsilon_i = \varepsilon_{(1)i} + \varepsilon_{(2)i}$ in which $\varepsilon_{(2)i}$ is a component of serial correlation suggesting that at least part of an indi-

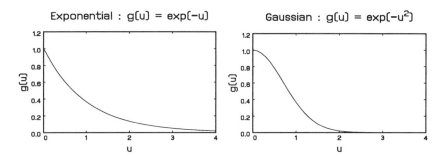

FIGURE 3.10. *Exponential and Gaussian serial correlation functions.*

vidual's observed profile is a response to time-varying stochastic processes operating within that individual. This type of random variation results in a correlation between serial measurements which is usually a decreasing function of the time separation between these measurements. Further, $\varepsilon_{(1)i}$ is an extra component of measurement error reflecting variation added by the measurement process itself, and assumed to be independent of $\varepsilon_{(2)i}$. The resulting linear mixed model can then be written as

$$
\begin{cases}
Y_i = X_i\beta + Z_i b_i + \varepsilon_{(1)i} + \varepsilon_{(2)i} \\[2mm]
b_i \sim N(\mathbf{0}, D), \\[2mm]
\varepsilon_{(1)i} \sim N(\mathbf{0}, \sigma^2 I_{n_i}), \\[2mm]
\varepsilon_{(2)i} \sim N(\mathbf{0}, \tau^2 H_i), \\[2mm]
b_1, \ldots, b_N, \varepsilon_{(1)1}, \ldots, \varepsilon_{(1)N}, \varepsilon_{(2)1}, \ldots, \varepsilon_{(2)N} \text{ independent,}
\end{cases}
\tag{3.32}
$$

and is completed by assuming a specific structure for the $(n_i \times n_i)$ correlation matrix H_i. Such structures are often borrowed from time-series analysis. One usually assumes that the serial effect $\varepsilon_{(2)i}$ is a population phenomenon, independent of the individual. The serial covariance matrix H_i then only depends on i through the number n_i of observations and through the time points t_{ij} at which measurements were taken. Further, it is assumed that the (j, k) element h_{ijk} of H_i is modeled as $h_{ijk} = g(|t_{ij} - t_{ik}|)$ for some decreasing function $g(\cdot)$ with $g(0) = 1$. This means that the correlation between $\varepsilon_{(2)ij}$ and $\varepsilon_{(2)ik}$ only depends on the time interval between the measurements y_{ij} and y_{ik}, and decreases if the length of this interval increases.

Two frequently used functions $g(\cdot)$ are the exponential and Gaussian serial correlation functions defined as $g(u) = \exp(-\phi u)$ and $g(u) = \exp(-\phi u^2)$ respectively ($\phi > 0$) and which are shown in Figure 3.10 for $\phi = 1$. The

most important qualitative difference between these functions is their behavior near $u = 0$. Extending the domain of the functions to all real u,
by requiring $g(-u) = g(u)$, we see that the exponential serial correlation
function is not differentiable at $u = 0$ while the Gaussian serial correlation function is infinitely differentiable. Note also that the corresponding
covariance matrices H_i are special cases of the so-called spatial covariance
structures, some of which have been shown in Table 3.3.

Verbeke, Lesaffre, and Brant (1997) and Verbeke and Lesaffre (1997b)
(see also Section 3.13.3) have shown that the residual components in the
prostate cancer model indeed contain a serial correlation component $\varepsilon_{(2)i}$,
which is probably of the Gaussian type. The linear mixed model with our
preliminary mean structure, with random intercepts and random slopes for
the linear as well as quadratic time effect, with measurement error and with
Gaussian serial correlation can now be fitted using the following program:

```
proc mixed data = prostate method = reml covtest;
class id group timeclss;
model lnpsa = group age group*time age*time
              group*time2 age*time2 / noint solution;
random intercept time time2 / type = un subject = id g;
repeated timeclss / type = sp(gau)(time) local subject = id;
run;
```

The option 'type=sp(gau)(time)' is used to specify the Gaussian serial correlation structure with the SAS variable *time* as the variable which needs
to be used to calculate the time-differences between the repeated measures.
The option 'local' is needed if a measurement error component $\varepsilon_{(1)i}$ should
be added to the serial correlation component $\varepsilon_{(2)i}$. The REML estimates
and estimated standard errors of all variance components in this model are
shown in Table 3.15. Note how SAS estimates $1/\sqrt{\phi}$ rather than ϕ itself.
This is to assure positiveness of ϕ and to allow testing whether $\phi = +\infty$,
under which H_i becomes equal to the identity matrix I_{n_i}, meaning that
no serial correlation would be present in the error components ε_i. Comparing minus twice the REML log likelihood of the above model with the
value obtained without the serial correlation component (see table 'Model
Fitting Information for LNPSA' on page 86) yields a difference of 12.896
indicating that adding the serial correlation component really improved
the covariance structure of our model. Further, note that the residual variability has now been split up into two components which are about equally
important (similar variance). Based on this extended covariance matrix, we
repeated our informal check presented in Section 3.12.2, comparing fitted
variances with sample variances in pre-specified time intervals. The fitted

TABLE 3.15. *REML estimates and estimated standard errors for all variance components in a linear mixed model with the preliminary mean structure defined in Section 3.12.1, with random intercepts and random slopes for the linear as well as quadratic time effect, with measurement error and with Gaussian serial correlation.*

Effect	Parameter	Estimate (s.e.)
Covariance of b_i:		
$\quad$ var(b_{1i})	d_{11}	0.389 (0.096)
$\quad$ var(b_{2i})	d_{22}	0.559 (0.206)
$\quad$ var(b_{3i})	d_{33}	0.059 (0.032)
$\quad$ cov(b_{1i}, b_{2i})	$d_{12} = d_{21}$	-0.382 (0.121)
$\quad$ cov(b_{2i}, b_{3i})	$d_{23} = d_{32}$	-0.175 (0.079)
$\quad$ cov(b_{3i}, b_{1i})	$d_{13} = d_{31}$	0.099 (0.043)
Measurement error variance:		
$\quad$ var$(\varepsilon_{(1)ij})$	σ^2	0.023 (0.002)
Gaussian serial correlation:		
$\quad$ var$(\varepsilon_{(2)ij})$	τ^2	0.032 (0.021)
$\quad$ rate of exponential decrease	$1/\sqrt{\phi}$	0.619 (0.202)
REML log-likelihood		-24.787
-2 REML log-likelihood		49.574

variances are now obtained from calculating

$$
\begin{pmatrix} 1 & t & t^2 \end{pmatrix} \widehat{D} \begin{pmatrix} 1 \\ t \\ t^2 \end{pmatrix} + \widehat{\sigma}^2 + \widehat{\tau}^2
$$

where the estimates $\widehat{D}$, $\widehat{\sigma}^2$ and $\widehat{\tau}^2$ are the ones reported in Table 3.15. The result is shown in Figure 3.11. As in Figure 3.9, we indicated the number of residuals r_{ij} used in the calculation of the sample variances above the corresponding interval. The Figures 3.9 and 3.11 are very similar except for large values of *time*, where the fitted variance is now closer to the sample variance.

Finally, it should be emphasized that for fitting complicated covariance structures as the one in model (3.32), one often needs to specify starting values (using the PARMS statement of PROC MIXED) in order for the iterative procedure to converge. Sometimes it is sufficient to use the Fisher scoring method (option 'scoring' in the PROC MIXED statement) in the iterative estimating procedure, which uses the expected Hessian matrix instead of the observed one. To illustrate this, we reparameterize the above

Variance function

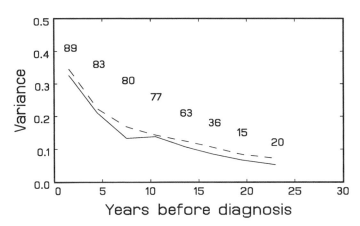

FIGURE 3.11. *Comparison of sample variances (solid line) to fitted variances (dashed line) obtained using the REML estimates in Table 3.15 for the variance components in model (3.7) extended with a Gaussian serial correlation component, at specific points in time. The numbers indicate the number of residuals r_{ij} used for the calculation of the corresponding sample variance.*

fitted model by defining the intercept successively at 0 years (= original parameterization), 5 years, 10 years, 15 years, and 20 years prior to diagnosis. The resulting estimates and standard errors for all variance components in the model are shown in Table 3.16.

Obviously, minus twice the maximized REML log-likelihood function is not affected by the reparameterization. The Fisher scoring algorithm was used in two cases in order to attain convergence. It is hereby important that the final steps in the iterative procedure are based on the default Newton-Raphson method since otherwise all reported standard errors are based on the expected rather than observed Hessian matrix, the consequences of which will be discussed in Section 5.8. Note that the variance components in the covariance structure of ε_i, as well as the variance d_{33} of the random slopes for the quadratic time-effect remain unchanged when the model is reparameterized. This is not the case for the other elements in the random-effects covariance matrix D. As was expected the random-intercepts variance d_{11} decreases as the intercept moves further away from the time of diagnosis, and the same holds for the overall variance $d_{11} + \sigma^2 + \tau^2$ at the time of the intercept. We therefore recommend to define random intercepts as the response value at the time where the random variation in the data is maximal. This facilitates the discrimination between the three sources of stochastic variability.

TABLE 3.16. *REML estimates and estimated standard errors for all variance components in a linear mixed model with the preliminary mean structure defined in Section 3.12.1, with random intercepts and random slopes for the linear as well as quadratic time effect, with measurement error and with Gaussian serial correlation. Each time, another parameterization of the model is used, based on how the intercept has been defined.*

Parameter	\multicolumn{5}{c}{Definition of intercept (time in years before diagnosis)}				
	$t = 0$	$t = 5$	$t = 10^{(1)}$	$t = 15$	$t = 20^{(2)}$
d_{11}	0.389 (0.096)	0.156 (0.039)	0.090 (0.032)	0.061 (0.027)	0.026 (0.025)
d_{22}	0.559 (0.206)	0.267 (0.085)	0.094 (0.027)	0.038 (0.026)	0.099 (0.091)
d_{33}	0.059 (0.032)	0.059 (0.032)	0.059 (0.032)	0.059 (0.032)	0.059 (0.032)
$d_{12} = d_{21}$	-0.382 (0.121)	-0.120 (0.042)	-0.033 (0.019)	-0.033 (0.017)	-0.030 (0.024)
$d_{23} = d_{32}$	-0.175 (0.079)	-0.116 (0.048)	-0.057 (0.021)	0.001 (0.023)	0.060 (0.051)
$d_{13} = d_{31}$	0.099 (0.043)	0.026 (0.023)	-0.018 (0.023)	-0.032 (0.020)	-0.016 (0.016)
σ^2	0.023 (0.002)	0.023 (0.002)	0.023 (0.002)	0.023 (0.002)	0.023 (0.002)
τ^2	0.032 (0.021)	0.032 (0.021)	0.032 (0.021)	0.032 (0.021)	0.032 (0.021)
$1/\sqrt{\phi}$	0.619 (0.202)	0.619 (0.202)	0.619 (0.202)	0.619 (0.202)	0.619 (0.202)
-2 log-lik	49.574	49.574	49.574	49.574	49.574

[1] Five initial steps of Fisher scoring

[2] One initial step of Fisher scoring

3.12.4   Model Reduction

Based on the residual covariance structure specified in the previous step, we can now investigate whether the random effects which we included in Section 3.12.2 are really needed in the model. As discussed in Section 3.12.2, Z_i should not contain a polynomial effect if not all hierarchically inferior terms are also included. Taking into account this hierarchy, one should test the significance of the highest order random effects first.

Finally, once the final covariance structure for the model has been selected, tests become available (see for example Sections 3.5.2 and 3.7) for the fixed effects in the preliminary mean structure. For the prostate cancer data, we then end up with the same model for the average profile as model (3.25) in Section 3.7.2. This model can now be fitted with the following program:

```
proc mixed data = test noclprint method = reml covtest;
class id group timeclss;
model lnpsa = group age bph*time loccanc*time metcanc*time
              cancer*time2 / noint solution;
random intercept time time2 / type = un subject = id g;
repeated timeclss / type = sp(gau)(time) local subject = id;
run;
```

TABLE 3.17. *Results from fitting the final model (3.25) to the prostate cancer data, using restricted maximum likelihood estimation. The covariance structure contains three random effects, Gaussian serial correlation and measurement error.*

Effect	Parameter	Estimate (s.e.)
Age effect	β_1	0.015 (0.006)
Intercepts:		
control	β_2	-0.496 (0.411)
BPH	β_3	0.320 (0.470)
L/R cancer	β_4	1.216 (0.469)
Met. cancer	β_5	2.353 (0.518)
Time effects:		
BPH	β_8	-0.376 (0.070)
L/R cancer	β_9	-1.877 (0.210)
Met. cancer	β_{10}	-2.274 (0.244)
Time^2 effects:		
cancer	$\beta_{14} = \beta_{15}$	0.484 (0.073)
Covariance of $\boldsymbol{b}_i$:		
var(b_{1i})	d_{11}	0.393 (0.093)
var(b_{2i})	d_{22}	0.550 (0.187)
var(b_{3i})	d_{33}	0.056 (0.028)
cov(b_{1i}, b_{2i})	$d_{12} = d_{21}$	-0.382 (0.114)
cov(b_{2i}, b_{3i})	$d_{23} = d_{32}$	-0.170 (0.070)
cov(b_{3i}, b_{1i})	$d_{13} = d_{31}$	0.098 (0.039)
Measurement error variance:		
var($\varepsilon_{(1)ij}$)	σ^2	0.023 (0.002)
Gaussian serial correlation:		
var($\varepsilon_{(2)ij}$)	τ^2	0.029 (0.018)
rate of exponential decrease	$1/\sqrt{\phi}$	0.599 (0.192)
Observations		463
REML log-likelihood		-13.704
-2 REML log-likelihood		27.407
Akaike's Information Criterion		-22.704
Schwarz's Bayesian Criterion		-41.235

The SAS variables *cancer*, *BPH*, *loccanc* and *metcanc* are as defined before in Section 3.7.2, while the other variables *id*, *group*, *time* and *timeclss* are as defined in Section 3.5.1. The parameter estimates and estimated standard errors are shown in Table 3.17, and they can be compared to the estimates shown in Table 3.11 which were obtained without assuming the presence of residual serial correlation. Note that adding this component to the model leads to smaller standard errors for all elements in the random-effects covariance matrix D.

3.13   Model Checks and Diagnostic Tools *

Although model (3.32) can be viewed as a direct extension of multiple regression to the case where the responses are no longer independent, it is not obvious how to generalize all diagnostic tools such as residual analysis, outlier detection, influence analysis, checking model assumptions,..., which are available in the classical regression situation (see for example Neter, Wasserman, and Kutner 1990). The aim of this section is therefore to discuss some results of recent research in this domain. It hereby should be emphasized that at this stage, none of the analyses which will be discussed in the sequel of this section are available in the SAS procedure PROC MIXED. Selected macros are available from the Web page listed in the Preface.

In general, residuals can be defined in several ways. For example, $y_i - X_i\beta$ represents the deviation of the observed profile for the ith subject from the overall mean regression surface (as in multiple regression). On the other hand, $y_i - X_i\widehat{\beta} - Z_i\widehat{b_i}$ describes how much the responses of the ith subject deviate from it's own subject-specific predicted profile. Note that these residual vectors yield different numbers of residuals for different subjects, depending on the number of repeated measurements available for each subject. This is not the case with the estimated random effects $\widehat{b_i}$, which can also be interpreted as residuals since they express how much the observed profile of the ith individual deviates from the fitted average profile $X_i\widehat{\beta}$. As discussed in Section 3.11, these 'residuals' are often of interest in practice. We will therefore investigate in Section 3.13.1, how the distributional assumption for these random effects can be checked, and what the impact is of possible non-normality on our inference results.

Also, it is not obvious how outliers and influential subjects should be defined or detected. For example, there are several possible ways of defining outliers. An individual might be considered as outlying if its observed profile (the vector y_i) is outlying in comparison with the measurements of the

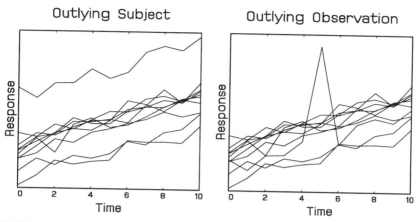

FIGURE 3.12. *Simulated longitudinal profiles for 10 subjects, with one outlying subject and one outlying observation respectively.*

other individuals. An observation on the other hand, could be viewed as outlying if it heavily deviates from the subject-specific regression line for the individual with that observation. The difference is graphically shown in Figure 3.12. In Section 3.13.2, we will use the local influence approach of Cook (1986) to measure the influence of a specific subject on the maximum likelihood estimates of all parameters in the marginal model, and to ascribe this influence to specific characteristics of the subject.

Finally, we have seen in Section 3.12.3 that the specification of an appropriate residual serial correlation structure may be seriously complicated by the dominating effect of the random effects previously included in the model. This calls for a general strategy to detect serial correlation in the presence of random effects, and to check whether a specified serial correlation function $g(\cdot)$ is appropriate. This will be discussed in Section 3.13.3.

3.13.1   Normality Assumption for the Random Effects   ✳

Our analyses of the prostate cancer data have revealed some significant differences between the control patients, patients with benign prostatic hyperplasia, local cancer cases and metastatic cancer cases, suggesting that repeated measures of PSA might be useful to detect prostate cancer in an early stage of the disease. Note that such a classification procedure cannot be based on a model for PSA which includes age at diagnosis and time before diagnosis as covariates (as in our final model (3.25) in Section 3.7.2) since these are only available in retrospective studies, such as the Baltimore Longitudinal Study of Aging, where classification of the individuals is superfluous. The indicator variables C_i, B_i, L_i and M_i are also not available for the same reason. The only possible adjustment of model (3.25) which could be used for our classification purposes is therefore given by

$$
\begin{aligned}
\ln(1 + PSA_{ij}) \;=\; & \beta_1 Age_i + (\beta_2 + b_{1i}) \\
& + (\beta_3 + b_{2i})\, t_{ij} + (\beta_4 + b_{3i})\, t_{ij}^2 + \varepsilon_{ij}, \quad (3.33)
\end{aligned}
$$

where Age_i is now the age of the ith subject at entry in the study (or at the time the first measurement was taken), and where the time points t_{ij} are now expressed as time since entry. The procedure would then be to first estimate all parameters in model (3.33), from which estimates for the random effects can be calculated, as explained in Section 3.11. These estimates could then be used to classify patients in either one of the diagnostic groups.

However, although this approach looks very appealing, it raises many problems with respect to the normality assumption for the random effects, which is automatically made by the linear mixed-effects model. For example, it follows from the results in Section 3.7.2 that the mean quadratic time effect is zero for the non-cancer cases, and positive for both cancer groups. Hence, the quadratic effects $\beta_4 + b_{3i}$ in model (3.33) should follow a normal distribution with mean zero for the non-cancer cases and with mean 0.484 (see Table 3.17) for the cancer cases. This means that the b_{3i} are no longer normally distributed, but follow a mixture of two normal distributions, i.e.,

$$
b_{3i} \;\sim\; p\, N(\mu_1, \sigma_1^2) \;+\; (1 - p)\, N(\mu_2, \sigma_2^2),
$$

in which μ_1, μ_2 and σ_1^2, σ_2^2 denote the means and variances of the b_{3i} in the non-cancer and cancer groups respectively, and where p is the proportion of patients in the data set which belong to the non-cancer group. Similar arguments hold for the random intercepts b_{1i} and for the random time slopes b_{2i}, which even may be sampled from mixtures of more than two normal distributions. Note that such mixtures reflect heterogeneity in the random-effects population, and that they may occur very often in practice. Whenever a categorical covariate has been omitted as fixed effect in a linear mixed-effects model, the random effects will follow a mixture of g normal distributions, where g is the number of categories of the missing covariate. It is therefore important to be aware of the impact of the normality assumption for the random effects on the inference results.

IMPACT ON THE ESTIMATION OF THE FIXED EFFECTS AND THE VARIANCE COMPONENTS

Using simulations and the analysis of a real data set, Butler and Louis (1992) have shown that wrongly specifying the random-effects distribution of univariate random effects has little effect on the fixed-effects estimates as well as on the estimates for the residual variance and the variance of the random effects. No evidence was found for any inconsistencies among these estimators. However, it was shown that the standard errors of all parameter estimators need correction in order to get valid inferences. Using theory on maximum likelihood estimation in misspecified models (White 1980, 1982), Verbeke and Lesaffre (1996b) extended this to the general model (3.8). As before, $\boldsymbol{\theta}$ denotes the vector of all parameters in our marginal linear mixed model. Let $N \times A_N(\boldsymbol{\theta})$ be minus the matrix of second-order derivatives of the log-likelihood function with respect to the elements of $\boldsymbol{\theta}$, and let $N \times B_N(\boldsymbol{\theta})$ be the matrix with cross-products of first-order derivatives of the log-likelihood function, also with respect to $\boldsymbol{\theta}$. Their estimated versions, obtained from replacing $\boldsymbol{\theta}$ by its MLE are denoted by $\widehat{A}_N$ and $\widehat{B}_N$ respectively. Verbeke and Lesaffre (1996b) then prove that, under general regularity conditions, the MLE $\widehat{\boldsymbol{\theta}}$ of $\boldsymbol{\theta}$ is asymptotically normally distributed with mean $\boldsymbol{\theta}$ and with asymptotic covariance matrix

$$\widehat{A}_N^{-1} \, \widehat{B}_N \, \widehat{A}_N^{-1}/N, \tag{3.34}$$

for $N \to \infty$.

It can easily be seen that the covariance matrix obtained from replacing $\boldsymbol{\alpha}$ in (3.13) by its MLE equals

$$\text{var}(\widehat{\boldsymbol{\beta}}) = \left(\sum_{i=1}^{N} X_i' V_i^{-1}(\widehat{\boldsymbol{\alpha}}) X_i \right)^{-1} = \widehat{A}_{N,11}^{-1}/N, \tag{3.35}$$

where $\widehat{A}_{N,11}$ is the leading block in $\widehat{A}_N$, corresponding to the fixed effects. Hence, we have that the asymptotic covariance matrix for $\widehat{\boldsymbol{\beta}}$, obtained from (3.34), adds extra variability to the 'naive' estimate (3.35), by taking into account the estimation of the variance components, but it also corrects for possible misspecification of the random-effects distribution. Note also that $\widehat{A}_N^{-1}\widehat{B}_N\widehat{A}_N^{-1}/N$ is of the same form as the so-called 'information sandwich' estimator for the asymptotic covariance matrix of fixed effects, estimated with quasi-likelihood methods (see Section 3.4.1 and e.g., Liang and Zeger 1986). However, the above asymptotic result relates to both the fixed effects and the parameters in the 'working correlation' model, and the model is incorrectly specified only through the random-effects distribution; the covariance structure is assumed to be correct.

As discussed in Section 3.4.2, one can use the inverse Fisher information matrix as asymptotic covariance matrix, if the assumed model is correct. Verbeke and Lesaffre (1997a) performed extensive simulations to compare this uncorrected covariance matrix with the above sandwich estimator, which corrects for possible non-normality of the random effects. In general, they conclude that, for the fixed effects, the corrected and uncorrected standard

True random intercepts

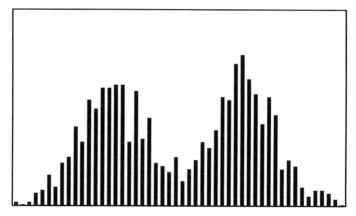

FIGURE 3.13. *Histogram (range $[-5, 5]$) of 1000 random intercepts drawn from the normal mixture $0.5N(-2, 1) + 0.5N(2, 1)$.*

errors are very similar. This is in agreement with the results of Sharples and Breslow (1992) who showed that, for correlated binary data, the sandwich estimator for the covariance matrix of fixed effects, is almost as efficient as the uncorrected model-based estimator, when the assumed form of the covariance matrix is correct, even under the correct model.

For the random components on the other hand, and more specifically for the elements in D, this is only true under the correct model (normal random effects). When the random effects are not normally distributed the corrected standard errors are clearly superior to the uncorrected ones. In some cases, the correction enlarges the standard errors to get confidence levels closer to the pursued level. In other cases, the correction results in smaller standard errors protecting against too conservative confidence intervals.

Verbeke and Lesaffre (1997a) calculated the corrected and uncorrected standard errors for all parameters in model (3.7). The ratio of the corrected over the uncorrected standard errors was between 0.52 and 1.72 for all parameters, while the same ratio was between 0.21 and 2.76 for any linear combination $\lambda'\theta$ of the parameters. They conclude that this might be used as an indicator for possible non-normality of the random effects b_i.

IMPACT ON THE ESTIMATION OF THE RANDOM EFFECTS

The above results have shown that the estimation of the parameters in the marginal linear mixed model are only slightly influenced by the normality

Empirical Bayes estimates

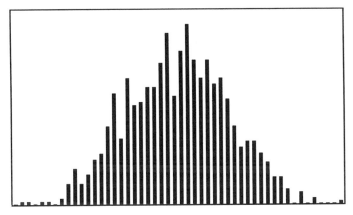

FIGURE 3.14. *Histogram (range* $[-5, 5]$*) of the Empirical Bayes estimates of the random intercepts shown in Figure 3.13, calculated under the assumption that the random effects are normally distributed.*

assumption for the random effects. This is no longer true for the estimation of the random effects themselves. To illustrate this, Verbeke and Lesaffre (1996a) simulated 1000 longitudinal profiles with 5 repeated measurements each, where univariate random intercepts b_i were drawn from the mixture distribution

$$\tfrac{1}{2}N(-2, 1) + \tfrac{1}{2}N(2, 1).$$

A histogram of the realized values is shown in Figure 3.13. They then fitted a linear mixed model, assuming normality for the random effects, and they calculated the EB estimates (3.28) for the random intercepts in the model. The histogram of these estimates is shown in Figure 3.14. Clearly, the normality assumption forces the estimates $\widehat{b}_i$ to satisfy the assumption of a homogeneous (normal) population.

Verbeke (1995) and Verbeke and Lesaffre (1996a) have shown that this will be the case as soon as the eigenvalues of $\sigma^2(Z_i'Z_i)^{-1}$ are sufficiently large. This means that both the error variance and the covariate structure play an important role in the shape of the distribution of $\widehat{b}_i$. First, if σ^2 is large, it will be difficult to detect heterogeneity in the random-effects population, based on the $\widehat{b}_i$. Thus, if the error variability σ^2 is large compared to the random-effects variability, the $\widehat{b}_i$ may not reflect the correct distributional shape of the random effects. For a linear mixed-effects model with only random intercepts, Crowder and Hand (1990, p.27) define the intraclass correlation ρ_I as $d_{11}/(d_{11} + \sigma^2)$, where d_{11} is the intercept variability. It represents the correlation between two repeated measurements within the same subject, i.e., $\rho_I = corr(Y_{ik}, Y_{il})$ for all $k \neq l$. We then have that subgroups in the random-effects population will be unrecognized when the within-subject correlation is small. On the other hand, the covariates Z_i are also important. For example, suppose that Z_i is a vector with elements $t_{i1}, t_{i2}, \ldots, t_{in_i}$. We then have that $Z_i'Z_i$ equals $\sum_{j=1}^{n_i} t_{ij}^2$. Hence, heterogeneity will be more likely to be detected when the b_i represent random slopes in a model for measurements taken at large time points t_{ij} than when the b_i are random intercepts (all t_{ij} equal to one). If Z_i contains both random intercepts and random slopes for time points t_{ij}, we have that $Z_i'Z_i$ equals

$$
Z_i'Z_i = \begin{pmatrix} n_i & \sum_{j=1}^{n_i} t_{ij} \\ \sum_{j=1}^{n_i} t_{ij} & \sum_{j=1}^{n_i} t_{ij}^2 \end{pmatrix}
$$

which has two positive eigenvalues λ_1 and λ_2, given by

$$
2\,\lambda_k = \sum_{j=1}^{n_i} t_{ij}^2 + n_i + (-1)^k \sqrt{\left(\sum_{j=1}^{n_i} t_{ij}^2 - n_i\right)^2 + 4\left(\sum_{j=1}^{n_i} t_{ij}\right)^2}.
$$

In a designed experiment with $Z_i = Z$ for all i, and where the time points t_j are centered, the eigenvalues are $\lambda_2 = \sum_{j=1}^{n} t_j^2$ and $\lambda_1 = n_i$, or vice versa. So, if we are interested in detecting subgroups in the random-effects population, we should take as many measurements as possible, at the beginning and at the end of the study (maximal spread of the time points).

CHECKING THE NORMALITY ASSUMPTION FOR THE RANDOM EFFECTS

Since the estimation of the random effects seems to depend heavily on the distributional assumptions for the b_i one really needs methods to check this underlying assumption. As discussed in Section 3.11, one here fore very often uses histograms and scatter plots of the random-effects estimates $\widehat{b}_i$. However, even when the assumed linear mixed model is correctly specified, the estimators $\widehat{b}_i$ will not have the same distribution unless all covariate matrices X_i and Z_i are the same, and therefore, it may be questioned whether or not histograms and scatter plots are interpretable. Also, it follows from the above section that one should not use EB estimates, obtained under the normality assumption, to check this assumption.

Lange and Ryan (1989) have proposed the use of weighted qq-plots of standardized linear combinations

$$
v_i = \frac{c'\widehat{b}_i}{\sqrt{c'\mathrm{Var}(\widehat{b}_i)c}},
$$

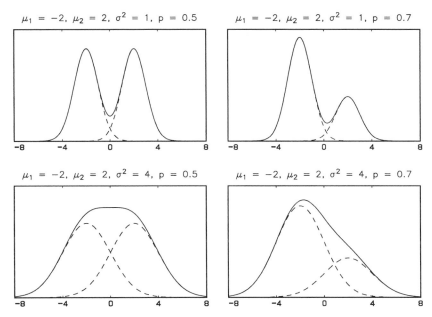

FIGURE 3.15. *Density functions of mixtures* $pN(\mu_1, \sigma^2) + (1-p)N(\mu_2, \sigma^2)$ *of two normal distributions, for varying values for p and σ^2. The dashed lines represents the densities of the normal components, the solid line represents the density of the mixture.*

of the estimates $\widehat{b_i}$, to check the normality assumption of the random effects. However, since the v_i are a function of the random effects b_i as well as of the error terms ε_i, these qq-plots can only indicate that the v_i do not have the distribution one expects under the assumed model, but the plots cannot differentiate a wrong distributional assumption for the random effects or the error terms, from a wrong choice of covariates. Therefore they are not suited for detecting e.g., a mixture of normal distributions as random-effects distribution.

Verbeke and Lesaffre (1996a) therefore relaxed the normality assumption for the random effects in the general linear mixed model (3.8). Instead they assume the b_i to be sampled from a mixture of g normal distributions with equal covariance matrix, i.e.

$$b_i \sim \sum_{j=1}^{g} p_j N(\mu_j, D),$$

with $\sum_{j=1}^{g} p_j = 1$. As discussed before, this extension naturally arises from assuming that there is unobserved heterogeneity in the random effects population. Each component in the mixture represents a cluster containing a proportion p_j of the total population. The model is therefore called the heterogeneity model and the linear mixed model discussed so far can then be called the homogeneity model. Also, as shown in Figure 3.15, it extends the assumption about the random-effects distribution to a very broad class of distributions: unimodal as well as multimodal, symmetric as well as very skewed. To assure that $E(\boldsymbol{Y_i}) = X_i\boldsymbol{\beta}$ (as before), the additional constraint

$$E(\boldsymbol{b_i}) \;=\; \sum_{j=1}^{g} p_j\,\boldsymbol{\mu}_j \;=\; \boldsymbol{0}$$

is needed.

The marginal distribution of the measurements $\boldsymbol{Y_i}$ under the heterogeneity model is now given by

$$\boldsymbol{Y_i} \sim \sum_{j=1}^{g} p_j N(X_i\boldsymbol{\beta} + Z_i\boldsymbol{\mu}_j, V_i(\boldsymbol{\alpha})), \tag{3.36}$$

where as before $V_i(\boldsymbol{\alpha})$ equals $Z_i D Z_i' + \Sigma_i = W_i^{-1}(\boldsymbol{\alpha})$. Note however that D is now the random-effects covariance matrix in each component of the mixture separately rather than the overall $\boldsymbol{b_i}$ covariance matrix. Let $\boldsymbol{\theta}$ again denote all parameters in this marginal distribution, i.e., $\boldsymbol{\theta}$ contains $\boldsymbol{\beta}$, $\boldsymbol{\alpha}$, D and all $\boldsymbol{\mu}_j$ and p_j. The vector $\boldsymbol{\theta}$ can then be estimated via maximum likelihood estimation. For this the EM algorithm has been advocated (Laird 1978). It is particularly useful for mixture problems since it often happens that a model is fitted with too many components (g too large) leading to a likelihood which is maximal anywhere on a ridge. As shown by Dempster, Laird and Rubin (1977), the EM algorithm is capable to converge to some particular point on that ridge. We refer to Section 5.9 for a discussion on the EM algorithm and to Verbeke (1995) for more details on how it can be applied within the framework of the heterogeneity model.

Once all parameters in the marginal model (3.36) have been estimated, we can calculate empirical Bayes estimates for the random effects $\boldsymbol{b_i}$. These are given by (Verbeke and Lesaffre 1996a)

$$\widehat{\boldsymbol{b_i}} \;=\; E(\boldsymbol{b_i}|\boldsymbol{y_i}, \widehat{\boldsymbol{\theta}})$$

$$=\; \widehat{D} Z_i' \widehat{W}_i (\boldsymbol{y_i} - X_i\widehat{\boldsymbol{\beta}}) \;+\; (I - \widehat{D} Z_i' \widehat{W}_i Z_i) \sum_{j=1}^{g} p_{ij}(\widehat{\boldsymbol{\theta}})\widehat{\boldsymbol{\mu}}_j,$$

where $p_{ij}(\widehat{\boldsymbol{\theta}})$ is equal to the estimated posterior probability for the ith subject to belong to the jth component of the mixture. Note how the first component of $\widehat{\boldsymbol{b_i}}$ is of exactly the same form as the estimator (3.28) obtained assuming normally distributed random effects. However, the overall covariance matrix of the $\boldsymbol{b_i}$ is now replaced by the within-component covariance

Empirical Bayes estimates

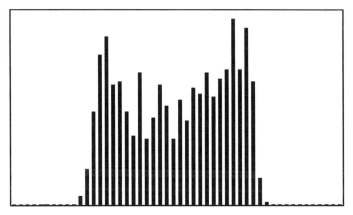

FIGURE 3.16. *Histogram (range $[-5, 5]$) of the Empirical Bayes estimates of the random intercepts shown in Figure 3.13, calculated under the assumption that the random effects are drawn from a two-component mixture of normal distributions.*

matrix D. The second component in the expression for $\widehat{b}_i$ can be viewed as a correction term towards the component means μ_j, with most weight on those means which correspond to components for which the subject has high posterior probability to belong to. As an illustration, Figure 3.16 shows the EB estimates of the 1000 simulated random intercepts previously shown in Figure 3.13, and obtained under a two-component heterogeneity model. In comparison to the histogram of the EB estimates under the normality assumption (Figure 3.14), the correct random-effects distribution is (much) better reflected. We do not claim that the $\widehat{b}_i$, calculated under the heterogeneity model perfectly reflect the correct mixture distribution, but at least, they suggest that the random effects certainly do not follow a normal distribution, as was suggested by the estimates obtained under the normality assumption.

Interest could also lie in the classification of the subjects into the different mixture components. It is natural in mixture models for such a classification to be based on the estimated posterior probabilities $p_{ij}(\widehat{\theta})$ (McLachlan and Basford 1988, Section 1.4). One then classifies the ith subject to the component to which it has the highest estimated posterior probability of belonging, i.e., to the $j(i)$th component, where $j(i)$ is the index for which $p_{i,j(i)}(\widehat{\theta}) = \max_{1 \leq j \leq g} p_{ij}(\widehat{\theta})$. Note how this technique can be used for cluster analysis within the framework of linear mixed-effects models: If the individual profiles are to be classified into g subgroups, fit a mixture model with g components and use the above rule for classification in either one of the g clusters.

The heterogeneity model can also be used to test the normality assumption for the random effects in linear mixed models. One then addresses the following question: Does the random-effects population consist of different subpopulations, or is one overall normal distribution sufficient to describe the between-subject variability ? Also, under heterogeneity, we haven't discussed yet how the number of components g should be chosen. A statistical test can be used to decide upon the presence of heterogeneity and, if so, upon the degree of heterogeneity. Verbeke and Lesaffre (1996a) consider the likelihood ratio test, and propose two approximate goodness-of-fit tests. As discussed by Ghosh and Sen (1985), testing for the number of components in a finite mixture is seriously complicated by boundary problems similar to the ones we discussed in Section 3.9.1 in the context of testing random effects. In order to briefly highlight the main problems, we consider testing $H_0 : g = 1$ versus $H_A : g = 2$. The null hypothesis can then be expressed as $H_0 : \mu_1 = \mu_2$. However, the same hypothesis is obtained by setting $H_0 : p_1 = 0$ or $H_0 : p_2 = 0$, which clearly illustrates that H_0 is on the boundary of the parameter space, and hence also that the usual regularity conditions for application of the classical maximum likelihood theory, are violated. In practice, one can fit several heterogeneity models, increasing g to the level where some of the subpopulations get very small weight (some p_j very small) or where some of the subpopulations coincide (some μ_j approximately the same). Also, if heterogeneity models are used only to allow a broader class of distributions for the b_i and not necessarily for classification purposes, it is usually sufficient to restrict g to be small (as is already suggested in Figure 3.15).

As an illustration of the heterogeneity model, Verbeke and Lesaffre (1996a) fitted several mixtures to the prostate cancer data. In order not to complicate the model too much at once, the prostatic benign hyperplasia patients (BPH) were excluded from the analyses. The main purpose was to investigate whether (1) the mixture approach detects the presence of heterogeneity in the random-effects population, which we know to be present, and whether (2) the classification procedure correctly classifies patients as being controls or cancer cases. As explained in Section 3.13.1 such an analysis should be based on model (3.33). A three-component mixture with estimated proportions 0.72, 0.19 and 0.09 was needed to describe the natural heterogeneity in the random-effects population. For each of these components the estimated mean profile is shown in Figure 3.17. Obviously, the first component represents the individuals who evolve mainly linearly: there is a constant increase of PSA over time. This is in contrast with the other two groups in the mixture which contain the subjects who evolve quadratically over time, for the second component after a period of small linear increase, for the last component immediately after enrollment in the study.

It will only be possible to use this model for the detection of prostate can-

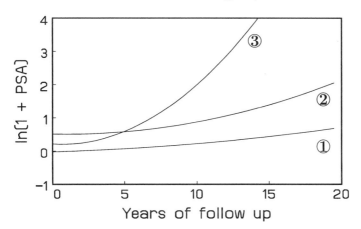

FIGURE 3.17. *Average mean profiles, estimated from a three-component hetero-geneity model.*

cer at early stages, if one or two of the components can be shown to represent the cancer cases, while the other component(s) then would represent the controls. We therefore compare classification by our mixture approach with the correct classification as control or cancer. The result is shown in Table 3.18. Except for one patient, all controls were classified in the first component, together with 10 cancer cases of which the profiles show hardly any difference from many profiles in the control group (only a moderate, linear increase over time). Three cancer cases were classified in the third component. These are those cases which have entered the study almost simultaneously with the start of the growth of the tumor. The 5 cancer cases, classified in the second component are these who were already in the study long before the tumor started to develop and therefore have profiles which hardly change in the beginning, but which start increasing quadratically after some period of time in the study. Apparently, the detection of the correct diagnostic group is hampered by the different onsets of observation periods. Further, the quadratic mixed-effects model is only a rough approximation to the correct model. For example, Carter *et al* (1992) and Pearson *et al* (1994) have fitted piecewise non-linear mixed-effects models to estimate the time when rapid increases in PSA were first observable. One could also think of extending the heterogeneity model to the case where the component probabilities p_j are modeled as functions over time. This would take into account the fact that the proportion of cancer cases increases with time. Note also that the fact that posterior classification of the subjects does not coincide with the prior diagnostic classification

TABLE 3.18. *Cross-classification of 34 patients according to the three-component mixture model and to their true disease status.*

		Mixture classification		
		1	2	3
Disease status	control	15	1	0
	cancer	10	5	3

may explain why we found some large discrepancies between the corrected and uncorrected standard errors of the MLE's for the parameters in the marginal model (3.7), suggesting that the random effects in that model are probably not normally distributed. In any case, this example has shown that the mixture approach not necessarily models what one might hope. There is no a priori reason why the mixture classification should exactly correspond to some pre-defined group-structure, which may not fully reflect the heterogeneity in growth-curves.

3.13.2   The Detection of Influential Subjects ∗

As explained in Section 3.4, fitting mixed models is often based on likelihood methods (maximum likelihood, restricted maximum likelihood), which are sensitive to peculiar observations. The data analyst should be aware of particular observations that have an unusually large influence on the results of the analysis. Such cases may be found to be completely appropriate and retained in the analysis, or they may represent inappropriate data and may be eliminated from the analysis, or they may suggest that additional data need to be collected or that the current model is inadequate. Of course, an extended investigation of influential cases is only possible once they have been identified.

Many diagnostics have been developed for linear regression models. See for example Cook and Weisberg (1982) and Chatterjee and Hadi (1988). Since the linear mixed model can be seen as a concatenation of several subject-specific regression models, it is most obvious to investigate how these diagnostics (residual analysis, leverage, Cook's distance,...) can be generalized to the models we consider. Still, it is not always clear how to do so. First, several kinds of residuals could be defined, as discussed on page 132. Further, the linear mixed model involves two kinds of covariates. The matrix X_i represents the design matrix for the fixed effects, Z_i is the design matrix for the random effects. Therefore, it is not clear how leverages should be defined, partially because the matrices X_i are not necessarily of the same dimension for all subjects, and the same is true for the matrices Z_i.

The final classification of subjects as influential or not influential can be based on the Cook's distance, first introduced by Cook (1977a, 1977b, 1979), which measures how much the parameter estimates change when a specific individual has been removed from the data set. In ordinary regression analysis, this can easily be calculated due to the availability of closed form expressions for the parameter estimates, which makes it also possible to ascribe influence to the specific characteristics of the subjects (leverage, outlying). Unfortunately, this is no longer the case in linear mixed models. For exact Cook's distances, the iterative estimation procedure has to be used $N + 1$ times, once to fit the model for all observations, and once for each individual that has been excluded from the analysis. This is not only extremely time-consuming, it also does not give any information on the reason why some individuals are more influential than others.

All these considerations suggest that an influence analysis for the linear mixed model should not be based on the same diagnostic procedures as ordinary least squares regression. DeGruttola, Ware and Louis (1987) described measures of influence and leverage for a generalized three-step least squares estimator for the regression coefficients in a class of multivariate linear models for repeated measurements. However, their method does not apply to maximum likelihood estimation, and it is also not clear how to extend their diagnostics to the case of unequal covariance matrices V_i.

Christensen, Pearson, and Johnson (1992) have noticed that, conditionally on the variance components $\boldsymbol{\alpha}$, there is an explicit expression for $\widehat{\boldsymbol{\beta}}$ (expression (3.11)), and hence it is possible to extend the Cook's distance to measure influence on the fixed effects in a mixed model. For known $\boldsymbol{\alpha}$, the so-obtained distances can be compared to a χ_p^2 distribution in order to decide which ones are exceptionally large. For estimated $\boldsymbol{\alpha}$, they still propose to use the χ^2 distribution as approximation. Further, they define Cook's distances, based on one-step estimates, for examining case influence on the estimation of the variance components. These one-step estimates are obtained from one single step in the Newton-Raphson procedure for the maximization of the log-likelihood corresponding to the incomplete data (ith case removed), starting from the estimates obtained for the complete data. Although these procedures seem intuitively appealing, they do not yield any influence diagnostic for the fixed effects and the variance components simultaneously. Further, no methods have been given to ascribe global influence on the estimation of the total parameter vector $\boldsymbol{\theta}$ to any of the subject's characteristics.

Since case-deletion diagnostics assess the effect of an observation by completely removing it, they fit into the framework of global influence analyses.

This is in contrast with a local influence analysis, first introduced by Cook (1986). Beckman, Nachtsheim, and Cook (1987) used the idea of local influence to develop methods for assessing the effect of perturbations from the usual assumptions in the mixed model analysis of variance with uncorrelated random components. They investigate how the parameters change under small perturbations of the error variances, the random-effects variances and the response vector. An alternative perturbation scheme, applied by Verbeke (1995) and Lesaffre and Verbeke (1997), is case-weight perturbation where it is investigated how much the parameter estimates are affected by changes in the weights of the log-likelihood contributions of specific individuals. One therefore proceeds as follows. It follows from expression (3.10) that the log-likelihood function maximized during maximum likelihood estimation can be rewritten as

$$\ell(\boldsymbol{\theta}) = \sum_{i=1}^{N} \ell_i(\boldsymbol{\theta}), \tag{3.37}$$

in which $\ell_i(\boldsymbol{\theta})$ is the contribution of the ith individual to the log-likelihood. In (3.37) each observation has the same weight, i.e., $w_i = 1$ for all i. We now define the following log-likelihood with different weights for different subjects:

$$\ell(\boldsymbol{\theta}|\boldsymbol{\omega}) = \sum_{i=1}^{N} w_i \ell_i(\boldsymbol{\theta}),$$

where the $N \times 1$ vector $\boldsymbol{\omega} = (w_1, w_2, \ldots, w_N)'$ expresses a case-weight perturbation scheme. The original log-likelihood (3.37) corresponds to $\boldsymbol{\omega_0} = (1, 1, \ldots, 1)'$, hence $\ell(\boldsymbol{\theta}) = \ell(\boldsymbol{\theta}|\boldsymbol{\omega_0})$. The log-likelihood with the ith case removed corresponds to the vector $\boldsymbol{\omega}$ with $w_i = 0$ and $w_j = 1$ for all $j \neq i$.

Let $\widehat{\boldsymbol{\theta}}$ be the maximum likelihood estimator for $\boldsymbol{\theta}$, obtained by maximizing $\ell(\boldsymbol{\theta})$, and let $\widehat{\boldsymbol{\theta}}_\omega$ denote the estimator for $\boldsymbol{\theta}$ under $\ell(\boldsymbol{\theta}|\boldsymbol{\omega})$. The local influence approach now compares $\widehat{\boldsymbol{\theta}}_\omega$ with $\widehat{\boldsymbol{\theta}}$. Similar estimates indicate that case-weight perturbations have little effect on the parameter estimates. Strongly different estimates suggest that the estimation procedure is highly sensitive to such perturbations. Cook (1986) proposed to measure the distance between $\widehat{\boldsymbol{\theta}}_\omega$ and $\widehat{\boldsymbol{\theta}}$ by the so-called likelihood displacement, defined by

$$LD(\boldsymbol{\omega}) = 2\left(\ell(\hat{\boldsymbol{\theta}}) - \ell(\hat{\boldsymbol{\theta}}_\omega)\right).$$

This way, the variability of $\widehat{\boldsymbol{\theta}}$ is taken into account. $LD(\boldsymbol{\omega})$ will be large if $\ell(\boldsymbol{\theta})$ is strongly curved at $\widehat{\boldsymbol{\theta}}$ (which means that $\boldsymbol{\theta}$ is estimated with high precision) and $LD(\boldsymbol{\omega})$ will be small if $\ell(\boldsymbol{\theta})$ is fairly flat at $\widehat{\boldsymbol{\theta}}$ (meaning that $\boldsymbol{\theta}$ is estimated with high variability). From this perspective, a graph of

$LD(\boldsymbol{\omega})$ versus $\boldsymbol{\omega}$, called the influence graph, contains essential information on the influence of case-weight perturbations.

Ideally, we would like a complete influence graph, i.e., a graph of $LD(\boldsymbol{\omega})$ for varying $\boldsymbol{\omega}$, to assess influence for a particular model and a particular data set. However, this is only possible in the simplest situation ($N = 2$) so that it becomes indispensable to consider methods for extracting the most relevant information from an influence graph. The approach used by Lesaffre and Verbeke (1997) is to measure the effect on $LD(\boldsymbol{\omega})$ of infinitesimal perturbations of particular w_i around 1, while the other weights are kept constant. This yields the so-called local influence C_i of the ith subject on the estimation of $\boldsymbol{\theta}$. C_i measures the effect of slightly giving less or more weight to the ith individual.

The main advantage of C_i as measure of influence is that it can be decomposed in 5 interpretable components which are functions of (1) the covariates X_i for the mean structure, (2) a vector of residuals which are large if the observed data for the ith subject are badly predicted by the mean structure $X_i\boldsymbol{\beta}$ of the model, (3) the covariates Z_i for the covariance structure, (4) a matrix of residuals which are large if the covariance structure for the ith subject is badly modeled by $V_i(\boldsymbol{\alpha})$, and (5) a measure of variability which is large if the measurements of the ith subject have small variability. It is also very straightforward to extend the approach to measure the local influences $C_i(\boldsymbol{\beta})$ and $C_i(\boldsymbol{\alpha})$ of the ith subject on the fixed effects and on the variance components respectively. They also contain the same 5 interpretable components in their decomposition as in C_i. Further, it follows from the asymptotic independence of the MLE's for the fixed effects and for the variance components (Verbeke and Lesaffre 1997a) that, asymptotically,

$$C_i \;=\; C_i(\boldsymbol{\beta}) \;+\; C_i(\boldsymbol{\alpha})$$

which means that the local influence for the fixed effects is independent of the local influence for the variance components, and that their sum equals the local influence for all parameters simultaneously. This implies that, for large samples, $C_i(\boldsymbol{\beta})$ can be decomposed using only the first two of the above interpretable components, while the other components are sufficient for the decomposition of $C_i(\boldsymbol{\alpha})$.

Lesaffre and Verbeke (1997) applied this local influence approach to the prostate cancer data which we have analyzed in the previous sections. In a first step, individuals which have a large impact on the parameter estimates, measured by C_i, are traced. In the second step, it is determined which part of the fitted model is affected by the influential cases, the mean structure, the covariance structure, or both. Finally, the cause of the influential character has to be established in order to get insight in the reasons why a case is peculiar.

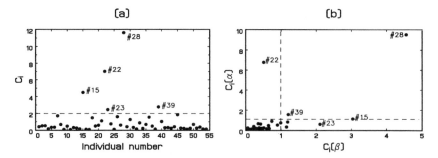

FIGURE 3.18. *(a) Plot of the local influences C_i versus the subject number i. Individuals with C_i larger than twice the average value (dashed line) are considered as influential.*
(b) Plot of $C_i(\alpha)$ versus $C_i(\beta)$. Subjects with $C_i(\alpha)$ or $C_i(\beta)$ larger than twice the average value (dashed lines) are considered as influential for the variance components or the fixed effects respectively.
The most influential subjects are indicated by their identification number.

Figure 3.18 (a) is an index plot of the total local influence C_i. The cut-off value used for C_i equals $2\sum_{i=1}^{N} C_i/N = 1.98$ and has been indicated in the figure by the dashed line. The participants #15, #22, #23, #28 and #39 are found to have a C_i value larger than 1.98 and are therefore considered to be influential for the estimation of the complete parameter vector θ. Pearson *et al* (1994) noticed that the subjects #22, #28 and #39 which were classified as local/regional cancer cases were probably misclassified metastatic cancer cases. It is therefore reassuring that this influence approach flagged these three cases as being special. In Figure 3.18(b), a scatter plot of $C_i(\alpha)$ versus $C_i(\beta)$ is given. Their respective cut-off values are 1.10 and 0.99. Obviously, subject #28, which is the subject with the largest C_i value, is highly influential for both the fixed effects and the variance components. The individuals #15 and #39 are also influential for both parts of the model, but to a much lesser extent. Finally, we have that subject #23 is influential, only for the fixed effects β and that, except for subject #28, subject #22 has the highest influence for the variance components α, but is not influential for β.

Figure 3.19 shows an index plot of each of the five interpretable components in the decomposition of the local influence measures C_i, $C_i(\beta)$ and $C_i(\alpha)$. These can now be used to ascribe the influence of the influential subjects to their specific characteristics. As an example, we will illustrate this for subject #22, which has been circled in Figure 3.19. As indicated by Figure 3.18, this subject is highly influential, but only for the estimation of the variance components. We therefore only need to consider the three last plots in Figure 3.19. Hence, although the residual component for the mean structure is the largest for subject #22, it is not the cause of the highly influential character of this subject on the variance components, and it is

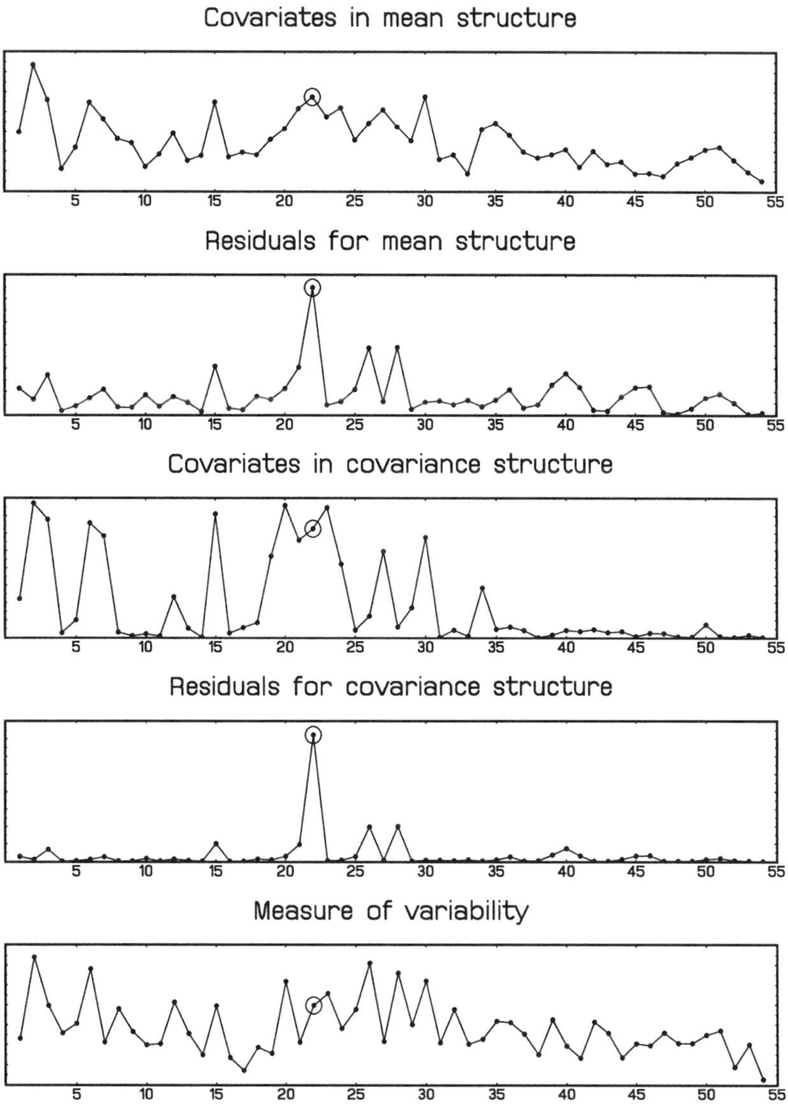

Covariates in mean structure

Residuals for mean structure

Covariates in covariance structure

Residuals for covariance structure

Measure of variability

FIGURE 3.19. *Index plot of the five interpretable components in the decomposition of the local influences C_i, $C_i(\beta)$ and $C_i(\alpha)$.*

not the cause of any large influence on the estimation of the fixed effects in the model. Note instead how this subject also has the largest residual for the covariance structure suggesting that the covariance matrix is badly predicted by the model-based covariance V_i. This is also illustrated in Figure 3.20 which shows the observed and fitted profiles for the subjects #22, #28 and #39 which are the metastatic cancer cases, wrongly classified as

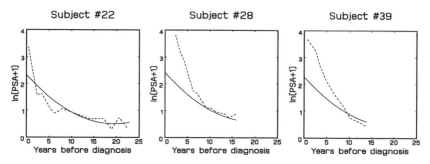

FIGURE 3.20. *Observed (dashed lines) and fitted (solid lines) profiles for 3 influential subjects which are metastatic cancer cases, but wrongly classified as local/regional cancer cases.*

local/regional cancer cases. Obviously, the large residual for the mean was caused by the bad prediction around the time of diagnosis. Further, a close look at the estimated covariance matrix V_{22} shows that only positive correlations are assumed between the repeated measurements, while the positive and negative residuals in Figure 3.20 suggest some negative correlations.

3.13.3 Checking the Covariance Structure ✻

In Section 3.12.3, we introduced the extended linear mixed-effects model (3.32) which allows to introduce residual serial correlation in addition to the random effects in the model. During the last decade, many papers have been published which discuss special cases of this model, which we denote by $M(\boldsymbol{b}_i, \boldsymbol{\varepsilon}_{(1)i}, \boldsymbol{\varepsilon}_{(2)i})$ to express that the covariance structure consists of the three sources of random variation. Similar notation will be used for models which are special cases of (3.32). For example, a random-effects model without serial correlation is denoted by $M(\boldsymbol{b}_i, \boldsymbol{\varepsilon}_{(1)i})$.

Mansour, Nordheim and Rutledge (1985) consider models $M(\boldsymbol{b}_i, \boldsymbol{\varepsilon}_{(2)i})$, where $\boldsymbol{b}_i$ is only a random intercept, and where $\boldsymbol{\varepsilon}_{(2)i}$ is assumed to follow a non-stationary(variance not constant over time) first-order autoregressive (AR(1)) model. They also propose to use the likelihood ratio test to test the presence of serial correlation. If the null hypothesis is accepted, their model reduces to a random-intercepts model with a measurement error component. Diem and Liukkonen (1988) discuss the use of $M(\boldsymbol{b}_i, \boldsymbol{\varepsilon}_{(1)i})$ models for non-stationary data, and of AR(1) $M(\boldsymbol{\varepsilon}_{(2)i})$ models for stationary data, not considering the aspect of goodness-of-fit. Diggle (1988) considered $M(\boldsymbol{b}_i, \boldsymbol{\varepsilon}_{(1)i}, \boldsymbol{\varepsilon}_{(2)i})$ models which incorporate all three sources of stochastic variation, but restricted attention to the case where $\boldsymbol{b}_i$ includes random intercepts only. Chi and Reinsel (1989) discuss the score test for comparing the $M(\boldsymbol{b}_i, \boldsymbol{\varepsilon}_{(1)i})$ model with the more general $M(\boldsymbol{b}_i, \boldsymbol{\varepsilon}_{(2)i})$ model.

They found that the $M(\boldsymbol{b_i}, \boldsymbol{\varepsilon}_{(2)i})$ model may sometimes overparameterize the covariance structure because the random effects are often able to represent the serial correlations among the measurements. They conclude that methods for determination of the best combination of serial correlation components and random effects are an important topic that deserves further consideration. Rochon (1992) considers $M(\boldsymbol{\varepsilon}_{(2)i})$ models in which $\boldsymbol{\varepsilon}_{(2)i}$ is assumed to follow an ARMA time-series model, adapted to allow non-stationarity, and he concludes that it may be of interest to extend the model with random effects. Another approach was suggested by Núñez-Antón and Woodworth (1994). They introduce an $M(\boldsymbol{\varepsilon}_{(2)i})$ model which assumes the correlation between two measurements to be a decreasing function of the distance between the power-transformed time points at which the measurements were taken. Finally, Diggle, Liang, and Zeger (1994) discuss several special cases of the general $M(\boldsymbol{b_i}, \boldsymbol{\varepsilon}_{(1)i}, \boldsymbol{\varepsilon}_{(2)i})$ model but do not include serial correlation as well as random effects other than intercepts simultaneously. Their most extensive model is the same as in Diggle (1988). They argue that, in applications, the effect of serial correlation is very often dominated by the combination of random effects and measurement error.

Obviously, there is a lot of interest in developing appropriate models for the covariance structure of longitudinal data, for reasons discussed in Section 3.12. As shown in Section 3.12.3, the SAS procedure MIXED allows the user to fit mixed models of the general form $M(\boldsymbol{b_i}, \boldsymbol{\varepsilon}_{(1)i}, \boldsymbol{\varepsilon}_{(2)i})$ but it only provides information criteria (Section 3.10) to discriminate between such models. This calls for methods to assess goodness-of-fit and to compare models with different covariance structures.

An explorative technique, developed for random-intercepts models (i.e., models $M(\boldsymbol{b_i}, \boldsymbol{\varepsilon}_{(1)i}, \boldsymbol{\varepsilon}_{(2)i})$ where the $\boldsymbol{b_i}$ are univariate random intercepts, implying that the variability in the data is assumed to be constant over time) is the so-called empirical semi-variogram, introduced by Diggle (1988). It is based on the fact that the residuals $\boldsymbol{y_i} - X_i\boldsymbol{\beta}$ satisfy

$$\frac{1}{2}\, E\left(r_{ij} - r_{ik}\right)^2 \;=\; \tau^2\left(1 - g(|t_{ij} - t_{ik}|)\right) \;=\; v(u_{ijk}), \qquad (3.38)$$

for all $i = 1, \ldots, N$ and for all $j \neq k$. The function $v(u)$ is called the semi-variogram, and it only depends on the time points t_{ij} through the time-lags $u_{ijk} = |t_{ij} - t_{ik}|$. Diggle then proposes to estimate $v(u)$, and hence also the unknown serial correlation function $g(u)$, via the sample semi-variogram which is a scatter plot of all half squared differences $v_{ijk} = (r_{ij} - r_{ik})^2/2$ versus the corresponding time differences $u_{ijk} = |t_{ij} - t_{ik}|$. The residuals r_{ij} are OLS residuals based on a preliminary mean structure (Section 3.12.1). The plot one then obtains contains $\sum_{i=1}^{N} n_i(n_i - 1)/2$ points, and smoothing methods are used to estimate the semi-variogram $v(u)$. This estimate, denoted by $\hat{v}(u)$, can now be used for deciding whether

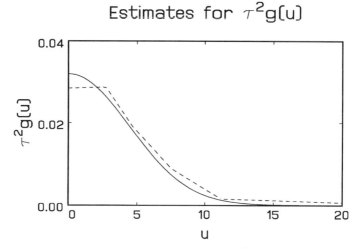

FIGURE 3.21. *Estimates for the residual serial covariance function $\tau^2 g(u)$. The dashed line represents the estimate obtained from the extended semi-variogram approach. The solid line shows the estimated Gaussian serial covariance function $\tau^2 \exp(-\phi u^2)$, where the parameter estimates of τ and ϕ are the ones reported in Table 3.15.*

or not the linear mixed model should include serial correlation, and if so, for selecting an appropriate function $g(u)$. Further, comparing $\widehat{v}(u)$ with a semi-variogram fitted using a specific linear mixed model, yields an informal check on the assumed covariance structure of this model.

Verbeke (1995) and Verbeke, Lesaffre and Brant (1997) extended the semi-variogram approach to models which contain other random effects additional to random intercepts. Because the effect of $\varepsilon_{(2)i}$ is often dominated by the random effects (Diggle, Liang, and Zeger 1994), they first remove the b_i-effect by transforming the OLS residuals orthogonal to the columns of the matrices Z_i. Similar to (3.38), one then calculates $E(\Re_{ij} - \Re_{ik})^2/2$, for the transformed residuals $\Re_i$, and based on this expression, one can estimate the unknown function $g(u)$. As for Diggle's semi-variogram, this estimate can be used for selecting an appropriate parametric model for the residual serial correlation in the data, or it can be compared to a fitted function $g(u)$ yielding a graphical check for the assumed covariance model.

As an illustration, we applied the above technique to check the appropriateness of the covariance structure derived in Section 3.12.3 for the prostate cancer data. The resulting estimate is shown by the dashed line in Figure 3.21. It clearly suggests the presence of serial correlation, which is probably Gaussian since there is no decrease for small u-values (compare to Figure 3.10). The solid line in Figure 3.21 is the estimate obtained from fitting a linear mixed model with Gaussian residual serial correlation, the results of which have been shown in Table 3.15. Since the two estimates are very similar, and because the variability in the data appears to be well described by this model (see Figure 3.11), we conclude that the covariance structure derived in Section 3.12.3 is appropriate.

4

Case Studies

Geert Verbeke
Geert Molenberghs

In this section, we will present four longitudinal data sets previously described in the medical or statistical literature. Each of them will be analyzed using linear mixed models, and we will illustrate how such models often yield additional insight into the data. All calculations will be performed with SAS procedures and therefore, none of the model checks or diagnostic tools discussed in Section 3.13 will be used.

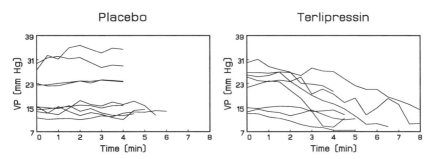

FIGURE 4.1. *Longitudinal trends of variceal pressure (VP) after intravenous administration of placebo or terlipressin.*

4.1   Example 1: Variceal Pressures

In this example, we use data reported by Nevens *et al* (1996) on the effect of intravenous administration of terlipressin and octreotide on variceal pressure. Patients with a stable variceal pressure were randomly assigned to either placebo or one of the two active drugs, and were then followed for 4 to 8 minutes. Repeated measures of variceal pressure were taken every thirty seconds. In order to simplify our analysis, we will exclude the patients treated with octreotide from our analyses. The individual profiles of the subjects in the other two groups are shown in Figure 4.1, while the crude data are given in the Tables 4.1 and 4.2. The objective of our analysis

TABLE 4.1. *Longitudinal measurements of variceal pressure in 9 placebo patients.*

Time	#1	#2	#3	#4	#5	#6	#7	#8	#9
0.0	11.6	22.5	29.7	15.4	27.6	14.3	23.0	13.7	15.3
0.5	11.1	22.6	31.6	13.3	32.4	14.6	22.2	13.2	15.0
1.0	11.3	23.1	32.1	12.7	31.2	15.1	22.3	15.4	14.7
1.5	11.4	23.5	31.3	14.9	35.0	15.4	23.1	13.7	15.7
2.0	11.0	23.9	31.7	17.4	35.8	15.9	23.9	12.4	13.8
2.5	11.5	23.8	30.0	16.1	34.5	15.7	23.2	13.4	14.7
3.0	12.3	24.2	28.4	15.6	33.2	14.9	24.3	12.8	13.3
3.5	12.0	23.9	29.2	16.9	34.9	15.7	24.1	11.7	12.5
4.0	13.2	23.6	28.9	16.1	34.5	15.8	23.8	11.0	12.4
4.5	13.6			17.2				14.1	13.0
5.0	13.5			15.7				14.4	
5.5	14.0			12.5					
6.0	13.8								

TABLE 4.2. *Longitudinal measurements of variceal pressure in 8 patients treated with terlipressin.*

Time	#10	#11	#12	#13	#14	#15	#16	#17
0.0	25.2	26.7	30.0	21.7	25.9	13.1	13.6	15.0
0.5	24.0	26.7	31.1	22.8	25.3	13.0	14.5	14.7
1.0	23.7	26.5	28.7	23.9	25.7	11.9	13.7	15.2
1.5	24.2	26.9	27.7	23.6	26.9	11.4	13.4	15.5
2.0	23.7	26.7	26.9	20.8	23.8	10.5	12.3	15.4
2.5	25.2	25.7	23.1	18.1	21.4	9.3	13.2	15.0
3.0	19.5	28.2	22.8	13.8	19.1	8.5	14.2	13.7
3.5	21.2	27.2	22.3	8.8	17.4	8.3		13.9
4.0	19.5	27.0	20.4	8.4	16.3	7.4	11.4	14.2
4.5	16.7	24.6		11.3	14.6	7.4	10.9	12.7
5.0	18.2	22.3			12.2	7.4	11.2	
5.5	12.6	21.1			9.4			
6.0	14.9	21.1			9.6			
6.5	18.1	18.6			8.6			
7.0	16.1	17.4						
7.5	9.5	16.1						
8.0	9.7	14.3						

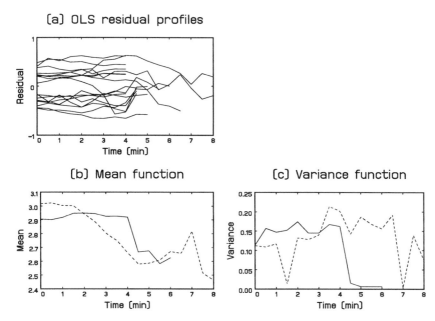

FIGURE 4.2. *(a) OLS residual profiles obtained from fitting a saturated mean structured to the variceal pressure data.*
(b) Evolution of the average variceal pressure over time, for the placebo (solid line) and terlipressin (dashed line) patients separately.
(c) Evolution of the variance of the OLS residuals over time, for the placebo (solid line) and terlipressin (dashed line) patients separately.

is to investigate the efficacy of the treatment, and to test whether change in variceal pressure is related to the baseline value. We refer to Nevens *et al* (1996) for more details on the data collection.

Since only measurements are taken at common points in time, we can use a saturated model as preliminary mean structure (see Section 3.12.1). Histograms of the OLS residuals at each time point separately, revealed some skewness in their distribution. We therefore decided to transform our response using a logarithmic transformation. The OLS residual profiles we then obtain are shown in panel (a) of Figure 4.2. The variance function of these residuals is shown in panel (c) of the same Figure. Note that the apparent drop in the variance function of the placebo group is based on very little data, and will therefore be ignored, assuming constant equal variance in both treatment groups. To explore the covariance structure, we fitted three models with a saturated mean structure and with random intercepts, but with different covariance models for the residual components ε_i. One model assumed exponential serial correlation, another model assumed Gaussian serial correlation, and the final model only included a measurement error component. Minus twice the resulting REML log-likelihood

TABLE 4.3. *Summary of the results of fitting three different random-intercepts models to the variceal pressure data. All models have a saturated mean structure.*

Model	$-2\ell_{\text{REML}}$	AIC	SBC	df
Exponential serial correlation	-217.750	105.875	101.272	3
Gaussian serial correlation	-198.326	96.163	91.560	3
Measurement error	-92.225	44.112	41.043	2

value is shown in Table 4.3, together with the Akaike and Schwarz information criteria, and with the number of parameters (degrees of freedom df) in the corresponding covariance model. Obviously, the exponential serial correlation model fits best.

Based on this covariance structure, we can now reduce the mean structure. Panel (b) in Figure 4.2 shows how the average variceal pressures evolve over time, for the two treatment groups separately. As for the variance function, the drop in average pressure for the placebo group after 4 minutes is based on very limited information, which is also the case for the means after 6 minutes in the terlipressin group. We therefore suggest a constant average profile for the placebo group, and a decreasing average profile for the treated patients, but only from the second minute on. Further, since the patients were randomly assigned to either placebo or terlipressin, and since the follow-up period started immediately after treatment, we assume that there are no systematic differences in average intercept between both treatment groups. The resulting mean structure can now be compared with the saturated mean structure, using the likelihood ratio test. Note that we then should fit the models using maximum likelihood estimation rather than restricted maximum likelihood estimation. Minus twice the difference in maximized log-likelihood value equals 39.297. The associated number of degrees of freedom is 28, implying that the reduced model is acceptable on the 5% level of significance ($p = 0.0763$).

This final, piecewise linear, model can now be written as

$$Y_i(t_{ij}) = \begin{cases} \beta_0 + b_{0i} + \varepsilon_{(2)ij} & \text{placebo} \\ \beta_0 + b_{0i} + \beta_1 \max[(t_{ij} - 1.5), 0] + \varepsilon_{(2)ij} & \text{terlipressin} \end{cases} \quad (4.1)$$

and with the usual distributional assumptions for all stochastic components. The residual vector $\varepsilon_{(2)i}$ is assumed to have an exponential serial correlation structure. REML estimation for all parameters in the above model can be performed by running the program:

```
data press;
```

TABLE 4.4. *Results from fitting the final model (4.1) using restricted maximum likelihood estimation.*

Effect	Parameter	Estimate (s.e.)
Mean structure:		
baseline	β_0	2.946 (0.084)
slope, terlipressin, time > 1.5	β_1	-0.132 (0.016)
Covariance structure		
$\text{var}(b_{0i})$	d_{11}	0.101 (0.044)
$\text{var}(\varepsilon_{(2)ij})$	τ^2	0.030 (0.015)
rate of exponential decrease	$1/\phi$	3.020 (1.623)
Observations		189
REML log-likelihood		152.541
-2 REML log-likelihood		-305.081
Akaike's Information Criterion		149.541
Schwarz's Bayesian Criterion		144.694

```
set press;
correct = (time>1.5)*(time-1.5)*(group=2);
timeclss = time;
run;

proc mixed data = press noclprint scoring = 5 covtest;
class group id timeclss;
model lresp = correct / s;
random intercept / type = un subject = id g;
repeated timeclss / type = sp(exp)(time) subject = id r;
estimate 'treat effect' correct -1 / cl alpha = 0.05;
run;
```

The ESTIMATE statement has been included such that a 95% confidence interval is calculated for the treatment effect and the option 'noclprint' in the PROC MIXED statement requests that printing of the levels of the CLASS variables be suppressed. The parameter estimates and associated estimated standard errors are given in Table 4.4. The model assumes constant variance over time, estimated to be equal to $0.101 + 0.030 = 0.131$, and of which 77% can be ascribed to between-subject variability. We further conclude that, on average, the treatment is effective from 2 minutes after administration on, and that it reduces the variceal pressure with an average rate of 0.132 mmHG per minute. A 95% confidence interval for this rate is $[0.101; 0.164]$.

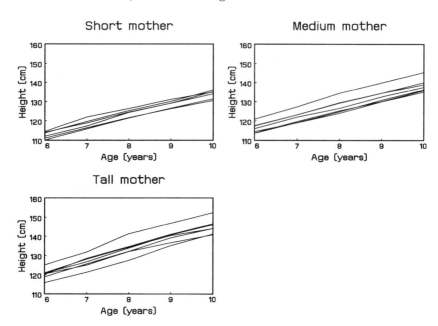

FIGURE 4.3. *Growth curves of 20 school girls from age 6 to 10, for girls with small, medium or tall mothers.*

4.2   Example 2: Growth Curves

Goldstein (1979, Table 4.3, p. 101) has analyzed growth curves of 20 pre-adolescent girls, measured on a yearly basis from age 6 to 10. The girls were classified according to the height of their mother (small: < 155 cm, medium: 155-164 cm, tall: > 164 cm). The individual profiles are shown in Figure 4.3, for each group separately. The measurements are given at exact years of age, some having been previously adjusted to these. The values Goldstein reports for the fifth girl in the first group are 114.5, 112, 126.4, 131.2, 135.0. This suggests that the second measurement is incorrect. We therefore replaced it by 122. Not using mixed models, Goldstein has found a significant (at the 5% level of significance) group effect as well as a significant interaction of age with group. Note that the individual profiles suggest that the variability is mainly due to between-subject variability. That is why we will now re-analyze the data using linear mixed models which allow us to use subject-specific regression coefficients.

As in the example in Section 4.1, we again have measurements at prespeci-fied points in time, allowing the use of a saturated mean structure to explore the covariance structure in the data. Based on this preliminary model for the average, OLS residuals were calculated indicating that the normality assumption is reasonable. The OLS residual profiles are shown in panel (a)

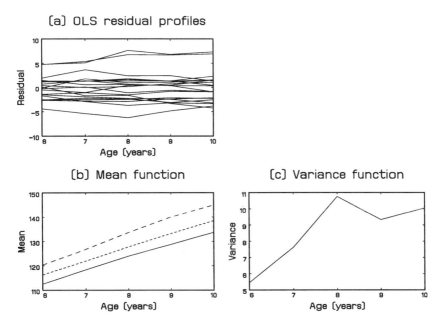

FIGURE 4.4. *(a) OLS residual profiles obtained from fitting a saturated mean structure to the growth data.*
(b) Evolution of the average growth over time, for the children with a short mother (solid line), medium mother (short dashes) or tall mother (long dashes) separately.
(c) Evolution of the variance of the OLS residuals over time.

of Figure 4.4. Panel (c) of the same figure shows how the variance of these residuals varies over time. In order to explore the covariance structure in the data, we fitted several models, all having the saturated mean structure. Table 4.5 shows minus twice the maximized REML log-likelihood value, the Akaike and Schwarz information criteria, and the number of parameters (degrees of freedom df) in the corresponding covariance model.

Since we have only a limited number of repeated measurements available for each subject, and since all subjects have their measurements taken at the same time points, we can fit an unstructured covariance matrix, i.e., a general 5×5 matrix $V_i = \Sigma_i = \Sigma$, which contains 15 covariance parameters that need to be estimated. The REML estimate for V_i equals

$$
\begin{pmatrix}
6.11 & 6.88 & 8.26 & 7.44 & 7.18 \\
6.88 & 8.53 & 9.78 & 9.01 & 8.70 \\
8.26 & 9.78 & 12.04 & 10.99 & 10.96 \\
7.44 & 9.01 & 10.99 & 10.42 & 10.56 \\
7.18 & 8.70 & 10.96 & 10.56 & 11.24
\end{pmatrix}
\tag{4.2}
$$

On the other hand, the OLS residual profiles in panel (a) of Figure 4.4

TABLE 4.5. *Summary of the results of fitting four different covariance models to the growth data. All models include a saturated mean structure.*

Model	$-2\ell_{\text{REML}}$	AIC	SBC	df
Unstructured	246.215	-138.107	-156.427	15
Random intercepts and slopes	281.807	-144.903	-149.789	4
Heterogeneous Toeplitz	261.669	-139.834	-150.826	9
Heterogeneous AR(1)	269.828	-140.914	-148.242	6

indicate that a random-effects model, assuming a linear residual trend for each subject separately, may fit the data well. We therefore also fitted a covariance structure consisting of random intercepts and random slopes for age minus 6. The transformation of age was used in order for the intercepts to be defined as the height measured at the first visit, i.e. the height at the age of 6 years. Note how the unstructured covariance matrix can be interpreted as a reparameterized random-effects covariance model with random intercepts, random slopes for age−6 and with three other random effects which are linearly independent of each other and of the first two. Hence, comparing our second covariance structure to the unstructured covariance model is a hypothesis of the same form as those described in case 4 of Section 3.9.1 and therefore, we cannot apply the usual asymptotic null-distribution for the likelihood ratio test. Instead, simulations would be needed to derive the correct null distribution. Still, we may conclude that twice the difference in maximized REML log likelihood value seems rather large in comparison with the difference in numbers of parameters involved in both covariance models. Also, our random-effects model implicitly assumes that the variance is a quadratic function over time, which seems not to be the case, considering the results in panel (c) of Figure 4.4 and the estimated variances in (4.2). Note also that the AIC criterion is in favor of the unstructured covariance matrix while the SBC criterion selects the random-effects model. The reason is that there is a big difference in number of parameters used in the two models. Since this number of degrees of freedom is multiplied by $\ln n^*$ in the SBC criterion (see Table 3.14), this criterion penalizes the use of many parameters much more severely than AIC. Therefore, it will more often select the model with the smallest number of parameters.

It seems that a good covariance structure should not restrict the variance function to be of any specific parametric form. A reduction of the number of covariance parameters can then only be based on a more parsimonious correlation structure. The correlation matrix corresponding to (4.2) equals

$$
\begin{pmatrix}
1.00 & 0.95 & 0.96 & 0.93 & 0.87 \\
0.95 & 1.00 & 0.97 & 0.96 & 0.89 \\
0.96 & 0.97 & 1.00 & 0.98 & 0.94 \\
0.93 & 0.96 & 0.98 & 1.00 & 0.98 \\
0.87 & 0.89 & 0.94 & 0.98 & 1.00
\end{pmatrix}. \tag{4.3}
$$

Since the correlations in bands along the main diagonal are rather similar, we fitted the heterogeneous Toeplitz model as well as the heterogeneous AR(1) model (denoted by ARH(1)), which both assume the correlations to be a function only of the time-distance between the measurements. The Toeplitz model assumes no relation among the correlations in different bands. The ARH(1) structure assumes all correlations to be of the form ρ^u where u is the time-lag between the measurements. Neither the Toeplitz nor the ARH(1) model is acceptable in comparison to the unstructured covariance matrix, based on the REML likelihood ratio test ($p = 0.017$ and $p = 0.005$ respectively). On the other hand, we have as before that the SBC criterion selects the model with the smallest number of parameters, i.e., the ARH(1) structure. The estimated covariance matrix, obtained from fitting the latter model equals

$$
\begin{pmatrix}
6.51 & 7.37 & 8.25 & 7.30 & 7.32 \\
7.37 & 8.88 & 9.94 & 8.80 & 8.82 \\
8.25 & 9.94 & 11.86 & 10.49 & 10.52 \\
7.30 & 8.80 & 10.49 & 9.89 & 9.92 \\
7.32 & 8.82 & 10.52 & 9.92 & 10.60
\end{pmatrix} \tag{4.4}
$$

and the corresponding correlation matrix equals

$$
\begin{pmatrix}
1.00 & 0.97 & 0.94 & 0.91 & 0.88 \\
0.97 & 1.00 & 0.97 & 0.94 & 0.91 \\
0.94 & 0.97 & 1.00 & 0.97 & 0.94 \\
0.91 & 0.94 & 0.97 & 1.00 & 0.97 \\
0.88 & 0.91 & 0.94 & 0.97 & 1.00
\end{pmatrix}. \tag{4.5}
$$

In view of the small sample size, and because there are no major differences between the fitted covariance matrices (4.4) and (4.2) or between the fitted correlation matrices (4.5) and (4.3), we propose to use the heterogeneous AR(1) structure for further inferences and for model reduction. To confirm that both models yield the same final conclusions, all tests will be performed based on the unstructured covariance matrix as well.

Table 4.6 shows minus twice the maximized ML log-likelihood function for four mean structures, and for the two covariance structures. The number of fixed effects (degrees of freedom df) are also shown. As before, we use the transformed version age-6 of age whenever linear models are fitted. Based

TABLE 4.6. *Summary of the results of fitting four different mean structures to the growth data, for models with a heterogeneous AR(1) covariance structure as well as for models with an unstructured (UN) covariance structure.*

	$-2\ell_{\mathrm{ML}}$		
Mean structure	ARH(1)	UN	df
Unstructured	267.760	239.979	15
Linear within each group	292.526	275.398	6
Piecewise linear within each group, (break point = 9 years)	274.385	247.635	9
Final model	278.888	253.577	6

on the ML likelihood ratio test, we conclude that a linear model within each group is not fitting well. We therefore propose to use a piecewise linear model for each group separately. We fitted three models, with break points at 7 years, 8 years and 9 years, yielding $-2\ell_{\mathrm{ML}} = 290.338$, $-2\ell_{\mathrm{ML}} = 279.369$ and $-2\ell_{\mathrm{ML}} = 274.385$ respectively. Because the model with break points at 9 years fits best, and is also acceptable when compared to the preliminary mean structure ($p = 0.3569$ and $p = 0.2644$ for ARH(1) and UN respectively), we reduce our model to

$$Y_i(t_{ij}) = \begin{cases} \beta_1 + \beta_2 t_{ij} + \beta_3 \max[(t_{ij} - 3), 0] + \varepsilon_{(2)ij} & \text{small,} \\ \beta_4 + \beta_5 t_{ij} + \beta_6 \max[(t_{ij} - 3), 0] + \varepsilon_{(2)ij} & \text{medium,} \\ \beta_7 + \beta_8 t_{ij} + \beta_9 \max[(t_{ij} - 3), 0] + \varepsilon_{(2)ij} & \text{tall,} \end{cases} \quad (4.6)$$

where t_{ij} equals $\text{age}_{ij} - 6$, and where $\varepsilon_{(2)ij}$ has a heterogeneous AR(1) covariance structure. The parameters β_1, β_4 and β_7, and the parameters β_2, β_5 and β_8 are the average heights at age 6, and the slopes for the children with small, medium and tall mothers respectively. The parameters β_3, β_6 and β_9 represent corrections to these slopes, which are effective from the age of 9 years on, and which indicate that the average growth has accelerated ($\beta > 0$) or has slowed down ($\beta < 0$).

The REML estimates for all fixed effects in model (4.6) are shown in Table 4.7. Using CONTRAST statements in combination with REML, we can now try to further reduce the mean structure of this model. First of all, we notice that the slopes as well as the corrections to these slopes are very similar for the children with small or medium mothers. Also, the correction terms for these two groups are not significantly different from zero. It is

TABLE 4.7. *REML estimates for the fixed effects in model (4.6), with a hetero-geneous AR(1) covariance structure.*

Effect	Parameter	Estimate (s.e.)
Intercepts:		
small mothers	β_1	111.426 (0.859)
medium mothers	β_4	115.991 (0.795)
tall mothers	β_7	119.946 (0.795)
Slopes :		
small mothers	β_2	5.339 (0.177)
medium mothers	β_5	5.624 (0.164)
tall mothers	β_8	6.492 (0.164)
Corrections to slopes		
small mothers	β_3	-0.411 (0.371)
medium mothers	β_6	-0.368 (0.344)
tall mothers	β_9	-1.493 (0.344)

therefore not surprising that the hypothesis

$$H_0 : \left\{ \begin{array}{l} \beta_2 = \beta_5 \\ \beta_3 = \beta_6 = 0 \end{array} \right.$$

was not rejected on the 5% level of significance ($p = 0.2416$ and $p = 0.1463$ for ARH(1) and UN respectively). Since there are highly significant pairwise differences at age 6, between the three groups (all p-values smaller than 0.005), and because the slopes β_2 and β_5 differ significantly from β_8 (p < 0.0001 under both covariance structures), no further model reduction is possible. Note that it follows from Table 4.6 that, when compared to the preliminary mean structure, our final model, given by

$$\boldsymbol{Y}_i(t_{ij}) = \left\{ \begin{array}{ll} \beta_1 + \beta_2 t_{ij} + \varepsilon_{(2)ij} & \text{small,} \\ \\ \beta_4 + \beta_2 t_{ij} + \varepsilon_{(2)ij} & \text{medium,} \quad (4.7) \\ \\ \beta_7 + \beta_8 t_{ij} + \beta_9 \max[(t_{ij} - 3), 0] + \varepsilon_{(2)ij} & \text{tall,} \end{array} \right.$$

is acceptable ($p = 0.2670$ and $p = 0.1374$ for ARH(1) and UN respectively). In this final model, $\varepsilon_{(2)ij}$ is assumed to have a ARH(1) covariance structure. The program needed to fit this model in SAS is

```
data grcurve;
set grcurve;
```

TABLE 4.8. *Results from fitting the final model (4.7) using restricted maximum likelihood estimation.*

Effect	Parameter	Estimate (s.e.)[1] (s.e.)[2]
Intercepts:		
small mothers	β_1	111.453 (0.856) (0.627)
medium mothers	β_4	115.819 (0.793) (0.740)
tall mothers	β_7	119.945 (0.800) (0.503)
Slopes:		
small & medium mothers	$\beta_2 = \beta_5$	5.403 (0.106) (0.085)
tall mothers	β_8	6.490 (0.166) (0.211)
Correction to slopes:		
tall mothers	β_9	-1.483 (0.350) (0.236)
Covariance structure :		
variance, age=6	$\sigma^2_{6,6}$	6.618 (2.285) (2.285)
variance, age=7	$\sigma^2_{7,7}$	9.075 (3.102) (3.102)
variance, age=8	$\sigma^2_{8,8}$	12.337 (4.197) (4.197)
variance, age=9	$\sigma^2_{9,9}$	10.267 (3.528) (3.528)
variance, age=10	$\sigma^2_{10,10}$	10.634 (3.572) (3.572)
correlation, time-lag=1	ρ	0.969 (0.011) (0.011)
Observations		100
REML log-likelihood		-139.962
-2 REML log-likelihood		279.925
Akaike's Information Criterion		-145.962
Schwarz's Bayesian Criterion		-153.592

[1] Default s.e.'s under the ARH(1) model.

[2] Sandwich s.e.'s, obtained from the 'empirical' option.

```
grp = (group=3);
grpclss = grp;
correct3 = (age>3)*(age-3);
run;

proc mixed data = grcurve noclprint covtest;
class child group grpclss ageclss;
model height = group grpclss*age grp*correct3 / noint s;
repeated ageclss / type = arh(1) subject = child r rcorr;
run;
```

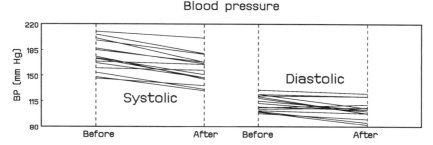

FIGURE 4.5. *Systolic and diastolic blood pressure in patients with moderate essential hypertension, immediately before and two hours after taking captopril.*

The REML estimates for all parameters in the marginal model are shown in Table 4.8. We conclude that there are highly significant differences in average height at age 6, between girls with small mothers, medium mothers and tall mothers respectively. The first two groups evolve linearly over time, and have the same average growth. The growth in the third group is significantly stronger than in the other groups, but is not linear since there is a slow-down from the age of 9 years on.

Because there is some doubt about the appropriateness of the ARH(1) covariance structure, we also included standard errors in Table 4.8 obtained from using the sandwich estimator (3.12) to estimate the covariance matrix for $\widehat{\beta}$. Recall that this estimator is robust for model deviations with respect to the specified covariance structure. The resulting standard errors can be requested in PROC MIXED by adding the option 'empirical' to the PROC MIXED statement. Note that this option does not affect the standard errors reported for the variance components in the model. For most fixed effects however, the robust standard errors tend to be somewhat smaller than the model-based standard errors, leading to less conservative inferences for the fixed effects in our final model (4.7).

4.3 Example 3: Blood Pressures

As an illustration of the use of linear mixed models for the analysis of repeated measures of a bivariate outcome, we analyze data reported by Hand *et al* (1994, data set #72). For 15 patients with moderate essential (unknown cause) hypertension, the supine (measured while patient is lying down) systolic and diastolic blood pressure was measured immediately before and two hours after taking the drug captopril. The individual profiles are shown in Figure 4.5. The objective of the analysis is to investigate the effect of treatment on both responses.

TABLE 4.9. *Summary of the results of fitting several covariance models to the blood pressure data. All models include a saturated mean structure. Notations RI_{dia}, RS_{dia}, RI_{sys}, RS_{sys}, RI and RS are used for random intercepts and slopes for the diastolic blood pressures, random intercepts and slopes for the systolic blood pressures, and random intercepts and slopes which are the same for both blood pressures.*

Model	$-2\ell_{\text{REML}}$	AIC	SBC	df
Unstructured	420.095	-220.047	-230.174	10
$RI_{dia} + RI_{sys} + RS_{dia} + RS_{sys}$	420.095	-221.047	-232.187	10
$RI_{dia} + RI_{sys} + RS$	420.656	-217.328	-224.417	7
$RI_{dia} + RI_{sys}$	433.398	-220.699	-224.749	4
$RI + RI_{sys} + RS$	420.656	-217.328	-224.417	7
$RI + RI_{sys} + RS$, uncorrelated	424.444	-216.222	-220.273	4

Note that, since we only have two measurements available for each response, there is no need for modeling the variance or the mean as continuous functions of time. Also, saturated mean structures and covariance structures can easily be fitted because of the balanced nature of the data. No transformation to normality is needed since none of the four responses has a distribution which shows clear deviations from normality.

In order to explore the covariance structure of our data, we fitted several linear mixed models with the saturated mean structure. Table 4.9 shows minus twice the maximized REML log-likelihood value, the Akaike and Schwarz information criteria, and the number of degrees of freedom in the corresponding covariance model. Our first model has a general unstructured covariance matrix. The REML-estimated covariance matrix and corresponding standard errors equal

$$\begin{pmatrix} 423\ (160) & 371\ (148) & 143\ (69) & 105\ (75) \\ 371\ (148) & 400\ (151) & 153\ (69) & 166\ (81) \\ 143\ (69) & 153\ (69) & 110\ (41) & 97\ (44) \\ 105\ (75) & 166\ (81) & 97\ (44) & 157\ (60) \end{pmatrix}, \tag{4.8}$$

for measurements ordered as indicated in Figure 4.5. Note that if one would model the diastolic and systolic blood pressures separately, a random-intercepts model would probably fit the data well. This would implicitly assume that for both responses, the variance before and after the treatment with captopril is the same, which is not unreasonable in view of the large standard errors shown in (4.8). We therefore reparameterize the unstructured covariance model as a random-effects model with random intercepts and random slopes for the two responses separately. The random slopes are random coefficients for the dummy covariate defined as 0 before the treatment and as 1 after the treatment, and therefore represent subject-specific deviations from the average effect of the treatment, for systolic and diastolic blood pressure respectively. Since this model includes 4 linearly independent covariates in the Z_i matrix, it is equivalent with the first model in Table 4.9, yielding the same maximized log-likelihood value. The advantage is that we now have expressed the model in terms of interpretable components. This will show to be convenient for reducing the number of variance components. As discussed before, SAS always adds a residual component $\varepsilon_{(1)i}$ of measurement error to any random-effects model. In our model this component is not identified. Still, the reported AIC and SBC values are based on 11 variance components and are therefore not the same as the ones found for the first model in Table 4.9.

In a first attempt to reduce the covariance structure, we fitted a linear mixed model assuming equal random slopes for diastolic and systolic blood pressure. This model, which is the third model in Table 4.9, assumes that for each subject, the treatment effect additional to the average effect is the same for both responses. Note that there is only a difference of 3 degrees of freedom when compared to the unstructured model, which is due to the estimation of the residual variance which was not included in the first model. Therefore, we can strictly speaking not apply the theory of Section 3.9 for testing random effects. However, the very small difference in twice the maximized REML log-likelihood clearly suggests that the random slopes may be assumed equal for both responses.

As a second step, we refit our model, not including the random slopes. This is the fourth model in Table 4.9. The p-value calculated using the theory of Section 3.9 on testing the significance of the random slopes, equals

$$
\begin{aligned}
P\left(\chi_{2:3}^2 \geq 12.742\right) &= 0.5\,P\left(\chi_2^2 \geq 12.742\right) + 0.5\,P\left(\chi_3^2 \geq 12.742\right) \\
&= 0.5 \times 0.0017 + 0.5 \times 0.0052 \\
&= 0.0035,
\end{aligned}
$$

indicating that the treatment effect is not the same for all subjects.

We therefore investigate our third model further. The REML-estimated random-effects covariance matrix D, and the corresponding estimated standard errors are

$$
\begin{array}{ll}
\mathrm{RI}_{sys} & \longrightarrow \\
\mathrm{RI}_{dia} & \longrightarrow \\
\mathrm{RS} & \longrightarrow
\end{array}
\left(
\begin{array}{rrr}
409\ (158) & 146\ (68) & -38\ (46) \\
146\ (68) & 92\ (39) & 4\ (22) \\
-38\ (46) & 4\ (22) & 51\ (25)
\end{array}
\right),
$$

where the random effects are ordered as indicated in front of the matrix. Clearly, there is no significant correlation between either one of the random intercepts on one side and the random slopes on the other side ($p = 0.8501$ and $p = 0.4101$ for the diastolic and systolic blood pressure respectively), meaning that the treatment-effect does not depend on the initial value. On the other hand, there is a significant positive correlation ($p = 0.0321$) between the random intercepts for the diastolic blood pressure and the random intercepts for the systolic blood pressure, meaning that a patient with an initial diastolic blood pressure higher than average, is likely to have an initial systolic blood pressure which is also higher than average.

This suggests that an overall subject-effect may be present in the data. We can easily reparameterize our fourth model such that an overall random intercept is included, but a correction term for either systolic or diastolic blood pressure is then needed. In view of the larger variability in systolic blood pressures than in diastolic blood pressures, we decided to reparameterize our model as a random-effects model, with overall random intercepts, random intercepts for systolic blood pressure, and random slopes. The overall random intercepts can then be interpreted as the random intercepts for the diastolic blood pressures. The random intercepts for systolic blood pressure are corrections to the overall intercepts indicating for each patient, what its deviation from the average initial systolic blood pressure is, additional to its deviation from the average initial diastolic blood pressure. These correction terms then explain the additional variability for systolic blood pressure, in comparison to diastolic blood pressure. Information on the model-fit for this fifth model is also shown in Table 4.9. Since this model is merely a reparameterization of our third model, we obtain the same results for both models. The REML-estimated random-effects covariance matrix D, and the corresponding estimated standard errors are now

$$
\begin{array}{ll}
\text{RI} & \longrightarrow \\
\text{RI}_{dia} & \longrightarrow \\
\text{RS} & \longrightarrow
\end{array}
\left(
\begin{array}{ccc}
92\ (39) & 54\ (42) & 4\ (22) \\
54\ (42) & 209\ (84) & -42\ (34) \\
4\ (22) & -42\ (34) & 51\ (25)
\end{array}
\right),
$$

suggesting that there are no pairwise correlations between the three random effects (all p-values larger than 0.19). We therefore fit a sixth model assuming independent random effects. The results are also shown in Table 4.9. Minus twice the difference in maximized REML log-likelihood between the sixth and fifth model equals 3.788 which is not significant when compared to a chi-squared distribution with 3 degrees of freedom ($p = 0.2853$). We will preserve this covariance structure (4 independent components of stochastic variability: a random subject effect, a random effect for the overall difference between the systolic and diastolic blood pressures, a random effect for the overall treatment effect, and a component of measurement error) in the models considered next. Note that this covariance structure is also the one selected by the AIC as well as the SBC criterion (see Table 4.9).

Using the above covariance structure, we can now try to reduce our saturated mean structure. The average treatment effect was found to be signif-

TABLE 4.10. *Results from fitting the final model (4.9), using restricted maximum likelihood estimation.*

Effect	Parameter	Estimate (s.e.)
Intercepts:		
diastolic, before	β_1	112.333 (2.687)
systolic, before	β_2	176.933 (4.648)
diastolic, after	β_3	103.067 (3.269)
systolic, after	β_4	158.000 (5.007)
Treatment effects:		
diastolic	$\beta_3 - \beta_1$	9.267 (2.277)
systolic	$\beta_4 - \beta_2$	18.933 (2.277)
Covariance of $\boldsymbol{b_i}$:		
var(b_{1i})	d_{11}	95.405 (39.454)
var(b_{2i})	d_{22}	215.728 (86.315)
var(b_{3i})	d_{33}	52.051 (24.771)
Measurement error variance:		
var($\varepsilon_{(1)ij}$)	σ^2	12.862 (4.693)
Observations		60
REML log-likelihood		-212.222
-2 REML log-likelihood		424.444
Akaike's Information Criterion		-216.222
Schwarz's Bayesian Criterion		-220.273

icantly different for the two blood pressure measurements, and we found significant treatment effects for the systolic as well as diastolic blood pressures (all p-values smaller than 0.0001). Our final model is now given by

$$
Y_{ij} = \begin{cases}
\beta_1 + b_{1i} + \varepsilon_{(1)ij} & \text{diastolic, before,} \\
\beta_2 + b_{1i} + b_{2i} + \varepsilon_{(1)ij} & \text{systolic, before,} \\
\beta_3 + b_{1i} + b_{3i} + \varepsilon_{(1)ij} & \text{diastolic, after,} \\
\beta_4 + b_{1i} + b_{2i} + b_{3i} + \varepsilon_{(1)ij} & \text{systolic, after.}
\end{cases} \tag{4.9}
$$

As before, we assume the random effects to be uncorrelated, and the $\varepsilon_{(1)ij}$ represent independent components of measurement error with equal variance σ^2. The program needed to fit this model in SAS is

```
data blood;
```

```
set blood;
slope = (time='after');
intsys = (meas='systolic');
run;

proc mixed data = blood covtest;
class time meas id ;
model bp = meas*time / noint s;
random intercept intsys slope / type = un(1) subject = id;
estimate 'trt_sys' meas*time 0 -1 0 1 / cl alpha = 0.05;
estimate 'trt_dia' meas*time -1 0 1 0 / cl alpha = 0.05;
contrast 'trt_sys = 2xtrt_dia' meas*time 2 -1 -2 1;
run;
```

The variables *meas* and *time* are factors with levels 'systolic' and 'diastolic' and with levels 'before' and 'after' respectively. The ESTIMATE statements are included to estimate the average treatment effect for the systolic and diastolic blood pressures separately. The CONTRAST statement is used to compare these two effects.

The REML estimates for all parameters in the marginal model are shown in Table 4.10. The 95% confidence intervals for the average treatment effect on diastolic and systolic blood pressure are $[4.383; 14.151]$ and $[14.050; 23.817]$ respectively. Further, the parameter estimates in Table 4.10 suggest that the average treatment effect on systolic blood pressure is twice the average treatment effect on diastolic blood pressure. This hypothesis, tested with the CONTRAST statement in the above program, was indeed accepted at the 5% level of significance ($p = 0.9099$).

4.4   Example 4: Growth Data

These data, introduced by Potthof and Roy (1964), contain growth measurements for 11 girls and 16 boys. For each subject the distance from the center of the pituitary to the maxillary fissure was recorded at the ages 8, 10, 12, and 14. The data were used by Jennrich and Schluchter (1986) to illustrate estimation methods for unbalanced data, where unbalancedness is now to be interpreted in the sense of an unequal number of boys and girls.

Little and Rubin (1987) deleted 9 of the $[(11 + 16) \times 4]$ measurements, rendering 9 incomplete subjects. Deletion is confined to the age 10 measurements. Little and Rubin (1987) describe the mechanism to be such that

TABLE 4.11. *Growth data for 11 girls and 16 boys. Measurements marked with* * *were deleted by Little and Rubin (1987).*

	Age (in years)					Age (in years)			
Girl	8	10	12	14	Boy	8	10	12	14
1	21.0	20.0	21.5	23.0	1	26.0	25.0	29.0	31.0
2	21.0	21.5	24.0	25.5	2	21.5	22.5*	23.0	26.5
3	20.5	24.0*	24.5	26.0	3	23.0	22.5	24.0	27.5
4	23.5	24.5	25.0	26.5	4	25.5	27.5	26.5	27.0
5	21.5	23.0	22.5	23.5	5	20.0	23.5*	22.5	26.0
6	20.0	21.0*	21.0	22.5	6	24.5	25.5	27.0	28.5
7	21.5	22.5	23.0	25.0	7	22.0	22.0	24.5	26.5
8	23.0	23.0	23.5	24.0	8	24.0	21.5	24.5	25.5
9	20.0	21.0*	22.0	21.5	9	23.0	20.5	31.0	26.0
10	16.5	19.0*	19.0	19.5	10	27.5	28.0	31.0	31.5
11	24.5	25.0	28.0	28.0	11	23.0	23.0	23.5	25.0
					12	21.5	23.5*	24.0	28.0
					13	17.0	24.5*	26.0	29.5
					14	22.5	25.5	25.5	26.0
					15	23.0	24.5	26.0	30.0
					16	22.0	21.5*	23.5	25.0

Source: Pothoff and Roy (1964), Jennrich and Schluchter (1986).

subjects with a low value at age 8 are more likely to have a missing value at age 10. The data are presented in Table 4.11. The measurements that were deleted are marked with an asterisk. Here, we will restrict attention to the analysis of the complete data. The analysis of the incomplete version of these data is the subject of Chapter 5.

Following guidelines in Section 3.12 and in Diggle, Liang, and Zeger (1994) model building should proceed by constructing an adequate description of the variability on an appropriate set of residuals. These residuals are preferably found by subtracting a saturated sex by time mean model from the measurements. When a satisfactory covariance model is found, attention would then shift to simplification of the mean structure. However, this insight is relatively recent and was certainly not the standard procedure in the mid eighties. Jennrich and Schluchter (1986) constructed 8 models where the first three concentrate on the mean model, leaving the 4 × 4 covariance matrix of the repeated measurements completely unstructured.

Once an adequate mean model is found, the remaining five models are fit to enable simplification of the covariance structure. Jennrich and Schluchter (1986) primarily wanted to illustrate their estimation procedures and did not envisage a comprehensive data analysis. Moreover, since this procedure can be considered legitimate in small balanced studies and also for reasons of comparability, we will, at first, adopt the same 8 models, in the same order. In this section, these models will be fitted to the original data, referred to henceforth as the *complete data set*. The results of Jennrich and Schluchter (1986) will be recovered and additional insight will be given. In Chapter 5, these solutions will be compared to the results for the same 8 models (possibly supplemented with a set of additional models) on the incomplete data, under a variety of missing data handling procedures.

Jennrich and Schluchter (1986) used Newton-Raphson, Fisher scoring, and generalized Expectation-Maximization (EM) algorithms to maximize the log-likelihood. We will show that the data can be analyzed relatively easy using PROC MIXED.

The models of Jennrich and Schluchter (1986) can be expressed in the general linear mixed models family (3.8):

$$Y_i = X_i\beta + Z_ib_i + \varepsilon_i, \qquad (4.10)$$

where

$$b_i \;\sim\; N(\mathbf{0}, D),$$
$$\varepsilon_i \;\sim\; N(\mathbf{0}, \Sigma),$$

and b_i and ε_i are statistically independent. As before (Section 3.4) Y_i is the (4×1) response vector, X_i is a $(4 \times p)$ design matrix for the fixed effects, β is a vector of unknown fixed regression coefficients, Z_i is a $(4 \times q)$ design matrix for the random effects, b_i is a $(q \times 1)$ vector of normally distributed random parameters, with covariance matrix D, and ε_i is a normally distributed (4×1) random error vector, with covariance matrix Σ. The random error ε_i encompasses both measurement error (as in a cross-sectional study), and serial correlation. In this study, the design will be a function of age, sex, and/or the interaction between both. Let us indicate boys with $x_i = 0$, girls with $x_i = 1$, and age with $t_i = 8, 10, 12, 14$.

4.4.1   Model 1

The first model we will consider assumes a separate mean for each of the eight age×sex combinations, together with an unstructured covariance. This is done by assuming that the covariance matrix Σ of the error vector ε_i is a completely general positive definite matrix.

This model can be expressed as

$$
\begin{aligned}
Y_{i1} &= \beta_0 + \beta_1 x_i + \beta_{0,8}(1 - x_i) + \beta_{1,8} x_i + \varepsilon_{i1}, \\
Y_{i2} &= \beta_0 + \beta_1 x_i + \beta_{0,10}(1 - x_i) + \beta_{1,10} x_i + \varepsilon_{i2}, \\
Y_{i3} &= \beta_0 + \beta_1 x_i + \beta_{0,12}(1 - x_i) + \beta_{1,12} x_i + \varepsilon_{i3}, \\
Y_{i4} &= \beta_0 + \beta_1 x_i + \varepsilon_{i4},
\end{aligned}
\tag{4.11}
$$

or, in matrix notation,

$$
\boldsymbol{Y}_i = X_i \boldsymbol{\beta} + \boldsymbol{\varepsilon}_i,
$$

with

$$
X_i = \begin{pmatrix}
1 & x_i & 1 - x_i & 0 & 0 & x_i & 0 & 0 \\
1 & x_i & 0 & 1 - x_i & 0 & 0 & x_i & 0 \\
1 & x_i & 0 & 0 & 1 - x_i & 0 & 0 & x_i \\
1 & x_i & 0 & 0 & 0 & 0 & 0 & 0
\end{pmatrix}
$$

and $\boldsymbol{\beta} = (\beta_0, \beta_1, \beta_{0,8}, \beta_{0,10}, \beta_{0,12}, \beta_{1,8}, \beta_{1,10}, \beta_{1,12})'$. With this parameterization, the means for boys are $\beta_0 + \beta_1 + \beta_{1,8}$; $\beta_0 + \beta_1 + \beta_{1,10}$; $\beta_0 + \beta_1 + \beta_{1,12}$; and $\beta_0 + \beta_1$ at ages 8, 10, 12, and 14, respectively. The corresponding means for girls are $\beta_0 + \beta_{0,8}$; $\beta_0 + \beta_{0,10}$; $\beta_0 + \beta_{0,12}$; and β_0. Of course, there are many equivalent ways to express the set of 8 means in terms of 8 linearly independent parameters.

This model can, for example, be fitted with the following SAS code:

```
proc mixed data = growth method = ml covtest;
title 'Growth Data, Model 1';
class idnr sex age;
model measure = sex age*sex / s;
repeated / type = un subject = idnr r rcorr;
run;
```

Let us discuss the fit of the model. The deviance (minus twice the log-likelihood at maximum) equals 416.5093, and there are 18 model parameters (8 mean, 4 variance, and 6 covariance parameters). This deviance will serve as a reference to assess the goodness-of-fit of simpler models. Parameter estimates and standard errors are reproduced in Table 4.12.

The estimated covariance matrix $\hat{\Sigma}$ of the error vector, based on this model, equals

$$
\begin{pmatrix}
5.0143 & 2.5156 & 3.6206 & 2.5095 \\
2.5156 & 3.8748 & 2.7103 & 3.0714 \\
3.6206 & 2.7103 & 5.9775 & 3.8248 \\
2.5095 & 3.0714 & 3.8248 & 4.6164
\end{pmatrix}
\tag{4.12}
$$

TABLE 4.12. *Maximum likelihood estimates and standard errors (model based and empirically corrected) for the fixed effects in Model 1, fitted to the growth data (complete data set).*

Parameter	MLE (s.e.)[1] (s.e.)[2]
β_0	24.0909 (0.6478) (0.7007)
β_1	3.3778 (0.8415) (0.8636)
$\beta_{0,8}$	-4.5938 (0.5369) (0.6468)
$\beta_{0,10}$	-3.6563 (0.3831) (0.4391)
$\beta_{0,12}$	-1.7500 (0.4290) (0.5358)
$\beta_{1,8}$	-2.9091 (0.6475) (0.3793)
$\beta_{1,10}$	-1.8636 (0.4620) (0.3407)
$\beta_{1,12}$	-1.0000 (0.5174) (0.2227)

[1] Default s.e.'s under Model 1.

[2] Sandwich s.e.'s, obtained from the 'empirical' option;
also obtained under Model 0.

with corresponding correlation matrix

$$
\begin{pmatrix}
1.0000 & 0.5707 & 0.6613 & 0.5216 \\
0.5707 & 1.0000 & 0.5632 & 0.7262 \\
0.6613 & 0.5632 & 1.0000 & 0.7281 \\
0.5216 & 0.7262 & 0.7281 & 1.0000
\end{pmatrix}. \tag{4.13}
$$

These quantities are easily obtained in PROC MIXED by using the options 'r' and 'rcorr' in the REPEATED statement. Apparently, the variances are close to each other, and so are the correlations.

Even though we opted to stick closely to the models discussed in Jennrich and Schluchter (1987), it is instructive to consider a more elaborate model, termed Model 0, where a separate unstructured covariance matrix is assumed for each of the two sex groups. This model has 10 extra parameters and can be fitted to the data using the following SAS code:

```
proc mixed data = growth method = ml covtest;
title 'Growth Data, Model 0';
class idnr sex  age;
model measure = sex age*sex / s;
repeated / type = un subject = idnr
          r = 1,12 rcorr = 1,12 group = sex;
run;
```

TABLE 4.13. *Predicted means for the growth data set.*

Model	Age	Boys Estimate	Boys SE	Girls Estimate	Girls Se
1	8	22.88	0.56	21.18	0.68
	10	23.81	0.49	22.23	0.59
	12	25.72	0.61	23.09	0.74
	14	27.47	0.54	24.09	0.65
2	8	22.46	0.49	21.24	0.59
	10	24.11	0.45	22.19	0.55
	12	25.76	0.47	23.14	0.57
	14	27.42	0.54	24.10	0.65
3	8	22.82	0.48	20.77	0.57
	10	24.16	0.45	22.12	0.55
	12	25.51	0.47	23.47	0.56
	14	26.86	0.52	24.82	0.60
4	8	22.64	0.53	21.22	0.64
	10	24.23	0.48	22.17	0.57
	12	25.83	0.48	23.12	0.57
	14	27.42	0.53	24.07	0.64
5	8	22.75	0.54	21.19	0.66
	10	24.29	0.44	22.16	0.53
	12	25.83	0.44	23.13	0.53
	14	27.37	0.54	24.09	0.66
6	8	22.62	0.51	21.21	0.61
	10	24.18	0.47	22.17	0.56
	12	25.75	0.48	23.13	0.58
	14	27.32	0.55	24.09	0.67
7	8	22.62	0.52	21.21	0.63
	10	24.18	0.47	22.17	0.57
	12	25.75	0.47	23.13	0.57
	14	27.32	0.52	24.09	0.63
8	8	22.62	0.46	21.21	0.56
	10	24.18	0.30	22.17	0.37
	12	25.75	0.30	23.13	0.37
	14	27.32	0.46	24.09	0.56

Source: Jennrich and Schluchter (1986).

These separate covariance matrices are requested by means of the 'group='
option.. These matrices and the corresponding correlation matrices are
printed using the 'r=' and 'rcorr=' options. The estimated covariance matrix for girls is

$$\begin{pmatrix} 4.1033 & 3.0496 & 3.9380 & 3.9607 \\ 3.0496 & 3.2893 & 3.6612 & 3.7066 \\ 3.9380 & 3.6612 & 5.0826 & 4.9690 \\ 3.9607 & 3.7066 & 4.9690 & 5.4008 \end{pmatrix}$$

with corresponding correlation matrix

$$\begin{pmatrix} 1.0000 & 0.8301 & 0.8623 & 0.8414 \\ 0.8301 & 1.0000 & 0.8954 & 0.8794 \\ 0.8623 & 0.8954 & 1.0000 & 0.9484 \\ 0.8414 & 0.8794 & 0.9484 & 1.0000 \end{pmatrix}.$$

The corresponding quantities for boys are

$$\begin{pmatrix} 5.6406 & 2.1484 & 3.4023 & 1.5117 \\ 2.1484 & 4.2773 & 2.0566 & 2.6348 \\ 3.4023 & 2.0566 & 6.5928 & 3.0381 \\ 1.5117 & 2.6348 & 3.0381 & 4.0771 \end{pmatrix}$$

and

$$\begin{pmatrix} 1.0000 & 0.4374 & 0.5579 & 0.3152 \\ 0.4374 & 1.0000 & 0.3873 & 0.6309 \\ 0.5579 & 0.3873 & 1.0000 & 0.5860 \\ 0.3152 & 0.6309 & 0.5860 & 1.0000 \end{pmatrix}.$$

From these we suspect that there is non-negligible difference between the
covariance structure between boys and girls, with in particular a weaker
correlation among the boys' measurements. This is indeed supported by a
deviance of 23.77 on 10 degrees of freedom ($p = 0.0082$). Nevertheless, the
point estimates for the fixed effects coincide exactly with the ones obtained
from Model 1 (see Table 4.12). However, even if attention is restricted to
fixed-effects inference, one still needs to address the quality of the estimates of precision. To this end, there are in fact two solutions. First, the
more elaborate Model 0 can be fitted, as was done already. A drawback is
that this model has 28 parameters altogether, which is quite a substantial
number for such a small dataset, implying that the asymptotic behavior
of, for example, the deviance statistic becomes questionable. As discussed
in Section 3.4.1, an alternative solution consists of retaining Model 1 and
estimating the standard errors by means of the so-called robust estimator
(equivalently termed 'sandwich' or 'empirically corrected' estimator; Liang
and Zeger 1986). To this end, the following code can be used:

```
proc mixed data = growth method = ml covtest empirical;
title 'Growth Data, Model 1, Empirically Corrected';
class idnr sex age;
model measure = sex age*sex / s;
repeated / type = un subject = idnr r rcorr;
run;
```

Here, the 'empirical' option is added to the PROC MIXED statement. This method yields a consistent estimator of precision, even if the covariance model is misspecified. In this particular case, both methods (Model 0 on the one hand and the empirically corrected Model 1 on the other hand) lead to *exactly* the same standard errors. This illustrates that the robust method can be advantageous if correct standard errors are required but finding an adequate covariance model is judged too involved. The robust standard errors are presented in Table 4.12 as the second entry in parentheses. It is seen that the naive standard errors are somewhat smaller than their robust counterparts, except for the parameters $\beta_{1,8}$, $\beta_{1,10}$, and $\beta_{1,12}$, where they are considerably larger. Even though the relation between the standard errors of the 'correct model' (here, Model 0) and the empirically corrected 'working model' (here, Model 1) will not always be a mathematical identity, the empirically corrected estimator option is a useful tool to compensate for misspecification in the covariance model.

Let us now return to our discussion of Model 1. It is useful to consider the means for each of the 8 categories explicitly. These means are presented in Table 4.13 for Models 1–8. The first panel of Figure 4.6 depicts the 8 individual group means, connected to form two profiles, one for each sex group. Clearly, there seems to be a linear trend in both profiles as well as a vague indication for diverging lines, and hence different slopes. These hypotheses will be assessed on the basis of likelihood ratio tests, using the simpler Models 2 and 3.

4.4.2 Model 2

The first simplification occurs by assuming a linear trend within each sex group. This implies that each profile can be described with two parameters (intercept and slope), instead of with four unstructured means. The error matrix Σ will be left unstructured. The model can be expressed as

$$Y_{ij} = \beta_0 + \beta_{01}x_i + \beta_{10}t_j(1 - x_i) + \beta_{11}t_jx_i + \varepsilon_{ij}, \qquad (4.14)$$

or, in matrix notation,

$$\boldsymbol{Y}_i = X_i\boldsymbol{\beta} + \boldsymbol{\varepsilon}_i,$$

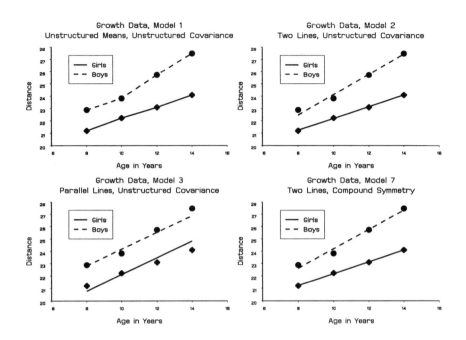

FIGURE 4.6. *Profiles for the complete growth data set, from a selected set of models.*

where the design matrix changes to

$$
X_i = \begin{pmatrix}
1 & x_i & 8(1 - x_i) & 8x_i \\
1 & x_i & 10(1 - x_i) & 10x_i \\
1 & x_i & 12(1 - x_i) & 12x_i \\
1 & x_i & 14(1 - x_i) & 14x_i
\end{pmatrix}.
$$

and $\boldsymbol{\beta} = (\beta_0, \beta_{01}, \beta_{10}, \beta_{11})'$. Here, β_0 is the intercept for boys and $\beta_0 + \beta_{01}$ is the intercept for girls. The slopes are β_{10} and β_{11} respectively.

The SAS code for Model 1 can be adapted simply by deleting age from the CLASS statement.

The likelihood ratio test comparing Model 2 to Model 1 does not reject the null hypothesis of linearity. A summary of model fitting information for this and subsequent models as well as for comparisons between models is given in Table 4.14. The first column contains the model number while a short description of the model is given in the second and third columns, in terms of the mean and covariance structures respectively. The number of

TABLE 4.14. *Growth data. Complete data set. Model fit summary.*

	Mean	Covar	par	-2ℓ	Ref	G^2	df	p
1	unstr.	unstr.	18	416.509				
2	$\neq$ slopes	unstr.	14	419.477	1	2.968	4	0.5632
3	$=$ slopes	unstr.	13	426.153	2	6.676	1	0.0098
4	$\neq$ slopes	banded	8	424.643	2	5.166	6	0.5227
5	$\neq$ slopes	AR(1)	6	440.681	2	21.204	8	0.0066
					4	16.038	2	0.0003
6	$\neq$ slopes	random	8	427.806	2	8.329	6	0.2150
7	$\neq$ slopes	CS	6	428.639	2	9.162	8	0.3288
					4	3.996	2	0.1356
					6	0.833	2	0.6594
					6	0.833	1:2	0.5104
8	$\neq$ slopes	simple	5	478.242	7	49.603	1	<0.0001
					7	49.603	0:1	<0.0001

parameters is given next, as well as the deviance (-2ℓ). The column labelled 'Ref' displays one (or more) numbers of models to which the current model is compared. The G^2 likelihood ratio statistic is the difference between -2ℓ of the current and the reference model. The final columns contain the number of degrees of freedom and the p-value corresponding to the likelihood ratio test statistic. Model 2 predicts the following mean growth curves:

$$\text{girls} \; : \; \hat{Y}_j = 17.43 + 0.4764t_j,$$
$$\text{boys} \; : \; \hat{Y}_j = 15.84 + 0.8268t_j.$$

These profiles are visualized in the second panel of Figure 4.6. The observed means are added to the graph. The mean model seems acceptable, consistent with the likelihood ratio test. The estimated covariance and correlation matrices of the measurements are similar to the ones found for Model 1.

4.4.3   Model 3

The next step is to investigate whether the two profiles are parallel. While the plot for Model 2 suggests that the profiles are diverging, the question remains whether this effect is statistically significant. The model can be described as follows:

$$Y_{ij} = \beta_0 + \beta_{01}x_i + \beta_1 t_j + \varepsilon_{ij}. \tag{4.15}$$

The design matrix X_i simplifies further:

$$X_i = \begin{pmatrix} 1 & x_i & 8 \\ 1 & x_i & 10 \\ 1 & x_i & 12 \\ 1 & x_i & 14 \end{pmatrix}$$

and $\beta = (\beta_0, \beta_{01}, \beta_1)'$. The two slopes in Model 2 have been replaced by β_1, a slope common to boys and girls.

Model 3 can be fitted in PROC MIXED by replacing the model statement in Model 2 with

```
model measure = sex age / s;
```

The predicted growth curves are:

$$\text{girls} \quad : \quad \hat{Y}_j = 15.37 + 0.6747t_j,$$
$$\text{boys} \quad : \quad \hat{Y}_j = 17.42 + 0.6747t_j.$$

Table 4.14 reveals that the likelihood ratio test statistic (comparing Models 2 and 3) rejects the common slope hypothesis ($p = 0.0098$). This is consistent with the systematic deviation between observed and expected means in the third panel of Figure 4.6.

Consistent with the choice of Jennrich and Schluchter (1986), the mean structure of Model 2 will be kept. We will now turn our attention to simplifying the covariance structure.

4.4.4 Graphical Exploration

Figure 4.7 presents the 27 individual profiles. The left hand panel shows the raw profiles, exhibiting the time trend found in the mean model. To obtain a rough idea about the covariance structure, it is useful to look at the right hand panel which gives the profiles after subtracting the means predicted by Model 2. Since these means agree closely with the observed means (see Figure 4.6), the corresponding sets of residuals are equivalent. A noticeable though not fully general trend is that a profile tends to be high or low *as a whole*, which points to a random intercept. Apparently, the variance of the residuals is roughly constant over time, implying that

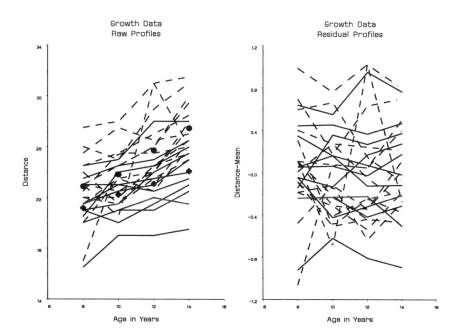

FIGURE 4.7. *Raw and residual profiles for the complete growth data set. (Girls are indicated with solid lines.)*

the random-effects structure is probably confined to the intercept. This observation is consistent with correlation matrix (4.13) of the unstructured Model 1. A more formal exploration can be done by means of the variogram (Diggle *et al* 1994, p. 51) or its extensions (Verbeke, Lesaffre, and Brant 1997). See also Section 3.13.3.

Jennrich and Schluchter (1986) considered several covariance structure models, which are all included in PROC MIXED as standard options.

4.4.5   Model 4

The first covariance structure model is the so-called *banded* or *Toeplitz* covariance matrix. Mean model formula (4.14) of Model 2 still applies, but the error vector ε_i is now assumed to follow a $\varepsilon_i \sim N(\mathbf{0}, \Sigma)$ distribution, where Σ is constrained to $\sigma_{ij} = \alpha_{|i-j|}$, i.e., the covariance depends on the measurement occasions through the lag between them only. In addition, Σ is assumed to be positive definite. For the growth data, there are only 4 free parameters: α_0, α_1, α_2, and α_3, instead of 10 in the unstructured case. The relationship between the α parameters is left unspecified. In the sequel, such additional constraints will lead to first-order autoregressive (Model 5) or exchangeable (Model 7) covariance structures.

To fit this model with PROC MIXED, the REPEATED statement needs to be changed, leading to the following program:

```
proc mixed data = growth method = ml covtest;
title 'Growth Data, Model 4';
class sex idnr;
model measure = sex age*sex / s;
repeated / type = toep subject = idnr r rcorr;
run;
```

Comparing the likelihood of this model to the one of the reference Model 2, shows that Model 4 is consistent with the data (see Table 4.14). The covariance matrix is

$$\begin{pmatrix} 4.9439 & 3.0507 & 3.4054 & 2.3421 \\ 3.0507 & 4.9439 & 3.0507 & 3.4054 \\ 3.4054 & 3.0507 & 4.9439 & 3.0507 \\ 2.3421 & 3.4054 & 3.0507 & 4.9439 \end{pmatrix},$$

and the derived correlation matrix is

$$\begin{pmatrix} 1.0000 & 0.6171 & 0.6888 & 0.4737 \\ 0.6171 & 1.0000 & 0.6171 & 0.6888 \\ 0.6888 & 0.6171 & 1.0000 & 0.6171 \\ 0.4737 & 0.6888 & 0.6171 & 1.0000 \end{pmatrix}.$$

The lag 2 correlation is slightly higher than the lag 1 correlation, while the lag 3 correlation shows a drop. In the light of the standard errors of the covariance parameters (0.9791, 0.9812, and 1.0358 respectively), this observation should not be seen as clear evidence for a particular trend. The standard errors are found from the 'Covariance Parameter Estimates' panel in the PROC MIXED output:

```
        Covariance Parameter Estimates (MLE)


    Cov Parm    Subject    Estimate      Std Error

    TOEP(2)     IDNR       3.05070312    0.97907984
    TOEP(3)     IDNR       3.40540527    0.98115569
    TOEP(4)     IDNR       2.34212396    1.03583358
    Residual    IDNR       4.94388956    0.98687143
```

Some issues with the use and interpretation of standard errors of variance components are discussed in Appendix B.

Note that this structure constrains the variance to be constant across time. Should this assumption be considered unrealistic, then heterogeneous versions can be fitted instead, combining the correlation matrix from the homogeneous version with variances that are allowed to change over time. Such covariance models will be discussed in Section 5.5.2.

At this point, Model 4 can replace Model 2 as the most parsimonious model, consistent with the data, found so far. Whether or not further simplifications are possible will be investigated next.

4.4.6   Model 5

A special case of the Toeplitz model is the first-order autoregressive model. This model is based on the assumption that the covariance between two measurements is a decreasing function of the time lag between them:

$$\sigma_{ij} = \sigma^2 \rho^{|i-j|}.$$

In other words, the variance of the measurements equals σ^2, and the covariance decreases with increasing time lag if $\rho > 0$. To fit this model with PROC MIXED, the REPEATED statement should include the option 'type=AR(1)'.

The estimated covariance matrix is

$$\begin{pmatrix} 4.8903 & 2.9687 & 1.8021 & 1.0940 \\ 2.9687 & 4.8903 & 2.9687 & 1.8021 \\ 1.8021 & 2.9687 & 4.8903 & 2.9687 \\ 1.0940 & 1.8021 & 2.9687 & 4.8903 \end{pmatrix}.$$

The correlation matrix is

$$\begin{pmatrix} 1.0000 & 0.6070 & 0.3685 & 0.2237 \\ 0.6070 & 1.0000 & 0.6070 & 0.3685 \\ 0.3685 & 0.6070 & 1.0000 & 0.6070 \\ 0.2237 & 0.3685 & 0.6070 & 1.0000 \end{pmatrix}.$$

Table 4.14 reveals that there is an apparent lack of fit for this model, when compared to Model 2. Jennrich and Schluchter (1986) compared Model 5 to Model 2 as well. Alternatively, we might want to compare Model 5 to Model 4. This more parsimonious test (2 degrees of freedom) yields $p = 0.0003$, strongly rejecting the AR(1) structure.

4.4.7 Model 6

An alternative simplification of the unstructured covariance Model 2 is given by allowing the intercept and slope parameters to be random. This is an example of model (4.10) with fixed-effects design matrix X_i as in Model 2 (equation (4.14)), random-effects design matrix

$$Z_i = \begin{pmatrix} 1 & 8 \\ 1 & 10 \\ 1 & 12 \\ 1 & 14 \end{pmatrix},$$

as well as measurement error structure $\Sigma = \sigma^2 I_4$.

An unstructured covariance matrix D for the random effects b_i will be assumed. The PROC MIXED code for this model is

```
proc mixed data = growth method = ml covtest;
title 'Jennrich and Schluchter, Model 6';
class sex idnr;
model measure = sex age*sex / s;
random intercept age / type = un subject = idnr g;
run;
```

The matrix D (requested by the 'g' option in the RANDOM statement) is estimated to be

$$\begin{pmatrix} 4.5569 & -0.1983 \\ -0.1983 & 0.0238 \end{pmatrix}. \tag{4.16}$$

One easily calculates the resulting covariance matrix of Y_i: $Z_i D Z_i' + \sigma^2 I_4$, which is estimated by

$$Z_i \hat{D} Z_i' + \hat{\sigma}^2 I_4 = \begin{pmatrix} 4.6216 & 2.8891 & 2.8727 & 2.8563 \\ 2.8891 & 4.6839 & 3.0464 & 3.1251 \\ 2.8727 & 3.0464 & 4.9363 & 3.3938 \\ 2.8563 & 3.1251 & 3.3938 & 5.3788 \end{pmatrix}, \tag{4.17}$$

where $\hat{\sigma}^2 = 1.7162$. Thus, this covariance matrix is a function of four parameters (three random-effects parameters and one measurement error parameter). The corresponding estimated correlation matrix is

$$\begin{pmatrix} 1.0000 & 0.6209 & 0.6014 & 0.5729 \\ 0.6209 & 1.0000 & 0.6335 & 0.6226 \\ 0.6014 & 0.6335 & 1.0000 & 0.6586 \\ 0.5729 & 0.6226 & 0.6586 & 1.0000 \end{pmatrix}. \tag{4.18}$$

This model is a submodel of Model 2, but not of Model 4 since the correlations increase within each diagonal, albeit only moderately since the variance of the random slope is very modest. From Table 4.14 we observe that this model is a plausible simplification of Model 2. It has the same number of degrees of freedom as Model 4, although the latter one has a slightly smaller deviance.

Since the variance of the random slope is small, it is natural to explore whether a random intercept model is adequate.

4.4.8 Model 7

A random intercept model is given by $Z_i = (1111)'$ with variance of the random intercepts equal to d. This variance is denoted by σ_c^2 in Section 2.1 (Example 2.4) and in Section 3.6. The resulting covariance matrix of Y_i is

$$Z_i d Z_i' + \sigma^2 I_4 = d J_4 + \sigma^2 I_4$$

where J_4 is a (4×4) matrix of ones. This covariance structure is called exchangeable or compound symmetry. All correlations are equal to $(d + \sigma^2)/\sigma^2$, implying that this model is a submodel of Models 4 and 6, as well as of Model 2. It can be fitted in PROC MIXED with two equivalent programs:

```
proc mixed data = growth method = ml covtest;
title 'Jennrich and Schluchter, Model 7';
class sex idnr;
model measure = sex age*sex / s;
random intercept / type = un subject = idnr g;
run;
```

and

```
proc mixed data = growth method = ml covtest;
title 'Jennrich and Schluchter, Model 7';
class sex idnr;
model measure = sex age*sex / s;
repeated / type = cs subject = idnr r rcorr;
run;
```

These two equivalent views towards the same model have been contrasted in Example 2.4 of Chapter 2 (page 18) and discussed in Section 3.6.

The estimated covariance matrix is

$$\begin{pmatrix} 4.9052 & 3.0306 & 3.0306 & 3.0306 \\ 3.0306 & 4.9052 & 3.0306 & 3.0306 \\ 3.0306 & 3.0306 & 4.9052 & 3.0306 \\ 3.0306 & 3.0306 & 3.0306 & 4.9052 \end{pmatrix},$$

with corresponding correlation matrix

$$\begin{pmatrix} 1.0000 & 0.6178 & 0.6178 & 0.6178 \\ 0.6178 & 1.0000 & 0.6178 & 0.6178 \\ 0.6178 & 0.6178 & 1.0000 & 0.6178 \\ 0.6178 & 0.6178 & 0.6178 & 1.0000 \end{pmatrix}.$$

Comparing the model to Model 2 yields $p = 0.3288$. Comparisons to Models 4 and 6 lead to the same conclusion. This implies that this model is currently the simplest one consistent with the data. It has to be noted that a comparison of Model 7 with Model 6 is slightly complicated by the fact that the null hypothesis implies that two of the three parameters in the D matrix of Model 6 are zero. For the variance of the random slope this null value lies on the boundary of the parameter space. As explained in Section 3.9.1, Stram and Lee (1994) show that the corresponding reference distribution is not χ_2^2, but a 50 : 50 mixture of a χ_1^2 and a χ_2^2. Such a mixture is indicated by $\chi_{1:2}^2$, or simply by 1 : 2. As a result, the corrected p-value would be 0.5104, not changing the conclusion. Similarly, comparing Models 2 and 6 as carried out before suffers from the same problem. Stram and Lee (1994) indicate that the asymptotic null distribution is even more complex, and involves projections of random variables on curved surfaces (Stram and Lee 1994). Therefore, the p-value is best determined by means of simulations. A simulation study of 500 samples yields $p = 0.046$, rather than $p = 0.215$, as reported in the table. To simulate the null distribution we generated 500 samples of 270 individuals rather than 27 individuals, to reduce small sample effects. While this choice reflects the desire to perform asymptotic inference, it is debatable since one might rightly argue that generating samples of size 27 would reflect small sample effects as well. Figure 4.8 shows the simulated as well as the inadequate χ_6^2 null distributions.

While such a correction is clearly necessary, it is hard to use in general practice in its current form. Additional work in this area is certainly required.

The profiles, predicted by Model 7, are

$$\text{girls} \quad : \quad \hat{Y}_j = 17.37 + 0.4795 t_j,$$
$$\text{boys} \quad : \quad \hat{Y}_j = 16.34 + 0.7844 t_j.$$

They are shown in the fourth panel of Figure 4.6. While not exactly the same, they are extremely similar to the profiles of Model 2.

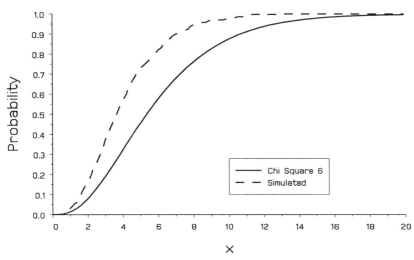

FIGURE 4.8. χ_6^2 and simulated null distributions for comparing Models 2 and 6.

4.4.9   Model 8

Finally, the independence model is considered in which the only source of variability is measurement error: $\Sigma = \sigma^2 I_4$. This model can be fitted in PROC MIXED using the 'type=simple' option in the REPEATED statement. Table 4.14 indicates that this model does not fit the data at all. Whether a χ_1^2 is used, or a $\chi_{0:1}^2$ does not affect the conclusion.

In summary, among the models presented, Model 7 is preferred to summarize the data. In Chapter 5, the trimmed version of the data will be used to assess the relative merits of several missing data handling procedures.

5

Linear Mixed Models and Missing Data

Geert Molenberghs
Luc Bijnens
David Shaw

5.1 Introduction

In virtually all longitudinal studies the issues of unbalancedness and missing data arise. Some studies, such as the Baltimore Longitudinal Study of Aging (Section 3.2) and the Variceal Pressures Study (Section 4.1) are designed such that the number of measurements per subject is variable or even random. The measurement times themselves can vary across subjects and can be random as well. We term these studies *unbalanced*. In such unbalanced studies it is usually not possible to identify non-response, unless measurement times have been recorded, even for occasions at which no measurement was actually taken. In contrast, in a *balanced* study the number of measurements per subject is fixed and the measurements are usually taken at an approximately common set of occasions. In this situation, missing observations can be identified without ambiguity. For this reason, we will focus attention on missing data in the balanced case. The specific case of *dropout* (i.e., a subject is completely observed until a certain point in time, where after no more measurements are taken) can be handled in the unbalanced case as well. The treatment of dropout in both balanced and unbalanced cases is very similar and therefore we will suffice with a balanced example of dropout (Section 5.11).

A potential source of confusion is the fact that in a part of the literature also the random effects are viewed as missing variables, which are then estimated using a generalization of the EM algorithm (Laird and Ware 1982). This use of the EM algorithm is also discussed in Section 3.4.5. It ought to be clear that this is *not* the type of missing data envisaged here. We are concerned with missing outcome variables, i.e., measurements that potentially could have been obtained, in contrast with the random effects, which are latent variables.

The missing data terminology, largely due to Little and Rubin (1987), is used as a standard framework to deal with missing data mechanisms and their effect on the analysis. This paradigm will be developed with particular attention for the general linear mixed model. The concepts and methods introduced are illustrated by means of the example analyzed in Section 4.4, to which we will refer as *the growth data*. Little and Rubin (1987) created a missing data problem by artificially deleting a fraction of the measurements. Therefore, the advantage of this example is that every missing data analysis can be contrasted with the analysis of the complete data, performed in Section 4.4.

Little and Rubin (1987) applied the EM algorithm to the trimmed data. Using general linear mixed model technology, quadratic (e.g., Newton-Raphson) or super-linear (e.g., Fisher scoring) algorithms can be applied. PROC MIXED is set up such that in many practically relevant situations no additional code is required when switching from complete to incomplete data problems.

In contrast to many other statistical software packages and procedures, PROC MIXED does not delete subjects with incomplete measurement sequences. Littell *et al* (1996) rightly assert that PROC MIXED is much easier to use when data are missing, at least under certain assumptions about the missingness mechanism. However, even though under these assumptions a satisfactory analysis is achievable, we must emphasize that care has to be taken when passing incomplete data to PROC MIXED. We will elaborate on this issue using the growth data. Since Little and Rubin (1987) created holes in this set of data, but the entire data collection is available as well (Potthof and Roy 1964 and Jennrich and Schluchter 1987), these data put us in the comfortable position that complete data analyses can be compared with incomplete data (or observed data) analyses on the trimmed version. These will be supplemented with analyses from 'classical' techniques, such as complete case and available case analyses and single imputation methods. Some of these simple methods have been subject to heavy criticism in the scientific literature (Little and Rubin, 1987) but are still commonly used in many areas of applied statistical research. For example, many clinical trial reports include a complete case analysis and a last observation carried forward (LOCF) analysis. We have tried to provide indications about the way in which such methods affect point and precision estimation, both in the fixed-effects parameters and in the various aspects of the association structure.

The validity of a method depends crucially on the inferential framework (see Section 5.2). We will focus on likelihood methods, thereby encompassing maximum likelihood (ML) and restricted maximum likelihood (REML) estimation.

This chapter divides naturally into two parts. Sections 5.2–5.7 contain the more fundamental material while Sections 5.8–5.11 are devoted to somewhat more advanced material. In the former sections a relatively strong emphasis is placed on PROC MIXED while also other software tools are illustrated in the later ones. A missing data formalism is given in Section 5.2. Section 5.3 gives an overview of methods for incomplete data, which are treated in more detail in subsequent sections. Sections 5.4, 5.5, and 5.6 are devoted to the relatively simple complete case analysis, single imputation analysis, and available case analysis respectively. A likelihood based ignorable analysis is discussed in Section 5.7. It is shown that PROC MIXED leads *nearly* to a valid analysis when the missing data are missing at random. In Section 5.8 it is established that there are still some remaining issues with the estimation of precision. We believe that the practicing statistician should be aware of these issues. The landmark expectation-maximization (EM) and multiple imputation techniques are reviewed in Sections 5.9 and 5.10. Finally, Section 5.11 discusses situations where the non-response mechanism needs to be considered explicitly, either because it is itself of scientific interest, or because the assumption of ignorability is not tenable. Here, focus is on the OSWALD software (Version 2.6), written for S-Plus (Smith, Robertson, and Diggle 1996). While most of Sections 5.8–5.10 are labelled with an asterisk, we do believe that the material covered in Section 5.8, especially in Section 5.8.4, should become integral part of the background knowledge of the applied statistician, even if he or she generally uses only standard software tools, such as PROC MIXED. The same remark is true for the informative dropout Section 5.11.

5.2 Missing Data

In this section we build on the standard framework for missing data, which is largely due to Rubin (1976) and Little and Rubin (1987).

In general, we assume that for subject i in the study a sequence of measurements Y_{ij} is designed to be measured at occasions $j = 1, \ldots, n_i$. As before, the outcomes are grouped into a vector $\boldsymbol{Y}_i = (Y_{i1}, \ldots, Y_{in_i})'$. In addition, for each time j define

$$R_{ij} = \left\{ \begin{array}{ll} 1 & \text{if } Y_{ij} \text{ is observed,} \\ 0 & \text{otherwise.} \end{array} \right.$$

The *missing data indicators* R_{ij} are grouped into a vector $\boldsymbol{R}_i$ which is, of course, of the same length as $\boldsymbol{Y}_i$.

Partition Y_i into two subvectors such that Y_i^o is the vector containing those Y_{ij} for which $R_{ij} = 1$ and Y_i^m contains the remaining components. These subvectors are referred to as the *observed* and *missing* components respectively. The following terminology is adopted:

Complete data Y_i: the scheduled measurements. This is the outcome vector that would have been recorded if there were no missing data.

Missing data indicators R_i. The process generating R_i is referred to as the missing data process.

Full data (Y_i, R_i): the complete data, together with the missing data indicators. Note that, unless all components of R_i equal 1, the full data components are never jointly observed.

Observed data Y_i^o.

Missing data Y_i^m.

Some confusion might arise between the terms *complete data* introduced here and *complete case analysis* of Section 5.4. While the former refers to the (hypothetical) data set that would arise if there were no missing data, 'complete cases' refers to deletion of all subjects for which at least one component is missing.

Note that one observes the measurements Y_i^o together with the dropout indicators R_i.

5.2.1   Missing Data Patterns

An hierarchy of missing data patterns can be considered. When missingness is due to *attrition*, all measurements for a subject from baseline onwards up to a certain measurement time are recorded, where after all data are missing. It is then possible to replace the information contained in the vector R_i by a single indicator variable. For example, R_i could indicate the last observed measurement occasion. The sample size decreases over time.

Attrition is a particular *monotone* pattern of missingness. In order to have monotone missingness there has to exist a permutation of the measurement components such that a measurement earlier in the permuted sequence is observed for at least those subjects that are observed at later measurements. Note that, for this definition to be meaningful, we need to have a balanced design in the sense of a common set of measurement occasions. Other patterns are called *non-monotone*.

5.2.2   Missing Data Mechanisms

First, one has to consider the density of the full data

$$f(\boldsymbol{y}_i, \boldsymbol{r}_i | X_i, Z_i, \boldsymbol{\theta}, \boldsymbol{\psi}),$$

where X_i and Z_i are the design matrices and $\boldsymbol{\theta}$ and $\boldsymbol{\psi}$ are vectors that parameterize the joint distribution. We will use $\boldsymbol{\theta} = (\boldsymbol{\beta}', \boldsymbol{\alpha}')'$ and $\boldsymbol{\psi}$ to describe the measurement and missingness processes respectively.

A useful taxonomy, constructed by Rubin (1976) and further developed in Little and Rubin (1987), is based on the factorization:

$$f(\boldsymbol{y}_i, \boldsymbol{r}_i | X_i, Z_i, \boldsymbol{\theta}, \boldsymbol{\psi}) = f(\boldsymbol{y}_i | X_i, Z_i, \boldsymbol{\theta}) f(\boldsymbol{r}_i | \boldsymbol{y}_i, X_i, \boldsymbol{\psi}), \qquad (5.1)$$

where the first factor is the marginal density of the measurement process and the second one is the density of the missingness process, conditional on the outcomes. Factorization (5.1) forms the basis of *selection modeling* as the second factor corresponds to the (self-)selection of individuals into 'observed' and 'missing' groups. An alternative taxonomy can be built based on so-called *pattern-mixture models* (Little 1993, Molenberghs *et al* 1997). These are based on the factorization

$$f(\boldsymbol{y}_i, \boldsymbol{r}_i | X_i, Z_i, \boldsymbol{\theta}, \boldsymbol{\psi}) = f(\boldsymbol{y}_i | \boldsymbol{r}_i, X_i, \boldsymbol{\theta}) f(\boldsymbol{r}_i | X_i, Z_i, \boldsymbol{\psi}). \qquad (5.2)$$

Indeed, (5.2) can be seen as a mixture of different populations, characterized by the observed pattern of missingness.

The natural parameters of selection models and pattern-mixture models have a different meaning, and transforming one probability model into one of the other framework is in general not straightforward, even not for normal measurement models. When a selection model is used, it is often mentioned that one has to make untestable assumptions about the relationship between dropout and missing data (discussion of Diggle and Kenward 1994, Molenberghs, Kenward, and Lesaffre 1997). In pattern-mixture models, it is explicit which parameters cannot be identified. Little (1993) suggests the use of identifying relationships between identifiable and non-identifiable parameters. Thus, even though these identifying relationships are also unverifiable (Little 1995), the advantage of pattern-mixture models is that the verifiable and unverifiable assumptions can easily be separated.

The selection model taxonomy is based on the second factor of (5.1):

$$f(\boldsymbol{r}_i | \boldsymbol{y}_i, X_i, \boldsymbol{\psi}) = f(\boldsymbol{r}_i | \boldsymbol{y}_i^o, \boldsymbol{y}_i^m, X_i, \boldsymbol{\psi}). \qquad (5.3)$$

If (5.3) is independent of the measurements, i.e., when it assumes the form $f(\boldsymbol{r}_i | X_i, Z_i, \boldsymbol{\psi})$, then the process is termed *missing completely at random* (MCAR).

If (5.3) is independent of the unobserved (missing) measurements $\boldsymbol{Y}_i^m$, but depends on the observed measurements $\boldsymbol{Y}_i^o$, thereby assuming the form $f(\boldsymbol{r}_i|\boldsymbol{y}_i^o, X_i, \boldsymbol{\psi})$, then the process is referred to as *missing at random* (MAR).

Finally, when (5.3) depends on the missing values $\boldsymbol{Y}_i^m$, the process is referred to as *informative missingness*. An informative process is allowed to depend on $\boldsymbol{Y}_i^o$.

It is important to note that above terminology is independent of the statistical framework chosen to analyze the data. This is to be contrasted with the terms *ignorable* and *non-ignorable* missingness. The latter terms depend crucially on the inferential framework (Rubin 1976).

5.2.3 Ignorability

Let us decide to use likelihood based estimation. The full data likelihood contribution for subject i assumes the form

$$L^*(\boldsymbol{\theta}, \boldsymbol{\psi}|X_i, Z_i, \boldsymbol{y}_i, \boldsymbol{r}_i) \propto f(\boldsymbol{y}_i, \boldsymbol{r}_i|X_i, Z_i, \boldsymbol{\theta}, \boldsymbol{\psi}).$$

Since inference has to be based on what is observed, the full data likelihood L^* has to be replaced by the observed data likelihood L:

$$L(\boldsymbol{\theta}, \boldsymbol{\psi}|X_i, Z_i, \boldsymbol{y}_i, \boldsymbol{r}_i) \propto f(\boldsymbol{y}_i^o, \boldsymbol{r}_i|X_i, Z_i, \boldsymbol{\theta}, \boldsymbol{\psi})$$

with

$$
\begin{aligned}
f(\boldsymbol{y}_i^o, \boldsymbol{r}_i|\boldsymbol{\theta}, \boldsymbol{\psi}) &= \int f(\boldsymbol{y}_i, \boldsymbol{r}_i|X_i, Z_i, \boldsymbol{\theta}, \boldsymbol{\psi}) d\boldsymbol{y}_i^m \\
&= \int f(\boldsymbol{y}_i^o, \boldsymbol{y}_i^m|X_i, Z_i, \boldsymbol{\theta}) f(\boldsymbol{r}_i|\boldsymbol{y}_i^o, \boldsymbol{y}_i^m, X_i, \boldsymbol{\psi}) d\boldsymbol{y}_i^m.
\end{aligned}
$$

Under an MAR process, we obtain

$$
\begin{aligned}
f(\boldsymbol{y}_i^o, \boldsymbol{r}_i|\boldsymbol{\theta}, \boldsymbol{\psi}) &= \int f(\boldsymbol{y}_i^o, \boldsymbol{y}_i^m|X_i, Z_i, \boldsymbol{\theta}) f(\boldsymbol{r}_i|\boldsymbol{y}_i^o, X_i, \boldsymbol{\psi}) d\boldsymbol{y}_i^m \\
&= f(\boldsymbol{y}_i^o|X_i, Z_i, \boldsymbol{\theta}) f(\boldsymbol{r}_i|\boldsymbol{y}_i^o, X_i, \boldsymbol{\psi}), \qquad (5.4)
\end{aligned}
$$

i.e., the likelihood factorizes into two components of the same functional form as the general factorization (5.1) of the complete data. If further $\boldsymbol{\theta}$ and $\boldsymbol{\psi}$ are disjoint in the sense that the parameter space of the full vector $(\boldsymbol{\theta}', \boldsymbol{\psi}')'$ is the product of the individual parameter spaces then inference can be based on the marginal observed data density only. This technical requirement is referred to as the separability condition. However, still some caution should be used when constructing precision estimators (see Section 5.8).

In conclusion, when the separability condition is satisfied, *within the likelihood framework*, ignorability is equivalent to the union of MAR and MCAR. Hence, non-ignorability and 'informativeness' are synonyms in this context. A formal derivation is given in Rubin (1976), where it is also shown that the same requirements hold for Bayesian inference, but that frequentist inference is ignorable only under MCAR. Of course, ignorability is unhelpful when at least part of the scientific interest is directed towards the missingness process.

Classical examples of the more stringent condition with frequentist methods are ordinary least squares (see also Section 5.6 and 5.7) and the generalized estimating equations approach of Liang and Zeger (1986). These GEE define an unbiased estimator only under MCAR. Robins, Rotnizky, and Zhao (1995) have established that some progress can be made under MAR and even under informative processes. Their method is based on including weights that depend on the missingness probability, proving the point that at least some information on the missingness mechanism should be included and thus that ignorability does not hold.

5.3   Approaches to Incomplete Data

Missing data nearly always entail problems for the practicing statistician. First, inference will often be invalidated when the observed measurements do not constitute a simple random subset of the complete set of measurements. Secondly, even when correct inference would follow, it is not always an easy task to trick standard software into operation on a ragged data structure.

Even in the simple case of a one-way ANOVA design and under an MCAR mechanism operating, problems occur since missingness destroys the balance between the sizes of the subsamples. This implies that a slightly more complicated least squares analysis has to be invoked. Of course, a regression module for the latter analysis is included in most statistical software packages. The trouble is that the researcher has to be aware which tool to choose for particular classes of incomplete data.

Little and Rubin (1987) give an extensive treatment of methods to analyze incomplete data, many of which are intended for continuous, normally distributed data. Some of these methods were proposed more than fifty years ago. Examples are Yates' (1933) iterated ANOVA and Bartlett's (1937)

ANCOVA procedures to analyze incomplete ANOVA designs. The former method is an early example of the Expectation-Maximization (EM) algorithm (Dempster, Laird, and Rubin 1977).

Section 5.4 discusses the computationally simplest technique, a *complete case* analysis, in which the analysis is restricted to the subjects for whom all intended measurements have been observed. A complete case analysis is popular because it maps a ragged data matrix into a rectangular one, by deleting incomplete cases. A second family of approaches, with a similar effect on the applicability of complete data software, is based on *imputing* missing values. One distinguishes between single imputation (Section 5.5) and multiple imputation (Section 5.10). In the first case, a single value is substituted for every 'hole' in the data set and the resulting data set is analyzed as if it represented the true complete data. Multiple imputation is used to account for the uncertainty in filling in missing values.

A third family is based on the principle of analyzing the incomplete data as such. A simple representative is so-called *available case* analysis. This simply means that every component of a parameter (e.g., made up of mean vector and covariance matrix elements for a multivariate normal sample) is estimated using the maximal amount of information available for that component. This technique is discussed in Section 5.6. While it makes use of more data than a corresponding complete case analysis, it still suffers from some drawbacks. For example, the method requires the missingness process to be MCAR. Section 5.7 describes a simple and convenient analysis, based on the more relaxed MAR assumption, that is consistent with factorization (5.4) and, importantly, can be carried out using PROC MIXED. A popular and very general technique to optimize incomplete data likelihoods under MAR is the EM algorithm (Dempster *et al* 1977). Little and Rubin (1987) used the EM algorithm to analyze their incomplete version of the growth data (Table 4.11). The principle ideas behind this method, and its connection to the MAR analysis of Section 5.7 will be given in Section 5.9.

Treatment of informative dropout is discussed in Section 5.11. Most of the analyses in this section are conducted using the OSWALD software (Version 2.6), written for S-Plus (Smith, Robertson, and Diggle 1996).

5.4   Complete Case Analysis

A complete case analysis includes only those cases for analysis, for which all n_i measurements were recorded. This method has obvious advantages. It is very simple to describe and, since the data structure is as would have resulted from a complete experiment, standard statistical software can be used. Further, since the complete estimation is done on the same subset of completers, there is a common basis for inference, unlike with the available case methods (see Section 5.6).

Unfortunately, the method suffers from severe drawbacks. First, there is nearly always a substantial loss of information. For example, suppose there are 20 measurements, with 10% of missing data on each measurement. Suppose further that missingness on the different measurements is independent, then the estimated percentage of incomplete observations is as high as 87%. The impact on precision and power is dramatic. Even though the reduction of the number of complete cases will be less dramatic in realistic settings where the missingness indicators R_i are correlated, the effect just sketched will often undermine a lot of complete case analyses. In addition, severe bias can result when the missingness mechanism is MAR but not MCAR. Indeed, should an estimator be consistent in the complete data problem, then the derived complete case analysis is consistent only if the missingness process is MCAR. Unfortunately, the MCAR assumption is much more restrictive than the MAR assumption.

A simple partial check on the MCAR assumption is as follows (Little and Rubin, 1987). Divide the observations on measurement j into two groups: (1) those subjects that are also observed on another measurement or set of measurements, (2) those missing on the other measurement(s). Should MCAR hold, then both groups should be random samples of the same population. Failure to reject equality of the distributional parameters of both samples increases the evidence for MCAR, but does not prove it.

5.4.1   Growth Data

In a complete case analysis of the growth data, the 9 subjects which lack one measurement are deleted, resulting in a working data set with 18 subjects. This implies that 27 available measurements will not be used for analysis, a quite severe penalty on a relatively small data set.

Let us first consider the eight models, described in Section 4.4. A summary of the model fit is given in Table 5.1. There are a few striking features. On the one hand, the common slope Model 3 is not rejected. The banded correlation structure on the other hand is marginally rejected when compared to Model 2, while the compound symmetry Model 7 is at the other side of the nominal 5% level. The auto-regressive structure is still not acceptable. The random slope and intercept Model 6 is marginally rejected. As before, Model 8 is strongly rejected. From this analysis we might conclude that Model 7 provides the most parsimonious description consistent with the data *among the eight models considered*, although this decision is less clear

TABLE 5.1. *Growth data. Complete case analysis. Model fit summary.*

	Mean	Covar	par	-2ℓ	Ref	G^2	df	p
1	unstr.	unstr.	18	256.756				
2	$\neq$ slopes	unstr.	14	263.681	1	6.925	4	0.1399
3	$=$ slopes	unstr.	13	265.185	2	1.504	1	0.2201
4	$\neq$ slopes	banded	8	277.488	2	13.807	6	0.0319
5	$\neq$ slopes	AR(1)	6	288.063	2	24.382	8	0.0020
					4	10.575	2	0.0051
6	$\neq$ slopes	random	8	276.834	2	13.153	6	0.0407
7	$\neq$ slopes	CS	6	278.127	2	14.446	8	0.0709
					4	0.639	2	0.7265
					6	1.293	2	0.5239
					6	1.293	1:2	0.3897
8	$\neq$ slopes	simple	5	306.163	7	28.036	1	<0.0001
					7	28.036	0:1	<0.0001

cut than in the analysis of the complete data set. Recall that we performed tests involving Model 6 both with the incorrect χ^2 null distributions, as well as with the asymptotic mixture null distributions (Stram and Lee 1994), discussed on page 188.

Let us now study the influence of the restriction to completers on the analysis. The estimated mean profiles for Models 2, 3, and 7 are as follows:

- Model 2:

$$\text{girls} \quad : \quad \hat{Y}_j = 18.81 + 0.4434t_j,$$
$$\text{boys} \quad : \quad \hat{Y}_j = 19.42 + 0.5842t_j.$$

- Model 3:

$$\text{girls} \quad : \quad \hat{Y}_j = 18.17 + 0.5203t_j,$$
$$\text{boys} \quad : \quad \hat{Y}_j = 19.95 + 0.5203t_j.$$

- Model 7:

$$\text{girls} \quad : \quad \hat{Y}_j = 18.29 + 0.4750t_j,$$
$$\text{boys} \quad : \quad \hat{Y}_j = 18.18 + 0.6750t_j.$$

Clearly, the separate slopes for boys and girls are closer to each other than in the analysis of the complete data set. This is true for both Models 2 and

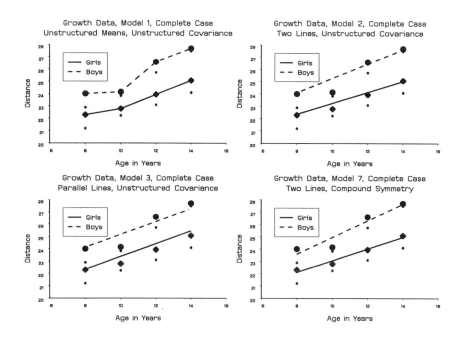

FIGURE 5.1. *Profiles for the growth data set, from a selected set of models. Complete case analysis. (The small dots are the observed group means for the complete data set.)*

7. Thus, the fact that Model 3 is not rejected is not only due to a reduced sample size, but also to convergence of the two profiles. This phenomenon is also seen in Figure 5.1. All observed group means have increased relative to the complete data set but mostly so at age 8. This is to be expected, since the probability of missingness at age 10 was modeled by Little and Rubin (1987) to depend directly on the measurement at age 8, such that lower measurements led to more non-response. As a consequence, those subjects deleted had low values at age 8. There is only indirect dependence on the measurements at ages 10 and 12, through the correlation with the measurement at age 8. The net effect is that the profiles overestimate the average length, and underestimate the difference in slopes between boys and girls. In addition, the average slope has decreased leading to flattened profiles, especially for boys.

The covariance matrix, estimated under Model 1, is equal to

$$
\begin{pmatrix}
2.2460 & 2.3155 & 2.3829 & 2.0754 \\
2.3155 & 4.2763 & 2.0420 & 2.5741 \\
2.3829 & 2.0420 & 5.4513 & 3.0752 \\
2.0754 & 2.5741 & 3.0752 & 3.8806
\end{pmatrix}.
\tag{5.5}
$$

Let us turn to the correlation matrices for a few models.

- Model 1 (unstructured):

$$
\begin{pmatrix}
1.0000 & 0.7471 & 0.6810 & 0.7030 \\
0.7471 & 1.0000 & 0.4229 & 0.6319 \\
0.6810 & 0.4229 & 1.0000 & 0.6686 \\
0.7030 & 0.6319 & 0.6686 & 1.0000
\end{pmatrix}
\tag{5.6}
$$

- Model 4 (Toeplitz):

$$
\begin{pmatrix}
1.0000 & 0.5499 & 0.5803 & 0.6794 \\
0.5499 & 1.0000 & 0.5499 & 0.5803 \\
0.5803 & 0.5499 & 1.0000 & 0.5499 \\
0.6794 & 0.5803 & 0.5499 & 1.0000
\end{pmatrix}
$$

- Model 5 (AR(1)):

$$
\begin{pmatrix}
1.0000 & 0.5013 & 0.2513 & 0.1260 \\
0.5013 & 1.0000 & 0.5013 & 0.2513 \\
0.2513 & 0.5013 & 1.0000 & 0.5013 \\
0.1260 & 0.2513 & 0.5013 & 1.0000
\end{pmatrix}
$$

- Model 7 (compound symmetry):

$$
\begin{pmatrix}
1.0000 & 0.5738 & 0.5738 & 0.5738 \\
0.5738 & 1.0000 & 0.5738 & 0.5738 \\
0.5738 & 0.5738 & 1.0000 & 0.5738 \\
0.5738 & 0.5738 & 0.5738 & 1.0000
\end{pmatrix}
$$

The first off-diagonal band in the unstructured version shows a moderate discrepancy between the (age 10, age 12) correlation and the other pairs of adjacent measurements. This phenomenon might explain why the banded and compound symmetry structures show a less satisfactory fit. Both correlations have decreased relative to the complete data set.

Inspecting Table 5.1, it is clearly unsatisfactory that the unequal slopes model is carried along Models 4–8, even though the comparison of Models

TABLE 5.2. *Growth data. Complete case analysis. Model fit summary for additional models.*

	Mean	Covar	par	-2ℓ	Ref	G^2	df	p
1	unstr.	unstr.	18	256.756				
2	$\neq$ slopes	unstr.	14	263.681	1	6.925	4	0.1399
3	= slopes	unstr.	13	265.185	2	1.504	1	0.2201
4b	= slopes	banded	7	279.778	3	14.593	6	0.0237
5b	= slopes	AR(1)	5	288.670	3	23.485	8	0.0028
6b	= slopes	random	7	278.780	3	13.595	6	0.0345
7b	= slopes	CS	5	280.044	3	14.859	8	0.0619
8b	= slopes	simple	4	306.990	3	41.805	9	<0.0001

2 and 3 does not reveal a departure from equality of the slopes. Alternatively, we might start simplifying the covariance structure from Model 3. A summary is presented in Table 5.2. There is evidence for lack of fit in the Toeplitz (banded), AR(1), random, and simple (uncorrelated) models. While the compound symmetry model does exhibit a better fit, the evidence in favor of this model is not overwhelming. It might be wiser to stick to Model 3. Its mean profile was given on page 200. The estimated mean profile for Model 7b is:

$$\text{girls} \quad : \quad \hat{Y}_j = 16.95 + 0.5972t_j,$$
$$\text{boys} \quad : \quad \hat{Y}_j = 19.03 + 0.5972t_j.$$

In conclusion, an analysis of the completers would lead to a linear profile with common slope but different intercepts (the difference in intercepts is 1.786 with standard error 0.717) and with an unstructured covariance matrix. This is in contrast with the analysis of the complete data set where we found a more complex mean model (different slopes) in conjunction with a very simple (exchangeable) covariance model.

5.5 Simple Forms of Imputation

An alternative way to obtain a data set on which complete data methods can be used is filling in the missing values, instead of deleting subjects with incomplete sequences. The principle of imputation is particularly easy. The observed values are used to impute values for the missing observations. There are several ways to use the observed information. First, one can use information on the same subject (e.g., last observation carried forward). Secondly, information can be borrowed from other subjects (e.g., mean imputation). Finally, both within and between subject information can be used (e.g., conditional mean imputation, hot deck imputation). Standard references are Little and Rubin (1987) and Rubin (1987). Imputation strategies have been very popular in sample survey methods.

However, great care has to be taken with imputation strategies. Dempster and Rubin (1983) write

> "The idea of imputation is both seductive and dangerous. It is seductive because it can lull the user into the pleasurable state of believing that the data are complete after all, and it is dangerous because it lumps together situations where the problem is sufficiently minor that it can be legitimately handled in this way and situations where standard estimators applied to the real and imputed data have substantial biases."

For example, Little and Rubin (1987) show that the method could work for a linear model with one fixed effect and one error term, but that it generally does not for hierarchical models, split-plot designs, repeated measures (with a complicated error structure), random-effects, and mixed-effects models. At the very least, different imputations for different effects would be necessary.

The user of imputation strategies faces several dangers. First, the imputation model could be wrong and hence the point estimates would be biased. Secondly, even for a correct imputation model, the uncertainty resulting from incompleteness is masked. Indeed, even when one is reasonably sure about the mean value the unknown observation would have, the actual stochastic realization, depending on both the mean structure as well as on the error distribution, is still unknown.

In this section, several mean imputation strategies will be described. Their relative merits and pitfalls will be exemplified by means of the growth data.

5.5.1   Last Observation Carried Forward

Whenever a value is missing, the last observed value is substituted. The technique can be applied to both monotone and non-monotone missing data. It is typically applied to settings where incompleteness is due to attrition.

Very strong and often unrealistic assumptions have to be made to ensure

TABLE 5.3. *Growth data. Last observation carried forward. Model fit summary.*

	Mean	Covar	par	-2ℓ	Ref	G^2	df	p
1	unstr.	unstr.	18	407.078				
2	$\neq$ slopes	unstr.	14	424.793	1	17.715	4	0.0014
3	$=$ slopes	unstr.	13	426.333	2	1.540	1	0.2146
4	$\neq$ slopes	banded	8	445.216	2	20.423	6	0.0023
5	$\neq$ slopes	AR(1)	6	449.640	2	24.847	8	0.0017
6	$\neq$ slopes	random	8	446.121	2	21.328	6	0.0016
7	$\neq$ slopes	CS	6	449.077	6	2.956	2	0.2281
					6	2.956	1:2	0.1568
8	$\neq$ slopes	simple	5	496.961	7	47.884	1	<0.0001
					7	47.884	0:1	<0.0001

validity of this method. First, one has to believe that a subjects' measurement stays at the same level from the moment of drop out onwards (or during the period they are unobserved in the case of intermittent missingness). In a clinical trial setting, one might believe that the response profile *changes* as soon as a patient goes off treatment and even that it would flatten. However, the constant profile assumption is even stronger. Further, this method shares with other single imputation methods that it overestimates the precision by treating imputed and actually observed values on equal footing.

GROWTH DATA

For this data set, the 9 subjects that lack a measurement at age 10 are completed by imputing the age 8 value. It is clear that this procedure will affect the linear but non-constant trend model discovered on the basis of the complete data set. We will also investigate the effect on the covariance model.

Let us first consider the 8 models, described in Section 4.4. A summary of the model fit is given in Table 5.3. Again, there are several noteworthy features. Both different (Model 2) and common (Model 3) slope profiles are inadequate. Inspecting Figure 5.2, the reason is immediately clear. The imputation procedure forces the means at ages 8 and 10 to be very similar, thereby destroying the linear relationship, as was anticipated.

The mean profiles for Models 2, 3, and 7 are estimated to be:

- Model 2:

$$\text{girls} \quad : \quad \hat{Y}_j = 18.53 + 0.3898t_j,$$
$$\text{boys} \quad : \quad \hat{Y}_j = 19.56 + 0.5483t_j.$$

- Model 3:

$$\text{girls} \quad : \quad \hat{Y}_j = 17.75 + 0.4632t_j,$$
$$\text{boys} \quad : \quad \hat{Y}_j = 20.46 + 0.4632t_j.$$

- Model 7:

$$\text{girls} \quad : \quad \hat{Y}_j = 16.79 + 0.5159t_j,$$
$$\text{boys} \quad : \quad \hat{Y}_j = 15.67 + 0.8266t_j.$$

There is more discrepancy between Models 2 and 7 here than in the complete data set. The slopes of Model 7 are considerably higher than those of Model 2; the slope for girls in Model 7 is almost as high as the slope for boys in Model 2. Of course, none of the models assuming a linear profile is consistent with these data and either further modeling, or restriction to the unstructured profiles of Model 1 seems necessary.

Let us consider the estimated correlation matrices.

- Unstructured:

$$\begin{pmatrix} 1.0000 & 0.9015 & 0.6613 & 0.5216 \\ 0.9015 & 1.0000 & 0.5567 & 0.5318 \\ 0.6613 & 0.5567 & 1.0000 & 0.7281 \\ 0.5216 & 0.5318 & 0.7281 & 1.0000 \end{pmatrix}$$

- Toeplitz:

$$\begin{pmatrix} 1.0000 & 0.6521 & 0.5833 & 0.3426 \\ 0.6521 & 1.0000 & 0.6521 & 0.5833 \\ 0.5833 & 0.6521 & 1.0000 & 0.6521 \\ 0.3426 & 0.5833 & 0.6521 & 1.0000 \end{pmatrix}$$

- AR(1):

$$\begin{pmatrix} 1.0000 & 0.6416 & 0.4117 & 0.2642 \\ 0.6416 & 1.0000 & 0.6416 & 0.4117 \\ 0.4117 & 0.6416 & 1.0000 & 0.6416 \\ 0.2642 & 0.4117 & 0.6416 & 1.0000 \end{pmatrix}$$

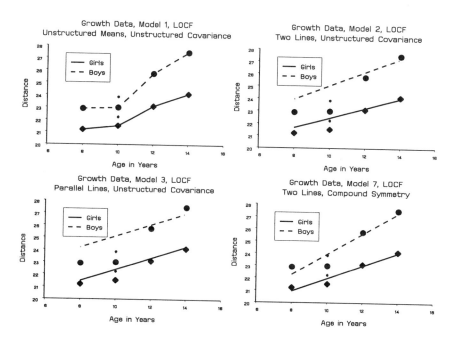

FIGURE 5.2. *Profiles for the growth data set, from a selected set of models. Last observation carried forward. (The small dots are the observed group means for the complete data set.)*

- Compound Symmetry:

$$\begin{pmatrix} 1.0000 & 0.6083 & 0.6083 & 0.6083 \\ 0.6083 & 1.0000 & 0.6083 & 0.6083 \\ 0.6083 & 0.6083 & 1.0000 & 0.6083 \\ 0.6083 & 0.6083 & 0.6083 & 1.0000 \end{pmatrix}$$

Clearly, none of the covariance Models 4–7 shows an acceptable fit, relative to Model 2. Of course, these comparisons have to be treated with great caution, since the reference Model 2 does not fit well and a further sequence of models will have to be constructed. The unstructured covariance matrix shows clearly the impact of the last observation carried forward (LOCF) approach. The measurements at ages 8 and 10 are made very similar, inducing a correlation as high as 0.9015, rather than 0.5707 in the complete data set. Thus, the three lag 1 correlations are more dissimilar, resulting in a bad fit for the Toeplitz model. Since Models 5, 6, and 7 simplify the Toeplitz structure, they show an equally bad fit. Let us take a closer look at the random-effects Model 6. The covariance matrix D of random intercept

TABLE 5.4. *Growth data. Last observation carried forward. Model fit summary for additional models.*

	Mean	Covar	par	-2ℓ	Ref	G^2	df	p
1	unstr.	unstr.	18	407.078				
2c	quadratic	unstr.	16	412.640	1	5.562	2	0.0620
4c	unstr.	banded	12	427.804	1	20.726	6	0.0021
5c	unstr.	AR(1)	10	433.714	1	26.636	8	0.0017
7c	unstr.	CS	10	437.394	1	30.216	8	0.0002

and slope is estimated to be

$$\begin{pmatrix} 13.5992 & -0.7910 \\ -0.7910 & 0.0616 \end{pmatrix}.$$

Further, $\hat{\sigma}^2 = 1.8741$.

The resulting correlation matrix is

$$\begin{pmatrix} 1.0000 & 0.6842 & 0.6135 & 0.5126 \\ 0.6842 & 1.0000 & 0.6430 & 0.5782 \\ 0.6135 & 0.6430 & 1.0000 & 0.6288 \\ 0.5126 & 0.5782 & 0.6288 & 1.0000 \end{pmatrix}.$$

Comparison with Model 6 on the complete data set suggests the following interpretation. Carrying the observations from age 8 forward to age 10 increases the similarity and thus the correlation between this pair of outcomes. This implies an increased variance of the random intercept over the complete data set version (4.18). This is at the expense of the variance σ^2.

Next, we consider a few additional models. Their fit is presented in Table 5.4. Figure 5.2 suggested that a linear profile is not appropriate, which was confirmed in the analysis. A quadratic time trend might seem more appropriate. Model 2c (Table 5.4) combines a quadratic time trend with an unstructured covariance matrix. It is marginally acceptable but it seems wiser to retain the unstructured Model 1. Simplifying the covariance structure (Toeplitz, AR(1), CS) does not seem possible.

In conclusion, the effect of an LOCF imputation is that both mean and covariance structure are severely distorted such that no obvious simplification is possible. Hence, a simple, intuitively appealing interpretation of the trends is rendered impossible. LOCF should be used with great caution. Of course, for the growth data there is a clear increasing trend over time. This is already seen from inspection of the completers. Therefore, LOCF seems particularly inappropriate. An alternative method, which might be better suited for intermittent missing data, would replace a missing observation with an average of the adjacent measurements. For example, a missing value at age 10 would be replaced with the average of the measurements at ages 8 and 12. For unequally spaced measurements a weighted average might be more appropriate. In certain settings, the principle underlying LOCF might better reflect the true mechanism generating the data (e.g., in a randomized clinical trial). We have to reemphasize that even in such cases, imputing a single value for missing measurements would still result in overestimation of the precision.

The LOCF depends uniquely on the measurements of the individual for which an imputation has to be generated. As such, we could term it *horizontal* imputation. Next, we will discuss a strategy where the imputed value depends uniquely on the other subjects, i.e., a *vertical* strategy.

5.5.2   Imputing Unconditional Means

The idea behind unconditional mean imputation (Little and Rubin, 1987) is to replace a missing value with the average of the observed values on the same variable over the other subjects. Thus, the term *unconditional* refers to the fact that one does not use (i.e., condition on) information on the subject for which an imputation is generated.

For example, in the growth data set, one could impute the grand mean from the observed measurement at age 10. Since earlier inspection of the data revealed that there is some evidence for a sex effect in the profiles, it might be prudent to calculate sex-specific means and to replace a missing value at age 10 with the proper sex group mean. In doing so, the principle of a purely vertical imputation scheme is relaxed. Both versions are contrasted, in terms of raw and residual profiles, in Figure 5.3. It is fair to say that the differences are not overwhelming, at least not from visual inspection. However, it is still obvious that the sex-specific imputation procedure might yield a less distorted picture. Hence, we will not consider the grand mean imputed data set for analysis.

GROWTH DATA

Let us again consider the eight models, described in Section 4.4. A summary of the model fit is given in Table 5.5. It is clear that the impact of this imputation strategy is less distorting than with last observation carried forward. The linear profile Model 2 is not rejected, but the equal slopes Model 3 is rejected, exactly as with the complete data set. Simplification of the covariance structure is slightly more cumbersome than with the original

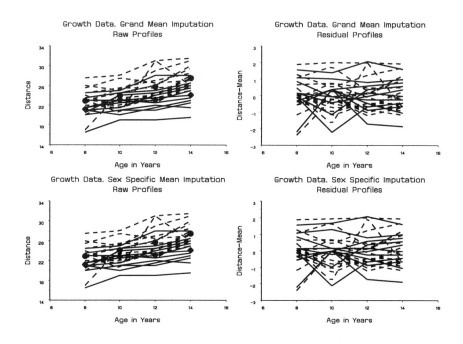

FIGURE 5.3. *Raw and residual profiles for the mean imputed growth data set.*
(Girls are indicated with solid lines.)

TABLE 5.5. *Growth data. Sex-specific mean imputation. Model fit summary.*

	Mean	Covar	par	-2ℓ	Ref	G^2	df	p
1	unstr.	unstr.	18	423.076				
2	$\neq$ slopes	unstr.	14	425.108	1	2.032	4	0.7299
3	= slopes	unstr.	13	430.108	2	5.000	1	0.0254
4	$\neq$ slopes	banded	8	437.264	2	12.156	6	0.0586
5	$\neq$ slopes	AR(1)	6	451.007	2	25.899	8	0.0011
6	$\neq$ slopes	random	8	437.851	2	12.743	6	0.0473
7	$\neq$ slopes	CS	6	438.574	2	13.466	8	0.0968
8	$\neq$ slopes	simple	5	472.550	2	47.442	9	<0.0001

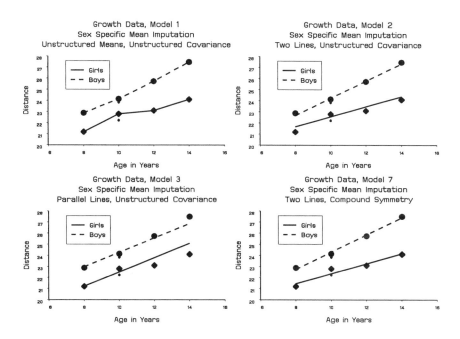

FIGURE 5.4. *Profiles for the growth data set, from a selected set of models. Sex-specific mean imputation. (The small dots are the observed group means for the complete data set.)*

data. Both Toeplitz Model 4 and random-effects Model 6 are suspect. Even though Model 4 is formally acceptable, we choose to keep Model 2 as the reference model. The auto-regressive Model 5 is unacceptable, exactly as before. Comparing compound symmetry (Model 7) to Model 2 shows an acceptable fit. However, care is required with this conclusion. Since Model 7 is a simplification of the very borderline Models 4 and 6, the test might be significant only by virtue of parsimony. Let us expand on this point. The assertion made here is that a clear lack of fit, concentrated in one part of the model, is diluted by the beneficial effect of removing some redundant model parameters. For example, the Toeplitz assumption might be violated, but the bands of the Toeplitz model could be sufficiently close to each other such that one might just as well replace the Toeplitz structure with the simpler exchangeable structure. Then, essentially the same misspecification is spread out over 8 rather than 6 degrees of freedom. We will reexamine this claim when studying the covariance structure in more detail.

Figure 5.4 shows the observed profiles (Model 1), and those predicted by Models 2, 3, and 7. The mean profiles for Models 2, 3, and 7 are as follows:

- Model 2:

$$\text{girls} \quad : \quad \hat{Y}_j = 18.05 + 0.4514t_j,$$
$$\text{boys} \quad : \quad \hat{Y}_j = 16.46 + 0.7759t_j.$$

- Model 3:

$$\text{girls} \quad : \quad \hat{Y}_j = 16.05 + 0.6442t_j,$$
$$\text{boys} \quad : \quad \hat{Y}_j = 17.82 + 0.6442t_j.$$

- Model 7:

$$\text{girls} \quad : \quad \hat{Y}_j = 17.82 + 0.4516t_j,$$
$$\text{boys} \quad : \quad \hat{Y}_j = 16.60 + 0.7682t_j.$$

The mean profiles are comparable to those found from the complete data set (Section 4.4). As argued before, there might be more reason to doubt the covariance structure. Let us consider the estimated correlation matrices:

- Model 1 (unstructured):

$$\begin{pmatrix} 1.0000 & 0.4083 & 0.6613 & 0.5216 \\ 0.4083 & 1.0000 & 0.3298 & 0.4730 \\ 0.6613 & 0.3298 & 1.0000 & 0.7281 \\ 0.5216 & 0.4730 & 0.7281 & 1.0000 \end{pmatrix} \tag{5.7}$$

- Model 4 (Toeplitz):

$$\begin{pmatrix} 1.0000 & 0.5114 & 0.5884 & 0.4331 \\ 0.5114 & 1.0000 & 0.5114 & 0.5884 \\ 0.5884 & 0.5114 & 1.0000 & 0.5114 \\ 0.4331 & 0.5884 & 0.5114 & 1.0000 \end{pmatrix}$$

- Model 5 (AR(1)):

$$\begin{pmatrix} 1.0000 & 0.4890 & 0.2391 & 0.1169 \\ 0.4890 & 1.0000 & 0.4890 & 0.2391 \\ 0.2391 & 0.4890 & 1.0000 & 0.4890 \\ 0.1169 & 0.2391 & 0.4890 & 1.0000 \end{pmatrix}$$

- Model 6 (random-effects):

$$\begin{pmatrix} 1.0000 & 0.4923 & 0.4983 & 0.5002 \\ 0.4927 & 1.0000 & 0.5275 & 0.5368 \\ 0.4992 & 0.5279 & 1.0000 & 0.5662 \\ 0.5015 & 0.5376 & 0.5666 & 1.0000 \end{pmatrix}$$

- Model 7 (compound symmetry):

$$\begin{pmatrix} 1.0000 & 0.5193 & 0.5193 & 0.5193 \\ 0.5193 & 1.0000 & 0.5193 & 0.5193 \\ 0.5193 & 0.5193 & 1.0000 & 0.5193 \\ 0.5193 & 0.5193 & 0.5193 & 1.0000 \end{pmatrix}$$

Since the LOCF technique is horizontal, it had the effect of increasing the correlation between ages 8 and 10 in the growth data. Unconditional mean imputation has exactly the opposite effect. Comparison of (4.13) with (5.7) shows that all correlations remain the same except for the (age 8, age 10) correlation which decreases from 0.5707 to 0.4083, the (age 10, age 12) correlation which decreases from 0.5632 to 0.3298, and the (age 10, age 14) correlation which decreases from 0.7262 to 0.4730. Thus, there is a change in each diagonal band of the correlation matrix, which explains why the banded structure and its simplifications are less appropriate.

There is another aspect of this imputation technique which requires careful consideration. By imputing the same value for all missing numbers at age 10, the variability at age 10 is reduced. This is seen from the estimated covariance matrix of Model 1:

$$\begin{pmatrix} 5.0143 & 1.5437 & 3.6206 & 2.5095 \\ 1.5437 & 2.8509 & 1.3614 & 1.7161 \\ 3.6206 & 1.3614 & 5.9775 & 3.8248 \\ 2.5095 & 1.7161 & 3.8248 & 4.6164 \end{pmatrix}.$$

The variance at age 10 is reduced from 3.87 in the complete data set to 2.85 here.

To assess whether the distorted correlation structure or rather the unequal variances lead to problems in finding a parsimonious model will be investigated by means of a few additional models.

Let us consider the Toeplitz model first. Assuming that the main cause for a bad fit is the unequal variance structure, we keep the banded correlation structure, but allow the variance to depend on the measurement occasion. The error vector ε_i is now assumed to follow a $\varepsilon_i \sim N(\mathbf{0}, \Sigma)$ distribution, where Σ is constrained to $\sigma_{ij} = \sigma_i \sigma_j \rho_{|i-j|}$. Here, σ_i is the standard deviation of the measurements at occasion i and $\rho_{|i-j|}$ is the correlation between

TABLE 5.6. *Growth data. Sex-specific mean imputation. Model fit summary for additional models.*

	Mean	Covar	par	-2ℓ	Ref	G^2	df	p
1	unstr.	unstr.	18	423.076				
2	$\neq$ slopes	unstr.	14	425.108	1	2.032	4	0.7299
3	$=$ slopes	unstr.	13	430.108	2	5.000	1	0.0254
4d	$\neq$ slopes	banded-H	11	434.672	2	9.565	3	0.0226
5d	$\neq$ slopes	ARH(1)	9	447.418	2	22.310	5	0.0005
7d	$\neq$ slopes	CSH	9	435.614	2	10.506	5	0.0621

two measurements with lag $|i-j|$. For the growth data, there are 7 free parameters: σ_i ($i = 1, 2, 3, 4$), and ρ_k ($k = 1, 2, 3$). For convenience, $\rho_0 \equiv 1$. This structure is called a *heterogeneous banded* or *heterogeneous Toeplitz* covariance. Heterogeneous counterparts for the AR(1) and compound symmetry models are defined in a similar fashion. Model fit information is summarized in Table 5.6. The model fit of the heterogeneous Models 4d, 5d, and 7d is inferior to the standard counterparts (Models 4, 5, and 7), suggesting that for this data set unconditional mean imputation affects the correlation structure more than the variance structure.

In conclusion, the linear but not parallel mean profile structure found in the complete data set analysis, is recovered with sex-specific mean imputation. The covariance structure poses more of a problem, since this form of imputation distorts the correlation structure by diluting some of the correlations and leaving others unchanged. This is bound to happen whenever the rate of incompleteness is different across measurement occasions. Note that a dilution of the correlation structure is an intrinsic feature of this approach, even if the rate of missingness is roughly constant across occasions.

Our next goal is to describe an imputation method which combines 'horizontal' and 'vertical' information in creating the imputations.

5.5.3   Buck's Method: Conditional Mean Imputation

This approach was suggested by Buck (1960) and reviewed by Little and Rubin (1987). The method is technically hardly more complex than mean imputation. Let us describe it first for a single multivariate normal sample. The first step is to estimate the mean vector μ and the covariance matrix Σ from the complete cases. This step builds on the assumption that $Y \sim N(\mu, \Sigma)$. For a subject with missing components, the regression of the missing components $(\boldsymbol{Y}_i^m)$ on the observed ones $(\boldsymbol{y}_i^o)$ is

$$\boldsymbol{Y}_i^m | \boldsymbol{y}_i^o \sim N(\boldsymbol{\mu}^m + \Sigma^{mo}(\Sigma^{oo})^{-1}(\boldsymbol{y}_i^o - \boldsymbol{\mu}_i^o), \Sigma^{mm} - \Sigma^{mo}(\Sigma^{oo})^{-1}\Sigma^{om}). \quad (5.8)$$

Superscripts o and m refer to 'observed' and 'missing' components respectively. The second step calculates the conditional mean from this regression and substitutes it for the missing values. In this way, 'vertical' information (estimates for $\boldsymbol{\mu}$ and Σ) is combined with 'horizontal' information $(\boldsymbol{y}_i^o)$.

Buck (1960) showed that under mild regularity conditions the method is valid for MCAR mechanisms. Little and Rubin (1987) added that the method is valid under certain types of MAR mechanisms. Even though the distribution of the observed components (e.g., the measurements at age 8, 12, and 14) is allowed to differ between complete and incomplete observations, it is very important that the regression of the missing components on the observed ones (e.g., the outcome at age 10, given the outcomes at the other ages) is constant across missingness patterns.

Again, this method shares with other single imputation strategies that, although point estimation may be consistent, the precision will be underestimated. Little and Rubin (1987, p. 46) indicated ways to correct the precision estimation for unconditional mean imputation.

GROWTH DATA

We applied a normal based conditional mean imputation as described above to the growth data set, with the sole modification that a separate mean vector and covariance matrix was calculated for the two sexes. Figure 5.5 displays raw and residual profiles. From the plots we infer that the conditional mean imputation does not seem to be able to fully recover the linear trend. Arguable, a couple of reasons could be responsible for this observation. First, the complete case sample size in each sex group is relatively small, leading to relatively imprecise parameter estimates. Secondly, the regression slope could vary between responders and non-responders at age 10. There is indeed some evidence to support a discrepancy between the covariance structure of the complete data set and the completers. Let us compare the unstructured covariance matrices (4.13) and (5.6). The correlations between age 10 on the one hand and ages 8, 12, and 14 on the other change from 0.5707 to 0.7471, 0.5632 to 0.4229, and 0.7262 to 0.6319 respectively. Thus, the correlations between age 10 and its adjacent measurements are virtually identical in the complete data set, but favor association between ages 8 and 10 when we restrict the sample to the completers. The influence of this shift will be discussed further.

Let us again consider the eight models, described in Section 4.4. A summary of the model fit is given in Table 5.7. Figure 5.6 depicts the estimated

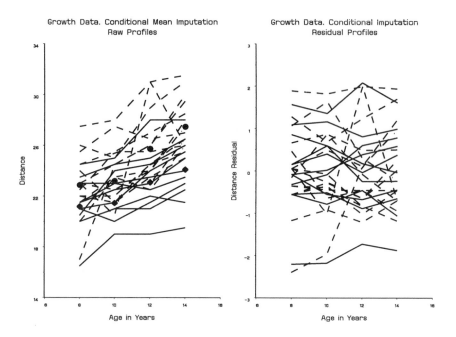

FIGURE 5.5. *Raw and residual profiles for the conditional mean imputed growth data set. (Girls are indicated with solid lines.)*

profiles from the unstructured Model 1 and the linear profiles Model 2. Both this figure and Table 5.7 show that there is an apparent non-linear trend induced by the imputation strategy, as was expected from graphical inspection of the data (Figure 5.5). Of course, Model 3 does not fit the data either.

For this reason, Models 4–8, based on linear mean profiles, do not fit the data. These models are omitted from Table 5.7. They are replaced with alternative covariance structures. Let us first consider the covariance matrix estimated from Model 1:

$$\begin{pmatrix} 5.0143 & 5.0105 & 3.6206 & 2.5095 \\ 5.0105 & 6.4156 & 3.4858 & 3.2186 \\ 3.6206 & 3.4858 & 5.9775 & 3.8248 \\ 2.5095 & 3.2186 & 3.8248 & 4.6164 \end{pmatrix},$$

TABLE 5.7. *Growth data. Conditional mean imputation. Model fit summary.*

	Mean	Covar	par	-2ℓ	Ref	G^2	df	p
1	unstr.	unstr.	18	406.435				
2	$\neq$ slopes	unstr.	14	423.307	1	16.872	4	0.0020
3	$=$ slopes	unstr.	13	425.740	1	19.305	5	0.0017
4c	unstr.	banded	12	422.477	1	16.042	6	0.0135
5c	unstr.	AR(1)	10	432.410	1	25.975	8	0.0011
7c	unstr.	CS	10	433.669	1	27.234	8	0.0006
4e	unstr.	banded-H	15	420.527	1	14.092	3	0.0028
5e	unstr.	ARH(1)	13	428.421	1	21.986	5	0.0005
7e	unstr.	CSH	13	432.181	1	25.746	5	0.0001

with corresponding correlation matrix

$$
\begin{pmatrix}
1.0000 & 0.8834 & 0.6613 & 0.5216 \\
0.8834 & 1.0000 & 0.5629 & 0.5914 \\
0.6613 & 0.5629 & 1.0000 & 0.7281 \\
0.5216 & 0.5914 & 0.7281 & 1.0000
\end{pmatrix}. \tag{5.9}
$$

As expected, the covariances and correlations in the second row and column all change relative to (4.13). Should the imputation model be entirely adequate, then the changes in the correlations would be due to random fluctuation. However, we observe a strongly increased correlation between the measurements at age 10 and age 8, with a decrease between age 10 and the other two. This implies that the regression model gives more weight to the age 8 measurement than to the age 10 and 12 measurements. For example, the regression coefficients for boys are 1.0167, -0.2677, and 0.4418 for age 8, age 12, and age 14 respectively. This picture is completely consistent with our earlier observation about the slightly distorted picture emerging from the correlation matrix (5.6) of the completers. As a consequence, the mean at age 10 will be pulled down, exactly as observed in Figure 5.5. The variance at age 10 is inflated by this process.

Above reasoning would suggest that there is again little hope to simplify the covariance structure. Indeed, none of the Models 4c, 5c, and 7c, combining an unstructured mean profile with a banded, AR(1), or CS correlation respectively, exhibit an acceptable fit. Models 4e, 5e, and 7e differ only in that they allow the variance to change over time. Again, these extra parameters seem to be redundant, resulting in a deteriorating overall fit.

In conclusion, while conditional mean imputation is quoted to be more promising than the previous forms of imputation (Little and Rubin, 1987),

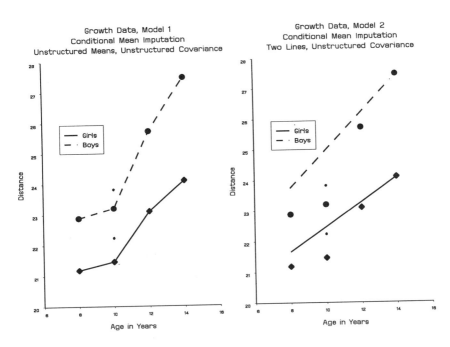

FIGURE 5.6. *Profiles for the growth data set, from a selected set of models. Conditional mean imputation. (The small dots are the observed group means for the complete data set.)*

it is outperformed by unconditional mean imputation in this particular example. The technique is recommendable when the sample size is sufficient to estimate the conditional regression from which imputations are calculated, and when the assumption of a constant regression slope is reasonable. In other words, the distribution of the missing components conditional on the observed components has to be approximately equal between responders and non-responders. Still, as with the other single imputation methods, the precision will be underestimated.

5.5.4   Discussion of Imputation Techniques

The imputation methods reviewed here are clearly not the only ones. Little and Rubin (1987) and Rubin (1987) mention several others. Several methods, such as hot deck imputation, are based on filling in missing values from 'matching' subjects, where an appropriate matching criterion is used.

Almost all imputation techniques suffer from the following limitations:

1. The performance of imputation techniques is unreliable. Situations where they do work are difficult to distinguish from situations were they prove misleading. For example, while conditional imputation is considered superior to unconditional imputation, we have seen that the latter performs better on the growth data.

2. Imputation often requires ad hoc adjustments to yield satisfactory point estimates.

3. The methods fail to provide simple correct precision estimators.

In addition, most methods require the MCAR assumption to hold. Methods such as last observation carried forward require additional and often unrealistically strong assumptions.

The main advantage, shared with complete case analysis, is that complete data software can be used. While a complete case analysis is even simpler since one does not need to address the imputation task, the imputation family uses all (and in fact too much) of the available information. With the availability of PROC MIXED, it is no longer necessary to stick to complete data software, since this procedure allows for measurement sequences of unequal length.

A discussion of multiple imputation is postponed until Section 5.10. In the next sections frequentist (valid under MCAR) and likelihood based (valid under MAR) available case methods will be studied. These methods operate on the observed data, neither deleting or imputing values.

5.6   Available Case Methods

Consider a single multivariate normal sample, based on $i = 1, \ldots, N$ subjects, for which $j = 1, \ldots, n$ variables are planned. In a longitudinal context the n variables would refer to n repeated measurements. The data matrix is $Y = (y_{ij})$.

Available case methods (Little and Rubin, 1987) use as much of the data as possible. Let us restrict attention to the estimation of the mean vector μ and the covariance matrix Σ. The jth component μ_j of the mean vector and the jth diagonal variance element σ_{jj} are estimated using all cases that are observed on the jth variable, disregarding their response status at the other measurement occasions. The (j, k)th element $(j \neq k)$ of the covariance matrix is computed using all cases that are observed on both the jth and the kth variable.

This method is more efficient than the complete case method, since more information is used. The number of components of the outcome vector has no direct effect on the sample available for a particular mean or covariance component.

The method is valid only under MCAR. In this respect it is no fundamental improvement over a complete case analysis. An added disadvantage is that, although more information is used and a consistent estimator is obtained under MCAR, it is not guaranteed that the covariance matrix is positive (semi-)definite. Of course, this is only a small sample problem and does not invalidate asymptotic results. However, for samples with a large number of variables and/or with fairly high correlations between pairs of outcomes, this nuisance feature is likely to turn up.

While a complete case analysis is possible for virtually every statistical method, and while single imputation is also fairly generally applicable, extending an available case analysis beyond multivariate means and co-variances can be tedious.

5.6.1   Growth Data

We will illustrate this method on the growth data. Specifically, the parameters for the unstructured mean and covariance Model 1 will be estimated.

The estimated mean vector for girls is

$$(21.1818, 22.7857, 23.0909, 24.0909)$$

while the vector for boys is

$$(22.8750, 24.1364, 25.7188, 27.4688).$$

The mean vector for girls is based on a sample of size 11, except for the second element which is based on the 7 complete observations. The corresponding sample sizes for boys are 16 and 11, respectively.

The estimated covariance matrix is

$$\begin{pmatrix} 5.4155 & 2.3155 & 3.9102 & 2.7102 \\ 2.3155 & 4.2763 & 2.0420 & 2.5741 \\ 3.9102 & 2.0420 & 6.4557 & 4.1307 \\ 2.7102 & 2.5741 & 4.1307 & 4.9857 \end{pmatrix}, \tag{5.10}$$

with correlation matrix

$$\begin{pmatrix} 1.0000 & 0.4812 & 0.6613 & 0.5216 \\ 0.4812 & 1.0000 & 0.3886 & 0.5575 \\ 0.6613 & 0.3886 & 1.0000 & 0.7281 \\ 0.5216 & 0.5575 & 0.7281 & 1.0000 \end{pmatrix} .$$

The elements of the covariance matrix are computed as

$$\hat{\sigma}_{jk} = \frac{1}{25} \left\{ \sum_{i=1}^{11} (y_{ij}^g - \overline{y}_j^g)(y_{ik}^g - \overline{y}_k^g) + \sum_{i=1}^{16} (y_{ij}^b - \overline{y}_j^b)(y_{ik}^b - \overline{y}_k^b) \right\}, \ j, k \neq 2,$$

$$\hat{\sigma}_{j2} = \frac{1}{18} \left\{ \sum_{i=1}^{7} (y_{ij}^g - \overline{y}_j^g)(y_{i2}^g - \overline{y}_2^g) + \sum_{i=1}^{11} (y_{ij}^b - \overline{y}_j^b)(y_{i2}^b - \overline{y}_2^b) \right\}.$$

The superscripts g and b refer to girls and boys respectively. It is assumed that, within each sex subgroup, the ordering is such that completers precede the incompletely measured children.

Looking at the available case procedure from the perspective of the individual observation, one might say that each observation contributes to the subvector of the parameter vector about which it contains information. For example, a complete observation in the growth data set contributes to 4 (sex specific) mean components as well as to all 10 variance-covariance parameters. In an incomplete observation, there is information about 3 mean components and 6 variance-covariance parameters (excluding those with a subscript 2).

Whether or not there is non-random selection of the incomplete observations does not affect those parameters without a subscript 2. For the ones involving a subscript 2, potential differences between completers and non-completers are not taken into account and hence biased estimation may result when an MAR mechanism is operating. In fact, the estimates for the parameters with at least one subscript 2 equal their complete case analysis counterparts, which is seen by comparing (5.10) with (5.5). Thus, MCAR is required. This observation is consistent with the theory in Rubin (1976), since the current available case method is frequentist rather than likelihood based.

A method which is consistent with the available case principle, makes use of likelihood based estimation, and is easily implemented in PROC MIXED, is discussed in the next section. It will also be shown that the well-known equality of the maximum likelihood and least squares estimators for a multivariate normal data does not hold for incomplete samples.

5.7   Likelihood-Based Ignorable Analysis and PROC MIXED

In Section 5.2.3 it was argued that likelihood based inference is valid, whenever the mechanism is MAR, and provided the technical condition holds that the parameters describing the non-response mechanism are distinct from the measurement model parameters. In other words, the missing data process should be ignorable in the likelihood inference sense, since then factorization (5.4) applies and the log-likelihood partitions into two functionally independent components.

This implies that a module with likelihood estimation facilities such as PROC MIXED manipulates the correct likelihood and leads to valid likelihood ratios. We will explore this method in detail. While this is an extremely important feature of PROC MIXED and in fact of any flexibly written linear mixed model likelihood optimization routine, a few cautionary remarks still apply.

1. Ignorability depends on the, often implicit, assumption that the scientific interest is directed towards the measurement model parameters θ and that the missing data mechanism parameters ψ are nuisance parameters. This is not always true. For instance, when the question of predicting a subject's measurement profile (individual or group averaged) is raised, past the time of dropout and *given that she dropped out*, then *both* parameter vectors θ and ψ need to be estimated. However, due to the ignorability and the resulting partitioning of the likelihood, one can construct a model for non-response, separately from the linear mixed measurement model. As a practical consequence, the software module to estimate the missingness model parameters, can be chosen independently from PROC MIXED. Often, categorical data analysis methods such as logistic regression will be a sensible choice in this respect.

2. Likelihood inference is often surrounded with references to the sampling distribution, e.g., to construct precision estimators and for statistical hypothesis tests (Kenward and Molenberghs 1997). This issue and its relationship to the PROC MIXED implementation will be discussed further in Section 5.8.

3. Even though the assumption of likelihood ignorability encompasses the MAR and not only the more stringent and often implausible MCAR mechanisms, it is difficult to exclude the option of a more general informative dropout mechanism. One solution is to fit an informative dropout model as proposed by Diggle and Kenward (1994). They

fitted models to the full data using the simplex algorithm (Nelder and Mead 1965). Alternatively, the EM algorithm can be used, as proposed by Molenberghs, Kenward, and Lesaffre (1997) for the longitudinal categorical data problem. A module for the linear mixed model with dropout is implemented in the OSWALD software, written for S-Plus (Smith, Robertson, and Diggle 1996). It is based on an extension of the Diggle and Kenward (1994) model and described in detail in Section 5.11. A SAS program for an EM algorithm for the linear model would consist of three parts. First, a macro to carry out the E step has to be written, where the incomplete data set is completed conditional on the current parameter vector and on the observed data. The M step consists of two substeps, where PROC MIXED might be used to maximize the measurement process likelihood and a different routine (e.g., logistic regression) could be called to maximize the non-response likelihood. Diggle and Kenward (1994) assumed a logistic model for the dropout process. The EM algorithm will be discussed further in Section 5.9.

5.7.1 Growth Data

As with the available case method of Section 5.6, a complete subject contributes to 'more parameters' than an incomplete subject. Whereas these contributions were direct in terms of parameter vector components in Section 5.6, in the current framework subjects contribute information through their factor of the likelihood function. For example, let us consider Model 1. A complete subject contributes by means of a four dimensional normal loglikelihood term with 4 out of 8 mean components (boys and girls have separate means) and a 4×4 positive definite covariance matrix. An incomplete observation contributes through the three dimensional marginal density, obtained by integrating over the second component. In practice, this is done by deleting the second component of the mean vector and the second row and the second column of the covariance matrix.

Little and Rubin (1987) fitted the same eight models as Jennrich and Schluchter (1986) to the incomplete growth data set. Whereas Little and Rubin made use of the EM algorithm, we set out to perform our analysis with direct maximization of the observed likelihood (with Fisher scoring or Newton-Raphson) in PROC MIXED. The results ought to coincide. Table 5.8 reproduces the findings of Little and Rubin. We added p-values. The PROC MIXED programs, constructed in Section 4.4 to analyze the complete data set, will be applied to the artificially incomplete data set. The structure of this data set is given in Table 5.9. While there would be four records for every subject in the complete data set, now there are 9 subjects

TABLE 5.8. *Growth data. MAR analysis (Little and Rubin). Model fit summary.*

	Mean	Covar	par	-2ℓ	Ref	G^2	df	p
1	unstr.	unstr.	18	386.957				
2	$\neq$ slopes	unstr.	14	393.288	1	6.331	4	0.1758
3	$=$ slopes	unstr.	13	397.400	2	4.112	1	0.0426
4	$\neq$ slopes	banded	8	398.030	2	4.742	6	0.5773
5	$\neq$ slopes	AR(1)	6	409.523	2	16.235	8	0.0391
6	$\neq$ slopes	random	8	400.452	2	7.164	6	0.3059
7	$\neq$ slopes	CS	6	401.313	6	0.861	2	0.6502
					6	0.861	1:2	0.5018
8	$\neq$ slopes	simple	5	441.583	7	40.270	1	<0.0001
					7	40.270	0:1	<0.0001

(e.g., subjects 3 and 27) with only three records.

Applying the models to the data yields some discrepancies, as seen from the model fit Table 5.10. Let us take a close look at these discrepancies. Although most of the tests performed lead to the same conclusion, there is one fundamental difference. In Table 5.8 the AR(1) model is rejected while it is not in Table 5.10. A puzzling difference is that the maximized log-likelihoods are different for Models 1–5, but not for Models 6–8. The same holds for the mean and covariance parameter estimates. To get a hold on this problem, let us consider the repeated statement (e.g., of Model 1):

```
repeated / type = un subject = idnr r rcorr;
```

This statement identifies the subject in terms of IDNR blocks but does not specify the ordering of the observations within a subject. Thus, PROC MIXED assumes the default ordering: 1, 2, 3, 4 for a complete subject and, erroneously, 1, 2, 3 for an incomplete one, while the correct incomplete ordering is 1, 2, 4. This means that, by default, dropout is assumed. Since this assumption is inadequate for the growth data, Models 1–5 in Table 5.10 are incorrect. The random-effects Model 6, on the other hand, uses the RANDOM statement

```
random intercept age / type = un subject = idnr g;
```

where the variable AGE conveys the information needed to correctly calculate the random-effects parameters. Indeed, for an incomplete observation,

TABLE 5.9. *Growth data. Extract of the incomplete data set.*

OBS	IDNR	AGE	SEX	MEASURE
1	1	8	2	21.0
2	1	10	2	20.0
3	1	12	2	21.5
4	1	14	2	23.0
5	2	8	2	21.0
6	2	10	2	21.5
7	2	12	2	24.0
8	2	14	2	25.5
9	3	8	2	20.5
10	3	12	2	24.5
11	3	14	2	26.0
...				
97	27	8	1	22.0
98	27	12	1	23.5
99	27	14	1	25.0

TABLE 5.10. *Growth data.* **Inadequate** *MAR analysis (Little and Rubin). Model fit summary.*

	Mean	Covar	par	-2ℓ	Ref	G^2	df	p
1	unstr.	unstr.	18	394.309				
2	$\neq$ slopes	unstr.	14	397.862	1	3.553	4	0.4699
3	$=$ slopes	unstr.	13	401.935	2	4.073	1	0.0436
4	$\neq$ slopes	banded	8	400.981	2	3.119	6	0.7938
5	$\neq$ slopes	AR(1)	6	408.996	2	11.134	8	0.1942
6	$\neq$ slopes	random	8	400.452	2	2.590	6	0.8583
7	$\neq$ slopes	CS	6	401.312	6	0.860	2	0.6505
					6	0.860	1:2	0.5021
8	$\neq$ slopes	simple	5	441.582	7	40.270	1	<0.0001
					7	40.270	0:1	<0.0001

the correct design

$$Z_i = \begin{pmatrix} 1 & 8 \\ 1 & 12 \\ 1 & 14 \end{pmatrix}$$

is generated. Finally, it remains to be discussed why Models 7–8 give a correct answer in spite of the fact that they also use the REPEATED statement rather than the RANDOM statement. It is best seen for Model 8, where we assume an independence covariance structure. This covariance structure is equivalent to assuming that the $99 = 108 - 9$ measurements form a simple random sample of size $n = 99$, rather than a longitudinal sample. Consequently, the actual position within a subject's sequence is irrelevant. The same holds for the compound symmetry or *exchangeable* model. The only difference with the simple model is that a *common* intra-class correlation between two measurements within the same sequence is assumed. Since this correlation is constant and thus independent of the actual distance between measurements, it can be determined from the full set of pairs of measurements within an individual (6 pairs for a complete observation and 3 pairs for an incomplete observation), with the order being immaterial.

There are two equivalent ways to overcome this problem. The first is to adapt the data set slightly. An example is given in Table 5.11. The effect of using this data set is, of course, that incomplete records are deleted from the analysis, but that the relative positions are correctly passed on to PROC MIXED. Running Models 1–8 on this data set yields exactly the same results as in Table 5.8.

It is also possible to use the data as presented in Table 5.9. Instead of passing on the position of the missing values through the data set, we have to specify explicitly the ordering by coding it properly into the PROC MIXED program. For Model 1, the following code can be used:

```
proc mixed data = growthav method = ml;
title 'Jennrich and Schluchter (MAR, Altern.), Model 1';
class sex idnr age;
model measure = sex age*sex / s;
repeated age / type = un subject = idnr r rcorr;
run;
```

The REPEATED statement now explicitly includes the ordering by means of the AGE variable. Note that any counter with the correct ordering (e.g., 1,2,3,4) would be suitable. The corresponding Model 2 program would be:

TABLE 5.11. *Growth data. Extract of the incomplete data set. The missing observations are explicitly indicated.*

OBS	IDNR	AGE	SEX	MEASURE
1	1	8	2	21.0
2	1	10	2	20.0
3	1	12	2	21.5
4	1	14	2	23.0
5	2	8	2	21.0
6	2	10	2	21.5
7	2	12	2	24.0
8	2	14	2	25.5
9	3	8	2	20.5
10	3	10	2	.
11	3	12	2	24.5
12	3	14	2	26.0
...				
105	27	8	1	22.0
106	27	10	1	.
107	27	12	1	23.5
108	27	14	1	25.0

```
proc mixed data = growthav method = ml;
title 'Jennrich and Schluchter (MAR, Altern.), Model 2';
class sex idnr;
model measure = sex age*sex / s;
repeated age / type = un subject = idnr r rcorr;
run;
```

However, this program generates an error since the variables in the RE-PEATED statement have to be *categorical* variables, termed CLASS variables in PROC MIXED. One of the tricks to overcome this issue is using the program:

```
data help;
set growthav;
agec = age;
run;

proc mixed data = help method = ml;
title 'Jennrich and Schluchter (MAR, Altern.), Model 2';
```

```
class sex idnr agec;
model measure = sex age*sex / s;
repeated agec / type = un subject = idnr r rcorr;
run;
```

Thus, there are two identical copies of the variable AGE, only one of which is treated as a class variable.

Let us now turn attention to the performance of the ignorable method of analysis and compare the results with the ones obtained earlier. First, the model comparisons performed in Tables 4.14 and 5.8 yield qualitatively the same conclusions. In both cases, linear profiles turn out to be consistent with the data, but parallel profiles do not. A banded correlation structure (Model 5) is acceptable, as well as a random intercepts and slopes model (Model 6). These models can be simplified further to compound symmetry (Model 7). The assumption of no correlation between repeated measures (Model 8) is untenable. This means that Model 7 is again the most parsimonious description of the data among the eight models considered. It has to be noted that the rejection of Models 3 and 5 is less compelling in the MAR analysis than it was in the complete data set. Of course, this is to be expected due to the reduction in the sample size, or rather in the number of available measurements. The likelihood ratio test statistic for a direct comparison of Model 5 to Model 4, is 11.494 on 2 degrees of freedom ($p = 0.0032$), which is again a clear indication of an unacceptable fit.

Figure 5.7 displays the fit of Models 1, 2, 3, and 7. Let us consider the fit of Model 1 first. As mentioned before, the complete observations at age 10 are those with a higher measurement at age 8. Due to the within subject correlation, they are the ones with a higher measurement at age 10 as well. This is seen by comparing the big dot with the corresponding small dot, reflecting the means for the complete data set and for those observed at age 10, respectively. Since the average of the observed measurements at age 10 is biased upwards, the fitted profiles from the complete case analysis and from unconditional mean imputation were too high. Clearly, the average observed from the data is the same for the complete case analysis, the unconditional mean imputation, the available case analysis, and for the present analysis. The most crucial difference is that the current Model 1, although saturated in the sense that there are 8 mean parameters (one for each age by sex combination), does *not* let the (biased) observed and fitted averages at age 10 coincide, in contrast to the means at ages 8, 12, and 14. Indeed, if the model specification is correct then an ignorable likelihood analysis is consistent for the correct complete data mean, rather than for the observed data mean. Of course, this effect might be blurred in relatively small data sets due to small sample variability.

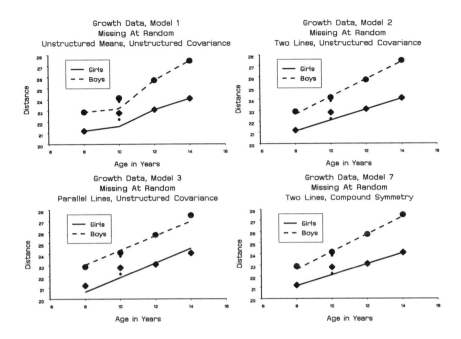

FIGURE 5.7. *Profiles for the growth data set, from a selected set of models. MAR analysis. (The small dots are the observed group means for the complete data set.)*

This discussion touches upon the key distinction between the frequentist available case analysis of Section 5.6 and the present likelihood based available case analysis. The method of Section 5.6 constructs an estimate for the age 10 parameters, irrespective of the (extra) information available for the other parameters. The likelihood approach implicitly constructs a correction, based on (1) the fact that the measurements at ages 8, 12, and 14 differ between the subgroups of complete and incomplete observations, and (2) the fairly strong correlation between the measurement at age 10 on the one hand, and the measurements at ages 8, 12, and 14 on the other hand. A detailed treatment of likelihood estimation in incomplete multivariate normal samples is given in Little and Rubin (1987, Chapter 6). Clearly, this correction leads to overshoot in the fairly small growth data set, whence the predicted mean at age 10 is actually *smaller* than the one of the complete data set. The means are reproduced in Table 5.12. All means coincide for ages 8, 12, and 14. Irrespective of the small sample behavior encountered here, the validity under MAR and the ease of implementation are good arguments to prefer this ignorable analysis over other techniques.

Note that a similar over correcting effect was seen for the conditional mean

TABLE 5.12. *Growth data. Means under unstructured Model 1.*

Age	Complete	Incomplete Obs.	Incomplete Pred.
		Girls	
8	21.18	21.18	21.18
10	22.23	22.79	21.58
12	23.09	23.09	23.09
14	24.09	24.09	24.09
		Boys	
8	22.88	22.88	22.88
10	23.81	24.14	23.17
12	25.72	25.72	25.72
14	27.47	27.47	27.47

imputation method of Section 5.5.3, where the correlation structure, and thus the regression of age 10 on the other ages, pulled the imputed value towards the age 8 measurement. In that analysis, the effect was more dramatic for two reasons. First, the regression model to impute from was based on the completers only. This is dangerous whenever any structure which is assumed to be equal between complete and incomplete observations actually differs systematically (e.g., the covariance matrix). Secondly, values are imputed explicitly and hence they are treated as if they were observed. In the ignorable analysis, there is no explicit imputation, in the sense that no values are filled in which then are allowed to contribute information to the likelihood function. Rather, an implicit imputation takes place in the sense that filling in the conditional means for a subject's missing measurements given its observed ones and given the parameters at convergence would lead to the same point estimates as the ones obtained from direct maximization of the observed data log-likelihood. This imputation is the same as the one obtained from conducting an E step of the EM algorithm *at convergence.* The conditional mean imputation procedure of Section 5.5.3 corresponds to performing a single *initial* E step of the EM algorithm, with starting values from the complete cases.

We now present the predicted mean curves for Models 2, 3, and 7:

- Model 2:

$$\text{girls} \quad : \quad \hat{Y}_j = 17.18 + 0.4917 t_j,$$
$$\text{boys} \quad : \quad \hat{Y}_j = 16.32 + 0.7886 t_j.$$

- Model 3:

$$\text{girls} \quad : \quad \hat{Y}_j = 15.40 + 0.6519t_j,$$
$$\text{boys} \quad : \quad \hat{Y}_j = 17.82 + 0.6519t_j.$$

- Model 7:

$$\text{girls} \quad : \quad \hat{Y}_j = 17.22 + 0.4890t_j,$$
$$\text{boys} \quad : \quad \hat{Y}_j = 16.30 + 0.7867t_j.$$

In contrast with earlier analyses, these profiles are fairly similar to their complete data counterparts. In the complete case analysis, the intercepts were overestimated but the slopes were underestimated. Last observation carried forward led to a similar conclusion, except for Model 7, where the slopes were slightly overestimated. Unconditional mean imputation exhibited an acceptable behavior, in contrast to conditional mean imputation, where the slopes were once again underestimated.

Let us now study this method in terms of the effect on the estimated covariance structure. The estimated covariance matrix of Model 1 is

$$\hat{\Sigma} = \begin{pmatrix} 5.0142 & 4.8796 & 3.6205 & 2.5095 \\ 4.8796 & 6.6341 & 3.3772 & 3.0621 \\ 3.6205 & 3.3772 & 5.9775 & 3.8248 \\ 2.5095 & 3.0621 & 3.8248 & 4.6164 \end{pmatrix}.$$

The variance at age 10 is inflated compared to its complete data set counterpart (4.12). The main reason is that the sample size at age 10 is only 2/3 of the original one, thereby making all estimators involved more variable. A correct analysis, such as the ignorable one considered here, should acknowledge this additional source of uncertainty. The correlation matrices are:

- Model 1 (unstructured):

$$\begin{pmatrix} 1.0000 & 0.8460 & 0.6613 & 0.5216 \\ 0.8460 & 1.0000 & 0.5363 & 0.5533 \\ 0.6613 & 0.5363 & 1.0000 & 0.7281 \\ 0.5216 & 0.5533 & 0.7281 & 1.0000 \end{pmatrix} \tag{5.11}$$

- Model 4 (Toeplitz):

$$\begin{pmatrix} 1.0000 & 0.6248 & 0.6688 & 0.4307 \\ 0.6248 & 1.0000 & 0.6248 & 0.6688 \\ 0.6688 & 0.6248 & 1.0000 & 0.6248 \\ 0.4307 & 0.6688 & 0.6248 & 1.0000 \end{pmatrix}$$

- Model 5 (AR(1)):

$$\begin{pmatrix} 1.0000 & 0.6265 & 0.3925 & 0.2459 \\ 0.6265 & 1.0000 & 0.6265 & 0.3925 \\ 0.3925 & 0.6265 & 1.0000 & 0.6265 \\ 0.2459 & 0.3925 & 0.6265 & 1.0000 \end{pmatrix}$$

- Model 6 (random effects):

$$\begin{pmatrix} 1.0000 & 0.6341 & 0.5971 & 0.5465 \\ 0.6341 & 1.0000 & 0.6302 & 0.6041 \\ 0.5971 & 0.6302 & 1.0000 & 0.6461 \\ 0.5465 & 0.6041 & 0.6461 & 1.0000 \end{pmatrix}$$

- Model 7 (compound symmetry):

$$\begin{pmatrix} 1.0000 & 0.6054 & 0.6054 & 0.6054 \\ 0.6054 & 1.0000 & 0.6054 & 0.6054 \\ 0.6054 & 0.6054 & 1.0000 & 0.6054 \\ 0.6054 & 0.6054 & 0.6054 & 1.0000 \end{pmatrix}$$

The unstructured model reveals an increased correlation between ages 10 and 8, but a decrease between ages 10 and 12, and also a decrease between ages 10 and 14. This picture is consistent with the conditional mean imputation correlation matrix (5.9). The only difference between the two matrices is that the correlations in column 2 are all slightly smaller here. As mentioned earlier, the effect of the explicit conditional imputation model is higher than the one seen in the ignorable analysis. While the differences in correlation between the complete data set and ignorable analyses are carried across the simplified correlation structures, they are in fact very modest. For example, the complete data exchangeable correlation of 0.6178 changes to 0.6054 here.

It is interesting to consider the covariance structure of random-effects Model 6 in a bit more detail. The matrix D is estimated to be

$$\begin{pmatrix} 6.7853 & -0.3498 \\ -0.3498 & 0.0337 \end{pmatrix}$$

and $\hat{\sigma}^2 = 1.7700$. Thus, all entries in the random-effects covariance matrix as well as the measurement error σ^2 seem to have increased slightly in absolute value in comparison to the complete data analysis version (4.16). The resulting covariance matrix is now

$$Z_i \hat{D} Z_i' + \hat{\sigma}^2 I_4 = \begin{pmatrix} 5.1140 & 3.1833 & 3.0226 & 2.8620 \\ 3.1833 & 4.9274 & 3.1315 & 3.1055 \\ 3.0226 & 3.1315 & 5.0103 & 3.3491 \\ 2.8620 & 3.1055 & 3.3491 & 5.3626 \end{pmatrix}.$$

5.7.2   Summary

In conclusion, a likelihood ignorable analysis is preferable since it uses all available information, without the need neither to delete nor to impute measurements or entire subjects. It is theoretically justified whenever the missing data mechanism is MAR, which is a more relaxed assumption than MCAR, necessary for simple analyses (complete case, frequentist available case, and single imputation based analyses, with the exception of Buck's method of conditional mean imputation). The statistical information is not distorted by considering imputed values as if they were observed. There is no additional programming involved to perform an ignorable analysis in PROC MIXED, provided the order of the measurements is correctly specified. This can be done either by supplying records with missing data in the input data set, or by properly indicating the order of the measurement in the REPEATED and/or RANDOM statements in PROC MIXED.

When the scientific interest is directed to the missing data mechanism as well, then a simple ignorable analysis is generally not sufficient and has to be supplemented with a model for missingness. Also, when the missingness mechanism is informative, then an ignorable analysis is not valid and more complex modeling (e.g., Diggle and Kenward 1994) is required. This topic is of vital importance and will be discussed further in Section 5.11.

There are still a few issues with the estimation of precision and with hypothesis testing, related to this type of analysis, that will be discussed in the next section. That section is of a somewhat more advanced level than the current and preceding sections. Readers who would like to skip the theoretical developments and are only interested in the implications for an analysis with PROC MIXED can go immediately to Section 5.8.4.

5.8   How Ignorable Is Missing At Random ?   *

For over two decades, following the pioneering work of Rubin (1976) and Little (1976), there has been a growing literature on incomplete data, with a lot of emphasis on longitudinal data. Following the original work of Rubin and Little, there has evolved a general view that 'likelihood methods' that ignore the missing value mechanism are valid under an MAR process, where likelihood is interpreted in a frequentist sense. The availability of flexible standard software for incomplete data, such as PROC MIXED, and the advantages quoted in Section 5.7, contribute to this point of view. This statement needs careful qualification however. Kenward and Molenberghs (1997) provided an exposition of the precise sense in which frequentist methods of inference are justified under MAR processes.

As discussed in Section 5.2.3, Rubin (1976) has shown that MAR (and parameter distinctness) is necessary and sufficient to ensure validity of *direct-likelihood* inference when ignoring the process that causes missing data. Here, direct-likelihood inference is defined as an 'inference that results solely from ratios of the likelihood function for various values of the parameter,' in agreement with the definition in Edwards (1972). In the concluding section of the same paper, Rubin remarks:

> "One might argue, however, that this apparent simplicity of likelihood and Bayesian inference really buries the important issues. (...) likelihood inferences are at times surrounded with references to the sampling distributions of likelihood statistics. Thus, practically, when there is the possibility of missing data, some interpretations of Bayesian and likelihood inference face the same restrictions as sampling distribution inference. The inescapable conclusion seems to be that when dealing with real data, the practicing statistician should explicitly consider the process that causes missing data far more often than he does."

In essence, the problem from a frequentist point of view is that of identifying and using the appropriate sampling distribution. This is obviously relevant for determining distributions of test statistics, expected values of the information matrix, and measures of precision.

Little and Rubin (1987) discuss several aspects of this problem and propose using the observed information matrix to circumvent problems associated with the determination of the correct expected information matrix. Laird (1988) makes a similar point in the context of incomplete longitudinal data analysis.

In a variety of settings, several authors have re-expressed this preference for the observed information matrix and derived methods to compute it: Meng and Rubin (1991), the supplemented EM algorithm; Baker (1992), composite link models; Fitzmaurice, Laird, and Lipsitz (1994), incomplete longitudinal binary data, and Jennrich and Schluchter (1986). A group of authors has used the observed information matrix, without reference to the problems associated with the expected information: Louis (1982), Meilijson (1989), and Kenward *et al* (1994).

However, others, while claiming validity of analysis under MAR mechanisms, have used expected information matrices, and other measures of precision that do not account for the missingness mechanism (Murray and Findlay 1988, Patel 1991). A number of references is given in Baker (1992). It is clear that the problem as identified in the initial work of Rubin (1976) is not fully appreciated in the more recent literature. An exception to this is Heitjan's (1994) clear restatement of the problem.

A recent exchange of correspondence (Diggle 1992, Heitjan 1993, and Diggle 1993) indicates a genuine interest in these issues and suggests a need for clarification. We will build on the framework of likelihood inference under an MAR process, sketched in Section 5.2. The difference between the expected information matrix with and without taking the missing data mechanism into account is elucidated and the relevance of this for Wald and score statistics is discussed. Analytic and numerical illustrations of this difference are provided using a bivariate Gaussian setting. A longitudinal example is used for practical illustration.

5.8.1 Information and Sampling Distributions *

In this section, we will drop the subject subscript i from notation. We assume that the joint distribution of the full data $(\boldsymbol{Y}, \boldsymbol{R})$ is regular in the sense of Cox and Hinkley (1974, p. 281). We are concerned here with the sampling distributions of certain statistics under MCAR and MAR mechanisms. Under an MAR process, the joint distribution of $\boldsymbol{Y}^o$ and $\boldsymbol{R}$ factorizes as in (5.4):

$$f(\boldsymbol{y}_i^o, \boldsymbol{r}_i | \boldsymbol{\theta}, \boldsymbol{\psi}) = f(\boldsymbol{y}_i^o | X_i, Z_i, \boldsymbol{\theta}) f(\boldsymbol{r}_i | \boldsymbol{y}_i^o, X_i, Z_i, \boldsymbol{\psi}).$$

In terms of the log-likelihood function we have

$$\ell(\boldsymbol{\theta}, \boldsymbol{\psi}; \boldsymbol{y}^o, \boldsymbol{r}) = \ell_1(\boldsymbol{\theta}; \boldsymbol{y}^o) + \ell_2(\boldsymbol{\psi}; \boldsymbol{r}, \boldsymbol{y}^o). \tag{5.12}$$

It is assumed that $\boldsymbol{\theta}$ and $\boldsymbol{\psi}$ satisfy the separability condition. This partition of the likelihood has, with important exceptions, been taken for granted to mean that, under an MAR mechanism, likelihood methods based on ℓ_1 alone are valid for inferences about $\boldsymbol{\theta}$ *even when interpreted in the broad frequentist sense.* We now consider more precisely the sense in which the different elements of the frequentist likelihood methodology can be regarded as valid in general under the MAR mechanism. It is now well-known that such inferences are valid under an MCAR mechanism (Rubin 1976, Section 6).

First we note that under the MAR mechanism $\boldsymbol{r}$ is *not* an ancillary statistic for $\boldsymbol{\theta}$ in the extended sense of Cox and Hinkley (1974, p. 35). (A statistic $S(\boldsymbol{Y}, \boldsymbol{R})$ is ancillary for $\boldsymbol{\theta}$ if its distribution does not depend upon $\boldsymbol{\theta}$.) Hence we are not justified in restricting the sample space from that associated with the pair $(\boldsymbol{Y}, \boldsymbol{R})$. In considering the properties of frequentist procedures below we therefore define the appropriate sampling distributions to be that determined by this pair. We call this the *unconditional* sampling framework. By working within this framework we do need to consider the missing value mechanism. We shall be comparing this with the sampling distribution that would apply if r were fixed by design, that is if we repeatedly sampled using the distribution $f(y^o; \theta)$. If this sampling distribution were appropriate, this would lead directly to the use of ℓ_1 as a basis for inference. We call this the *naive* sampling framework.

Little (1976), in a comment on the paper by Rubin (1976) mentions explicitly the role played by the non-response pattern. He argues: "For sampling based inferences, a first crucial question concerns when it is justified to condition on the observed pattern, that is on the event $R = r$ (...). A natural condition is that R should be ancillary (...). Otherwise the pattern on its own carries at least some information about θ, which should in principle be used."

Certain elements of the frequentist methodology can be justified immediately from (5.12). The maximum likelihood estimator obtained from maximizing $l_1(\theta; y^o)$ alone is identical to that obtained from maximizing the complete log-likelihood function. Similarly the maximum likelihood estimator of ψ is functionally independent of θ and so any maximum likelihood ratio concerning θ, with common ψ, will involve ℓ_1 only. Because these statistics are identical whether derived from ℓ_1 or the complete log-likelihood it follows at once that they have the required properties under the naive sampling framework. See for example Rubin (1976), Little (1976), and Little and Rubin (1987, Section 5.2).

An important element of likelihood based frequentist inference is the derivation of measures of precision of the maximum likelihood estimators from the information. For this either the observed information, i_O, can be used where

$$i_O(\theta_j, \theta_k) = -\frac{\partial^2 \ell(\cdot)}{\partial \theta_j \partial \theta_k}$$

or the expected information, i_E, where

$$i_E(\theta_j, \theta_k) = E\{i_O(\theta_j, \theta_k)\}. \tag{5.13}$$

The argument above justifying the use of the maximum likelihood estimators from $\ell_1(\theta; y^o)$ applies equally well to the use of the inverse of the *observed* information derived from ℓ_1 as an estimate of the asymptotic variance-covariance matrix of these estimators. This has been pointed out by Little and Rubin (1987, Section 8.2.2) and Laird (1988, p. 307). In addition, there are other reasons for preferring the observed information matrix (Efron and Hinkley 1978).

The use of the expected information matrix is more problematic. The expectation in (5.13) needs to be taken over the *unconditional* sampling distribution (the *unconditional information* i_U) and consequently the use of the naive sampling framework (producing the *naive information* i_N) can lead to inconsistent estimates of precision. In the next section we give an example of the bias resulting from the use of the naive framework. It is possible however, as we show below, to calculate the unconditional information by taking expectations over the appropriate distribution and so correct this bias. Although this added complication is generally unnecessary in practice, given the availability of the observed information, it does allow a direct examination of the effect of ignoring the missing value mechanism on the expected information.

As part of the process of frequentist inference we also need to consider the sampling distribution of the test statistics. Provided that use is made of the likelihood ratio, or Wald and score statistics based on the observed information, then reference to a null asymptotic χ^2 distribution will be appropriate because this is derived from the *implicit* use of the unconditional sampling framework. Only in those situations in which the sampling distribution is explicitly constructed must care be taken to ensure that the unconditional framework is used, that is, account must be taken of the missing data mechanism.

5.8.2   Illustration $*$

For an incomplete multivariate normal sample Little and Rubin (1987) state: "If the data are MCAR, the expected information matrix of $\theta = (\mu, \Sigma)$ represented as a vector is block diagonal. (...) The observed information matrix, which is calculated and inverted at each iteration of the Newton-Raphson algorithm, is not block diagonal with respect to μ and Σ, so this simplification does not occur if standard errors are based on this matrix. On the other hand, the standard errors based on the observed information matrix are more conditional and thus valid when the data are MAR but not MCAR, and hence should be preferable to those based on [the expected information] in applications."

Suppose now that we have N independent pairs of observations, (Y_{i1}, Y_{i2}) each with a bivariate Gaussian distribution with mean vector $\mu = (\mu_1, \mu_2)'$ and variance-covariance matrix

$$\Sigma = \begin{pmatrix} \sigma_{11} & \sigma_{12} \\ \sigma_{12} & \sigma_{22} \end{pmatrix}.$$

It is assumed that m complete pairs, and only the first member (Y_{i1}) of the remaining pairs, are observed. This implies that the dropout process can be represented by a scalar indicator R_i which is 1 if the second component is observed and 0 otherwise. The log-likelihood can be expressed as the sum of the log-likelihoods for the complete and incomplete pairs:

$$\ell = \sum_{i=1}^{m} \ln f(y_{i1}, y_{i2} \mid \mu_1, \mu_2, \sigma_{11}, \sigma_{12}, \sigma_{22}) + \sum_{i=m+1}^{N} \ln f(y_{i1} \mid \mu_1, \sigma_{11}),$$

which, in the Gaussian setting, has kernel,

$$\ell = -\frac{n-m}{2} \ln \sigma_{11} - \frac{m}{2} \ln \mid \Sigma \mid -\frac{1}{2\sigma_{11}} \sum_{i=m+1}^{N} (y_{i1} - \mu_1)^2$$

$$-\frac{1}{2} \sum_{i=1}^{m} \begin{pmatrix} y_{i1} - \mu_1 \\ y_{i2} - \mu_2 \end{pmatrix}' \begin{pmatrix} \sigma_{11} & \sigma_{12} \\ \sigma_{12} & \sigma_{22} \end{pmatrix}^{-1} \begin{pmatrix} y_{i1} - \mu_1 \\ y_{i2} - \mu_2 \end{pmatrix}.$$

Straightforward differentiation produces the elements of the observed information matrix that relate to μ:

$$i_O(\mu, \mu) = (n - m) \begin{pmatrix} \sigma_{11}^{-1} & 0 \\ 0 & 0 \end{pmatrix} + m\Sigma^{-1},$$

and

$$i_O(\mu_j, \sigma_{k\ell}) = \begin{cases} \displaystyle\sum_{i=m+1}^{n} \frac{y_{i1} - \mu_1}{\sigma_{11}^2} \\ \displaystyle + \sum_{i=1}^{m} e_1' \Sigma^{-1} E_{11} \Sigma^{-1} \begin{pmatrix} y_{i1} - \mu_1 \\ y_{i2} - \mu_2 \end{pmatrix}, & j = k = \ell = 1, \\ \displaystyle \sum_{i=1}^{m} e_j' \Sigma^{-1} E_{k\ell} \Sigma^{-1} \begin{pmatrix} y_{i1} - \mu_1 \\ y_{i2} - \mu_2 \end{pmatrix}, & \text{otherwise,} \end{cases}$$

$$\tag{5.14}$$

for

$$e_1 = \begin{pmatrix} 1 \\ 0 \end{pmatrix}, \ e_2 = \begin{pmatrix} 0 \\ 1 \end{pmatrix}$$

and

$$E_{11} = \begin{pmatrix} 1 & 0 \\ 0 & 0 \end{pmatrix}, \ E_{12} = \begin{pmatrix} 0 & 1 \\ 1 & 0 \end{pmatrix}, \ E_{22} = \begin{pmatrix} 0 & 0 \\ 0 & 1 \end{pmatrix}.$$

For the naive information we just take expectations of these quantities over $(Y_{i1}, Y_{i2})' \sim N(\mu, \Sigma)$ for $i = 1, \dots m$ and $Y_{i1} \sim N(\mu_1, \sigma_{11})$ for $i = m+1, \dots, n$. It follows at once that the cross-terms linking the mean and variance-covariance parameters vanish, establishing the familiar orthogonality property of these sets of parameters in the Gaussian setting. We now examine the behavior of the expected information under the actual sampling process implied by the MAR mechanism.

We need to consider first the conditional expectation of these quantities given the occurrence of R, the dropout pattern. Because $(\boldsymbol{Y}, R)$ enters the expression for $i_U(\boldsymbol{\mu}, \boldsymbol{\mu})$ only through m, the naive and unconditional information matrices for $\boldsymbol{\mu}$ are effectively equivalent. However we show now that this is not true for the cross-term elements of the information matrices. Define $\alpha_j = \mathrm{E}(Y_{i1} \mid r_i = j) - \mu_1$, $j = 0, 1$. For the conditional expectation of Y_{i2} in the complete subgroup we have

$$\mathrm{E}(Y_{i2} \mid r_i = 1) = \int \left\{ y_{i2} \int f(y_{i2} \mid y_{i1}) dy_{i2} \right\} f(y_{i1} \mid r_i = 1) dy_{i1}$$

$$= \mu_2 - \sigma_{12} \sigma_{11}^{-1} \mu_1 + \frac{\sigma_{12}}{\sigma_{11} \mathrm{P}(r_i = 1)} \int y_{i1} f(y_{i1}, r_i = 1) dy_{i1}$$

$$= \mu_2 + \sigma_{12} \sigma_{11}^{-1} \{\mathrm{E}(Y_{i1} \mid r_i = 1) - \mu_1\}$$

or

$$\mathrm{E}_{Y|R}(Y_{i2} - \mu_2) = \beta \alpha_1$$

for $\beta = \sigma_{12} \sigma_{11}^{-1}$. Hence

$$\mathrm{E}_{Y|R} \left\{ \left(\begin{array}{c} Y_{i1} - \mu_1 \\ Y_{i2} - \mu_2 \end{array} \right) \right\} = \alpha_1 \left(\begin{array}{c} 1 \\ \beta \end{array} \right).$$

Noting that

$$\Sigma^{-1} \left(\begin{array}{c} 1 \\ \beta \end{array} \right) = \left(\begin{array}{c} \sigma_{11}^{-1} \\ 0 \end{array} \right) = \sigma_{11}^{-1} \boldsymbol{e_1},$$

we then have from (5.14)

$$\mathrm{E}_{Y|R} \{i_O(\mu_j, \sigma_{kl})\} = \left\{ \begin{array}{ll} (n - m) \frac{\alpha_0}{\sigma_{11}^2} + m \frac{\alpha_1}{\sigma_{11}} \boldsymbol{e_1}' \Sigma^{-1} \boldsymbol{E_{11}} \boldsymbol{e_1} & j = k = \ell = 1, \\ m \frac{\alpha_1}{\sigma_{11}} \boldsymbol{e_j}' \Sigma^{-1} \boldsymbol{E_{k\ell}} \boldsymbol{e_1} & \text{otherwise.} \end{array} \right.$$

Finally, taking expectations over R, we get for the cross-terms of the unconditional information matrix:

$$i_U(\boldsymbol{\mu}, \sigma_{11}) = \frac{n}{\sigma_{11}} \left\{ \frac{(1 - \pi) \alpha_0}{\sigma_{11}} \left(\begin{array}{c} 1 \\ 0 \end{array} \right) + \frac{\pi \alpha_1}{\sigma_{11} \sigma_{22} - \sigma_{12}^2} \left(\begin{array}{c} \sigma_{22} \\ -\sigma_{12} \end{array} \right) \right\} \quad (5.15)$$

$$i_U(\boldsymbol{\mu}, \sigma_{12}) = \frac{n \pi \alpha_1}{\sigma_{11} \sigma_{22} - \sigma_{12}^2} \left(\begin{array}{c} -\beta \\ 1 \end{array} \right), \quad (5.16)$$

$$i_U(\boldsymbol{\mu}, \sigma_{22}) = \left(\begin{array}{c} 0 \\ 0 \end{array} \right), \quad (5.17)$$

for $\pi = \mathrm{P}(r_i = 1)$. In contrast to the naive information these cross-terms do not all vanish, and the orthogonality of mean and variance-covariance parameters is lost under the MAR mechanism. One implication of this is that although the information relating to the linear model parameters alone is not affected by the move from an MCAR to an MAR mechanism, the asymptotic variance-covariance matrix *is* affected due to the induced non-orthogonality and therefore the dropout mechanism cannot be regarded as ignorable as far as the estimation of precision of the estimators of the linear model parameters is concerned. It can also be shown that the expected information for the variance-covariance parameters is not equivalent under the MCAR and MAR dropout mechanisms, but the expressions are more involved. Assuming that π is non-zero, it can be seen that the necessary and sufficient condition for the terms in (5.15) and (5.16) to be equal to zero is that $\alpha_0 = \alpha_1 = 0$, the condition defining, as expected, an MCAR mechanism.

We now illustrate these findings with a few numerical results. The off-diagonal unconditional information elements (5.15)–(5.17) are computed for sample size $n = 1000$, mean vector $(0,0)'$ and two covariance matrices: (1) $\sigma_{11} = \sigma_{22} = 1$ and correlation $\rho = \sigma_{12} = 0.5$, and (2) $\sigma_{11} = 2$, $\sigma_{33} = 3$, and $\rho = 0.5$ leading to $\sigma_{12} = \sqrt{6}/2$. Further, two MAR dropout mechanisms are considered. They are both of the logistic form

$$P(R_1 = 0|y_{i1}) = \frac{\exp(\gamma_0 + \gamma_1 y_{i1})}{1 + \exp(\gamma_0 + \gamma_1 y_{i1})}.$$

We choose $\gamma_0 = 0$ and (a) $\gamma_1 = 1$ or (b) $\gamma_1 = -\infty$. The latter mechanism implies $r_i = 0$ if $y_{i1} \geq 0$ and $r_i = 1$ otherwise. Both dropout mechanisms yield $\pi = 0.5$. In all cases $\alpha_1 = -\alpha_0$, with α_1 in the four possible combinations of covariance and dropout parameters: (1a) 0.4132, (1b) 0.7263, (2a) $\sqrt{2/\pi}$, (2b) $2/\sqrt{\pi}$. Numerical values for (5.15)–(5.17) are presented in Table 5.13, as well as the average from the observed information matrices in a simulation with 500 replicates.

Obviously, these elements are far from zero, as would be found with the naive estimator. They are of the same order of magnitude as the upper left block of the information matrix (pertaining to the mean parameters), which are

$$\begin{pmatrix} 1166.67 & -333.33 \\ -333.33 & 666.67 \end{pmatrix}.$$

We performed a limited simulation study to verify the coverage probability for the Wald tests under the unconditional and a selection of conditional frameworks. The hypotheses considered are $H_{01} : \mu_1 = 0$, $H_{02} : \mu_2 = 0$, and $H_{03} : \mu_1 = \mu_2 = 0$. The simulations have been restricted to the first covariance matrix used in Table 5.13 and to the second dropout mechanism ($\gamma_1 = -\infty$). Results are reported in Table 5.14. The coverages for the unconditional framework are in good agreement with a χ^2 reference distribution, the first naive framework (500 complete cases) leads to a conservative procedure, whereas the second and the third lead to extreme

TABLE 5.13. *Bivariate normal data. Computed and simulated values for the off-diagonal block of the unconditional information matrix. Sample size is $n = 1000$ (500 replications). (The true model has zero mean vector. Two true covariances Σ and two dropout parameters γ_1 are considered.)*

parameters			uncond. $i_U(\boldsymbol{\mu}, .)$			simulated $\widehat{i_O}(\boldsymbol{\mu}, .)$		
Σ		γ_1	σ_{11}	σ_{12}	σ_{22}	σ_{11}	σ_{12}	σ_{22}
1	0.5	1	-68.87	137.75	0.00	-69.36	137.95	-0.04
0.5	1		137.75	-275.49	0.00	137.88	-276.83	-0.04
2	$\sqrt{6}/2$	1	-30.26	49.42	0.00	-30.21	49.54	0.04
$\sqrt{6}/2$	3		49.42	-80.70	0.00	49.52	-81.31	0.06
1	0.5	$-\infty$	132.98	-265.96	0.00	135.67	-267.66	0.16
0.5	1		-265.96	531.92	0.00	-267.73	537.58	-0.02
2	$\sqrt{6}/2$	$-\infty$	47.02	-76.78	0.00	49.52	-78.73	-0.02
$\sqrt{6}/2$	3		-76.78	125.38	0.00	-78.58	126.91	0.02

TABLE 5.14. *Bivariate normal data. True values are as in the third model of Table 5.13. Coverage probabilities ($\times 1000$) for Wald test statistics. Sample size is $n = 1000$ (500 replications). The null hypotheses are $H_{01} : \mu_1 = 0$, $H_{02} : \mu_2 = 0$, $H_{03} : \mu_1 = \mu_2 = 0$. For the naive sampling frameworks, m denotes the fixed number of complete cases.*

hypothesis	uncond.	$m = 500$	$m = 450$	$m = 400$
H_{01}	933	996	187	0
H_{02}	953	952	913	830
H_{03}	952	992	338	0

liberal behavior, that is most marked for hypotheses H_{01} and H_{03}. This is to be expected, because by fixing $m = 500$, the proportion of positive first outcomes is constrained to be equal to its predicted value. This has the effect of reducing the variability of $\hat{\mu}_1$. The second and the third framework also suppress the variability, but introduce bias at the same time. The comparative insensitivity of the behavior of the test for H_{02} to the sampling framework is because μ_1 has only an indirect influence through the correlation between the outcomes on both occasions. It should be noted that due to numerical problems, not all simulations led to 500 successful estimations. On average, 489 convergencies were observed, the lowest value being 460 for H_{02} in the first naive sampling frame.

5.8.3 Example *

We will now consider a relatively small example with a continuous response, analyzed in Crépeau et al (1985). 54 rats were divided into five treatment groups corresponding to exposure to increasing doses of halothane (0%, 0.25%, 0.5%, 1% and 2%). The groups were of sizes 11, 10, 11, 11, and 11 rats respectively. Following an induced heart attack in each rat the blood pressure was recorded on nine unequally spaced occasions. A number of rats died during the course of the experiment, including all rats from group 5 (2% halothane). Following the original authors we omit this group from the analysis since they contribute no information at all, leaving 43 rats, of which 23 survived the experiment.

Examination of the data from these four groups does not provide any evidence of an MAR dropout process, although this observation must be considered in the light of the small sample size. A Gaussian multivariate linear model with an unconstrained covariance matrix was fitted to the data. There was very little evidence of a treatment-by-time interaction and the following results are based on the use of a model with additive effects for treatment and time. The Wald statistics for the treatment main effect on 3 degrees of freedom are equal to 46.95 and 30.82 respectively using the expected and observed information matrices. Although leading to the same qualitative conclusions the figures are notably discrepant. A first reaction may be to attribute this difference to the incompleteness of the data. However, the lack of evidence for an MAR process together with the relatively small sample size points to another cause. The equivalent analysis of the 24 completers produces Wald statistics of 45.34 and 26.35 respectively. That is, the effect can be attributed to a combination of small sample variation and possible model misspecification. A theoretical reason for this difference might be that the expected value of the off-diagonal block of the information matrix of the maximum likelihood estimates (describing covariance between mean and covariance parameters) has expectation zero but is likely to depart from this in small samples. As a consequence, the variances of the estimated treatment effects will be higher when derived from the observed information, hereby reducing the Wald statistic.

To summarize, this example provides an illustration of an alternative source of discrepancy between the expected and observed information matrices, which is likely to be associated with the use, in smaller samples, of covariance matrices with many parameters.

5.8.4   Implications for PROC MIXED

The literature indicates an early awareness of problems with conventional likelihood-based frequentist inference in the MAR setting. Specifically, several authors point to the use of the observed information matrix as a way to circumvent issues with the expected information matrix. In spite of this, it seems that a broad awareness of this problem has diminished while the number of methods formulated to deal with the MAR situation has risen dramatically in recent years. We therefore feel that a restatement and exposition of this important problem is timely, especially since PROC MIXED allows routine fitting of ignorable models with likelihood based methods.

The MIXED procedure allows both Newton-Raphson and Fisher scoring algorithms. Specifying the 'scoring' option in the PROC MIXED statement requests the Fisher scoring algorithm in conjunction with the method of estimation for a specified number of iterations (1 by default). If convergence is reached before scoring stopped, then the expected Hessian is used to compute approximate standard errors rather than the observed Hessian. In both cases, the standard errors for the fixed effects are based on inverting a single block of the Hessian matrix. Since we have shown in Section 5.8.2 that the off-diagonal block, pertaining to the covariance between the fixed effects and covariance parameters, does not have expectation zero, this procedure is, strictly speaking, incorrect. Correction factors to overcome this problem have been proposed (e.g., Prasad and Rao 1990) but they tend to be small for fairly well balanced data sets. It has to be noted that a substantial amount of (randomly) missing data will destroy this balance. The extent to which all this is problematic is illustrated in Table 5.15. Model 7 for the growth data is reconsidered for both the complete data set, as well as for the incomplete data on the basis of an ignorable analysis. The fixed-effects parameters are as in (4.14), while the covariance structure consists of the residual variance σ^2 and the variance of the random intercept d. Apart from the parameter estimates, two sets of standard errors are shown: (1) taken from inverting the fixed-effects block from the observed Hessian and (2) taken from inverting the entire observed Hessian. The first set is found from the MIXED output, while the second one was constructed using the numerical optimizer OPTMUM of GAUSS (Edlefsen). Clearly, there are only minor differences between the two sets of standard errors and the analysis on an incomplete set of data does not seem to widen the gap.

We can conclude from this that, with the exception of the expected information matrix, conventional likelihood-based frequentist inference, including standard hypothesis testing, is applicable in the MAR setting. Standard errors based on inverting the *entire* Hessian are to be preferred and in this sense it is a pity that this option is presently not available in PROC MIXED.

TABLE 5.15. *Maximum likelihood estimates and standard errors (in parentheses) for the parameters in Model 7, fitted to the growth data (complete data set and ignorable analysis).*

	Complete Data	Ignorable
Parameter	Estimate (s.e.)[1] (s.e.)[2]	Estimate (s.e.)[1] (s.e.)[2]
β_0	17.3727 (1.1615,1.1645)	17.2218 (1.2220,1.2207)
β_{01}	-1.0321 (1.5089,1.5156)	-0.9188 (1.5857,1.5814)
β_{10}	0.4795 (0.0923,0.0925)	0.4890 (0.0969,0.0968)
β_{11}	0.7844 (0.0765,0.0767)	0.7867 (0.0802,0.0801)
σ^2	1.8746 (0.2946,0.2946)	2.0173 (0.3365,0.3365)
d	3.0306 (0.9552,0.9550)	3.0953 (1.0011,1.0011)

[1] Standard error based on the Newton-Raphson algorithm of PROC MIXED
[2] Standard error obtained from inverting the entire observed information matrix.

5.9   The Expectation-Maximization Algorithm ✳

While the models in Table 5.8 are fitted using direct observed data likelihood maximization in PROC MIXED, Little and Rubin (1987) obtained these results using the *expectation-maximization* algorithm. Special forms of the algorithm, designed for specific applications, had been proposed for about half a century (e.g., Yates 1933), but the first unifying and formal account was given by Dempster *et al* (1977). McLachlan and Krishnan (1997) devoted a whole volume to the EM algorithm and its extensions.

We will first give a brief description of the algorithm. Suppose we are interested in maximizing the ignorable observed data log-likelihood $\ell(\boldsymbol{\theta}; \boldsymbol{y}^o)$. Let $\boldsymbol{\theta}^{(0)}$ be an initial guess, which can be found from, e.g., a complete case analysis, an available case analysis, single imputation, or any other convenient method.

The EM algorithm consists of an *expectation* and a *maximization* step.

The E Step. Given the current value $\boldsymbol{\theta}^{(t)}$ of the parameter vector, the E step computes the expected value of the complete data log-likelihood, given the observed data and the current parameters, which is called the *objective function*:

$$Q(\boldsymbol{\theta}|\boldsymbol{\theta}^{(t)}) \;=\; \int \ell(\boldsymbol{\theta}, \boldsymbol{y}) f(\boldsymbol{y}^m|\boldsymbol{y}^o, \boldsymbol{\theta}^{(t)}) d\boldsymbol{y}^m$$

$$= E\left\{\ell(\boldsymbol{\theta}|\boldsymbol{y})|\boldsymbol{y}^o,\boldsymbol{\theta}^{(t)}\right\}.$$

In case the log-likelihood is linear in the sufficient statistics, this procedure comes down to substituting the expected value of the sufficient statistics, given $\boldsymbol{Y}^o$ and $\boldsymbol{\theta}^{(t)}$. In particular, for exponential family models, the E step reduces to the computation of complete data sufficient statistics.

The M Step. Next, the M step determines $\boldsymbol{\theta}^{(t+1)}$, the parameter vector maximizing the log-likelihood of the completed data (i.e., the complete data log-likelihood). Formally, $\boldsymbol{\theta}^{(t+1)}$ satisfies

$$Q(\boldsymbol{\theta}^{(t+1)}|\boldsymbol{\theta}^{(t)}) \geq Q(\boldsymbol{\theta}|\boldsymbol{\theta}^{(t)}), \qquad \text{for all } \boldsymbol{\theta}.$$

One then iterates between the E and M steps until convergence.

Consider for example a multivariate normal sample. Then $\boldsymbol{\theta} = (\boldsymbol{\mu}, \Sigma)$. The E step computes

$$E\left(\sum_{i=1}^n Y_{ij}|\boldsymbol{y}^o,\boldsymbol{\theta}^{(t)}\right) \quad \text{and} \quad E\left(\sum_{i=1}^n Y_{ij}Y_{ik}|\boldsymbol{y}^o,\boldsymbol{\theta}^{(t)}\right).$$

From these, computation of $\boldsymbol{\mu}^{(t+1)}$ and $\Sigma^{(t+1)}$ is straightforward.

When the covariance matrix is structured or patterned, the E step remains the same, but the M step is slightly modified. This situation arose when Little and Rubin (1987) fitted the incomplete growth data Models 5–7 using the EM algorithm. Let us sketch their procedure. Emphasis is placed on the patterns in the covariance matrix. The outcomes $\boldsymbol{Y}_i$ are assumed to follow a normal model $\boldsymbol{Y}_i \sim N(\boldsymbol{\mu}_i, \Sigma)$ where $\boldsymbol{\mu}_i = X_i\boldsymbol{\beta}$ and $\Sigma = \Sigma(\boldsymbol{\alpha})$, a known function of $\boldsymbol{\alpha}$, such as a banded, AR(1), or exchangeable model, or a model induced by random effects. The complete data log-likelihood is linear in $\boldsymbol{y}_i$ and $\boldsymbol{y}_i'\boldsymbol{y}_i$. The E step is restricted to computing

$$E\left(\boldsymbol{Y}_i|\boldsymbol{y}_i^o, X_i, Z_i, \boldsymbol{\theta}\right) \quad \text{and} \quad E\left(\boldsymbol{Y}_i'\boldsymbol{y}_i|\boldsymbol{y}_i^o, X_i, Z_i, \boldsymbol{\theta}\right).$$

These computations can easily be done using the *sweep* operator (Little and Rubin 1987).

The M step consists of a standard estimation procedure for complete data. While for simple and unstructured covariance models the M step may be available in closed form, it is usually iterative for patterned covariance matrices, turning the EM algorithm into a doubly iterative scheme. To make the M step non-iterative, a GEM (generalized EM) algorithm can be used. A GEM algorithm merely increases the likelihood in the M step, rather than maximizing it. For example, a single scoring step can be used rather than full convergence. Under general conditions, the convergence of the GEM is the same as for the EM (Dempster *et al* 1977).

Let us write Σ as a function of α for the covariance matrices in the growth example.

Unstructured: $\Sigma = \alpha$.

Banded: $\sigma_{jk} = \alpha_r$ with $r = |j - k| + 1$.

Autoregressive: $\sigma_{jk} = \alpha_1 \alpha_2^{|j-k|}$.

Compound symmetry: $\Sigma = \alpha_1 J_4 + \alpha_2 I_4$ with J_4 a matrix of ones.

Random-effects: $\Sigma = Z\alpha Z' + \sigma^2 I$ with α the covariance matrix of the random effects.

Independence: $\Sigma = \alpha I_4$.

The mean structure design matrices X_i are as discussed in Section 4.4.

The main drawbacks of the EM algorithm are its typically slow rate of convergence. The double iterative structure of many implementations adds to the problem. Further, the algorithm does not automatically provide precision estimators. Proposals for overcoming these limitations have been made by e.g., Louis (1982), Meilijson (1989), Meng and Rubin (1991) and Baker (1992).

In the light of these observations, one might argue that the existence of PROC MIXED, enabling the use of Newton-Raphson or Fisher scoring algorithms to maximize the observed data likelihood is fortunate. While this statement is certainly warranted for a wide range of applications, there may be situations where the EM algorithm is beneficial. Baker (1994) mentions advantages of starting with an EM algorithm and then switching to Newton-Raphson, if necessary, including less sensitivity to poor starting values and more reliable convergence to a boundary when the maximum likelihood estimators is indeed a boundary value. In the latter situation, Newton-Raphson and Fisher scoring algorithms exhibit a tendency to converge to values outside the allowable parameter space. Further, the EM algorithm can be easily extended for use with non-ignorable problems, such as discussed by Diggle and Kenward (1994). This route was explicitly chosen by Molenberghs, Kenward, and Lesaffre (1997) for a comparable categorical data setting. Non-ignorable missing data will be discussed further in Section 5.11. The next section is devoted to a method which combines the ease of single imputation with the ability to reach valid inferences.

5.10   Multiple Imputation ✳

Multiple imputation was formally introduced by Rubin (1978). The concept refers to replacing each missing value by more than one imputed value. The goal is to combine the simplicity of imputation strategies, with unbiasedness in both point estimates and measures of precision. In Section 5.5 we have seen that some simple imputation procedures may yield inconsistent point estimates as soon as the missingness mechanism surpasses MCAR. This could be overcome to a large extent with conditional mean imputation, but the problem of underestimating the variability of the estimators was common to all methods since they all treat imputed values as observed values. By imputing several values for a single missing component, this uncertainty is explicitly acknowledged.

Rubin (1987), who gives a comprehensive treatment of the subject, points to another very useful application of multiple imputation. Rather than merely accounting for *sampling uncertainty*, the method can be used to incorporate *model uncertainty*. Indeed, when a measurement is missing but the researcher has a good idea about the probabilistic measurement and missingness mechanisms, then constructing the appropriate distribution to draw imputations from is, at least in principle, relatively straightforward. In practice there may be considerable uncertainty about some parts of the joint model. In that case, several mechanisms for drawing imputations might seem equally plausible. They can be combined in a single multiple imputation analysis. As such, multiple imputation can be used as a tool for sensitivity analysis.

In this section, we will review the general theory of multiple imputation. It has been presented extensively by Rubin (1987). Several other sources, such as Rubin and Schenker (1986), Little and Rubin (1987), and Tanner and Wong (1987) give excellent descriptions of the technique. Efron (1994) discusses connections between multiple imputation and the bootstrap. Then, applications to the linear mixed model are discussed. There are two quite distinct reasons for including multiple imputation in this text. First, the ignorable analysis of Section 5.7 based on PROC MIXED, which coincides with the corresponding EM algorithm analysis (Section 5.9) as performed by Little and Rubin (1987) can be usefully contrasted with multiple imputation. It will be seen that applying this method sheds additional light on certain aspects of the missing data process. It will serve as an easy introduction to the principles of multiple imputation. Of course, since PROC MIXED is very flexible in dealing with missing *outcomes*, there is most often no compelling reason to apply multiple imputation, except for reasons of comparison and confirmation. The second reason to discuss it here is that in more complex applications one might be confronted not only with missing outcomes but also with missing *covariates*. Then, multiple imputation could be used to create a number of versions of the completed covariate information, where after PROC MIXED can be run on each of these, say M, completed data bases. The multiple imputation methodology allows combination of the M inferences into a single one.

5.10.1   General Theory   ✱

Suppose we have a sample of N, i.i.d. $n \times 1$ random vectors $\boldsymbol{Y}_i$. Our interest lies in estimating some parameter vector $\boldsymbol{\theta}$ of the distribution of $\boldsymbol{Y}_i$.

Group the observed and missing parts for the N subjects as follows:

$$\boldsymbol{Y}^o = (\boldsymbol{Y}_1^o, \ldots, \boldsymbol{Y}_N^o) \quad \text{and} \quad \boldsymbol{Y}^m = (\boldsymbol{Y}_1^m, \ldots, \boldsymbol{Y}_N^m).$$

Multiple imputation fills in $\boldsymbol{Y}^m$ using the observed data $\boldsymbol{Y}^o$, and then the completed data are used to estimate $\boldsymbol{\theta}$.

As discussed by Rubin and Schenker (1986), the theoretical justification for multiple imputation is most easily understood using Bayesian concepts, but a likelihood-based treatment of the subject is equally possible. If we knew the joint distribution of $\boldsymbol{Y}_i = (\boldsymbol{Y}_i^o, \boldsymbol{Y}_i^m)$ with parameter vector $\boldsymbol{\gamma}$ say, then we could impute $\boldsymbol{Y}_i^m$ by drawing a value of $\boldsymbol{Y}_i^m$ from the conditional distribution

$$f(\boldsymbol{y}_i^m | \boldsymbol{y}_i^o, \boldsymbol{\gamma}). \tag{5.18}$$

Note that we explicitly distinguish the parameter of scientific interest $\boldsymbol{\theta}$ from the parameter $\boldsymbol{\gamma}$ in (5.18). Since $\boldsymbol{\gamma}$ is unknown, we must estimate it from the data, say $\hat{\boldsymbol{\gamma}}$, and presumably use

$$f(\boldsymbol{y}_i^m | \boldsymbol{y}_i^o, \hat{\boldsymbol{\gamma}}) \tag{5.19}$$

to impute the missing data. In Bayesian terms, $\boldsymbol{\gamma}$ in (5.18) is a random variable of which the distribution is a function of the data. In particular, we first obtain the distribution of $\boldsymbol{\gamma}$ from the data, and this distribution is a function of $\hat{\boldsymbol{\gamma}}$. The construction of model (5.18) is referred to by Rubin (1987) as the Modeling Task.

After formulating the distribution of $\boldsymbol{\gamma}$, the imputation algorithm is:

1. Draw $\boldsymbol{\gamma}^*$ from the distribution of $\boldsymbol{\gamma}$.

2. Draw $\boldsymbol{Y}_i^{m*}$ from $f(\boldsymbol{y}_i^m | \boldsymbol{y}_i^o, \boldsymbol{\gamma}^*)$.

3. Using the completed data, $(\boldsymbol{Y}^o, \boldsymbol{Y}^{m*})$, and the method of choice (i.e., maximum likelihood, restricted maximum likelihood, method

of moments, partial likelihood), estimate the parameter of interest $\hat{\boldsymbol{\theta}} = \hat{\boldsymbol{\theta}}(\boldsymbol{Y}) = \hat{\boldsymbol{\theta}}(\boldsymbol{Y}^o, \boldsymbol{Y}^{m*})$ and its variance (called *within*-imputation variance) $\boldsymbol{U} = \widehat{\text{Var}}(\hat{\boldsymbol{\theta}})$.

4. Independently repeat steps 1–3 M times. The M data sets give rise to $\hat{\boldsymbol{\theta}}^{(m)}$ and $\boldsymbol{U}^{(m)}$, for $m = 1, ..., M$.

Steps 1 and 2 are referred to as the Imputation Task. Step 3 is the Estimation Task. Of course, one wants to combine the M inferences into a single one. This will be discussed next.

The M within-imputation estimates for $\boldsymbol{\theta}$ are pooled to give the multiple imputation estimate:

$$\hat{\boldsymbol{\theta}}^* = \frac{1}{M} \sum_{m=1}^{M} \hat{\boldsymbol{\theta}}^{(m)}.$$

Suppose that complete data inference about $\boldsymbol{\theta}$ would be made by $(\boldsymbol{\theta} - \hat{\boldsymbol{\theta}}) \sim N(\boldsymbol{0}, \boldsymbol{U})$. Then, one can make normal based inferences for $\boldsymbol{\theta}$ based upon $(\boldsymbol{\theta} - \hat{\boldsymbol{\theta}}^*) \sim N(\boldsymbol{0}, \boldsymbol{V})$, where

$$V = \hat{W} + \left(\frac{M+1}{M} \right) \hat{B}, \tag{5.20}$$

$$\hat{W} = \frac{\sum_{m=1}^{M} \boldsymbol{U}^{(m)}}{M} \tag{5.21}$$

is the average within-imputation variance, and

$$\hat{B} = \frac{\sum_{m=1}^{M} (\hat{\boldsymbol{\theta}}^{(m)} - \hat{\boldsymbol{\theta}}^*)(\hat{\boldsymbol{\theta}}^{(m)} - \hat{\boldsymbol{\theta}}^*)'}{M - 1} \tag{5.22}$$

is the between-imputation variance (Rubin 1987). Rubin and Schenker (1986) report that a small number of imputations ($M = 2, 3$) already yields a major improvement over single imputation. Upon noting that the factor $(M + 1)/M$ approaches 1 for large M, (5.20) is approximately the sum of the within and the between imputations variability. In the next section, the technique will be illustrated on the basis of 5 and 25 imputations.

Multiple imputation is most useful in situations where $\boldsymbol{\gamma}$ is an easily estimated set of parameters characterizing the distribution of $\boldsymbol{Y}_i$, while $\boldsymbol{\theta}$ is complicated to estimate in the presence of missing data. In the next section, we will indicate how to proceed when $\boldsymbol{\gamma}$ and $\boldsymbol{\theta}$ refer at least partly to the same parameters.

TABLE 5.16. *Growth data. Parameter estimates (standard errors) for the imputation model (Model 1 on the complete cases).*

Mean Model		Covariance Model	
Parameter	Estimate (s.e.)	Parameter	Estimate (s.e.)
girls 8	22.286 (0.566)	σ_{11}	2.246 (0.749)
girls 10	22.786 (0.782)	σ_{12}	2.316 (0.912)
girls 12	23.929 (0.883)	σ_{13}	2.383 (0.998)
girls 14	25.071 (0.745)	σ_{14}	2.075 (0.851)
boys 8	24.000 (0.452)	σ_{22}	4.276 (1.426)
boys 10	24.136 (0.624)	σ_{23}	2.042 (1.236)
boys 12	26.591 (0.704)	σ_{24}	2.574 (1.136)
boys 14	27.682 (0.594)	σ_{33}	5.451 (1.817)
		σ_{34}	3.075 (1.304)
		σ_{44}	3.881 (1.294)

5.10.2   Illustration: Growth Data   ✳

Let us illustrate the performance of multiple imputation on the growth data set. Our aim is to estimate the parameters of Model 7, assuming a linear trend with separate slopes for boys and girls, and an exchangeable covariance matrix. This model has 6 parameters: the 4 mean model parameters of (4.14), $\boldsymbol{\beta} = (\beta_0, \beta_{01}, \beta_1, \beta_{11})'$ are supplemented with d and σ^2 of the covariance matrix $H = dJ_4 + \sigma^2 I_4$. These parameters form the vector

$$\boldsymbol{\theta} = (\beta_0, \beta_{01}, \beta_{10}, \beta_{11}, \sigma^2, d)$$

of Section 5.10.1.

In Section 5.5.3 it was argued that conditional mean imputation, following the conditional model (5.8) leads to valid point estimates, although it might overestimate the precision. The parameters of (5.8) are grouped into the vector $\boldsymbol{\gamma}$ of Section 5.10.1. To avoid misspecification for the imputation model, it is wise to keep it as general as possible. A possible candidate is Model 1, with a separate mean for each age by sex combination, and a common unstructured covariance matrix. In this way, $\boldsymbol{\gamma}$ is made up of 18 parameters. As in conditional mean imputation Section 5.5.3, $\hat{\boldsymbol{\gamma}}$ will be determined using the complete cases. Since we have to draw $\boldsymbol{\gamma}^*$ from its distribution, we also need the (18×18) covariance matrix of $\hat{\boldsymbol{\gamma}}$, $\hat{C}$ say. Table 5.16 displays the parameter estimates and their standard errors. The covariances are not shown. Even though these parameter estimates can be obtained from PROC MIXED we have chosen to write a single GAUSS

(Edlefsen and Jones) program with which the entire multiple imputation process can be completed. This GAUSS program, together with a SAS macro, are available from the Web page listed in the Preface.

The first step is to draw a vector γ^* from a $N(\hat{\gamma}, \hat{C})$ distribution. Should the normal approximation be questionable, in particular for the covariance parameters, then a normal distribution for the mean parameters can be combined with a Wishart distribution for the covariance parameters.

Plugging in γ^* in (5.8) yields

$$Y_i^m | y_i^o \sim N(\mu_{\text{IMP}}, \Sigma_{\text{IMP}}), \tag{5.23}$$

with

$$\mu_{\text{IMP}} = \mu^m + \Sigma^{mo*}(\Sigma^{oo*})^{-1}(y_i^o - \mu_i^{o*}),$$

$$\Sigma_{\text{IMP}} = \Sigma^{mm*} - \Sigma^{mo*}(\Sigma^{oo*})^{-1}\Sigma^{om*}).$$

In our case, for the 9 incomplete observations of the growth data set, m refers to age 10, while o refers to ages 8, 12, and 14. Next, rather than merely plugging in the conditional mean, a draw is made from conditional distribution (5.23). Let us choose to construct $M = 5$ imputations. For instance, for the second boy, with true profile (21.5, 22.5, 23.0, 26.5) but where 22.5 had been deleted, the 5 imputed values are 21.815, 19.793, 20.223, 23.400, 23.145. Even though Little and Rubin (1987) suggest that a moderate number of imputations ($M = 2, 3$) often gives very satisfactory results, the size of the data problem is modest and we consider a somewhat larger number of imputations.

Model 7 will be fitted to each of the $M = 5$ imputed data sets. This is done using the same GAUSS program. One of the reasons to do so is that it is very convenient to retain from each analysis not only the 6 parameter estimates, but also the corresponding (6×6) covariance matrix. Technically, a Newton-Raphson optimization of the four dimensional normal log-likelihood function is done using the GAUSS routine OPTMUM. The 5 sets of parameter estimates are shown in Table 5.17.

We now construct the covariance estimator (5.20). The within variability (5.21), obtained by pooling the variance estimates of each imputed data set, is

$$\begin{pmatrix}
1.4971 & -1.4941 & -0.1059 & -0.0002 & 0.0000 & -0.0001 \\
-1.4941 & 2.5206 & 0.1057 & -0.0726 & -0.0001 & 0.0001 \\
-0.1059 & 0.1057 & 0.0096 & 0.0000 & -0.0000 & 0.0000 \\
-0.0002 & -0.0726 & 0.0000 & 0.0066 & 0.0000 & -0.0000 \\
0.0000 & -0.0001 & -0.0000 & 0.0000 & 0.1413 & -0.0353 \\
-0.0001 & 0.0001 & 0.0000 & -0.0000 & -0.0353 & 1.2125
\end{pmatrix}.$$

TABLE 5.17. *Growth data. Parameter estimates for multiply imputed data sets (Model 7).*

m	β_0	β_{01}	β_{10}	β_{11}	σ^2	d
1	16.7006	-0.6727	0.5216	0.8039	1.9909	3.5437
2	16.4536	-1.4221	0.5370	0.8662	3.6931	4.0140
3	16.4708	-0.8952	0.5359	0.8322	2.4969	3.8124
4	16.4513	-0.2093	0.5371	0.7905	2.0342	3.5680
5	16.7223	-1.1114	0.5202	0.8300	2.5198	3.8945

The 'off-diagonal block', pertaining to the covariance between the 4 mean and 2 covariance parameters, is close to zero, as expected. The between variability (5.22), measuring the variance of the 5 estimated parameter vectors, and hence the additional uncertainty due to incompleteness, is

$$
\begin{pmatrix}
0.0193 & -0.0056 & -0.0012 & -0.0009 & -0.0361 & -0.0049 \\
-0.0056 & 0.2097 & 0.0003 & -0.0128 & -0.2684 & -0.0859 \\
-0.0012 & 0.0003 & 0.0001 & 0.0001 & 0.0023 & 0.0003 \\
-0.0009 & -0.0128 & 0.0001 & 0.0009 & 0.0190 & 0.0057 \\
-0.0361 & -0.2684 & 0.0023 & 0.0190 & 0.4722 & 0.1259 \\
-0.0049 & -0.0859 & 0.0003 & 0.0057 & 0.1259 & 0.0422
\end{pmatrix}.
$$

Note that the between variability is orders of magnitude smaller than the within variability for the β parameters, in particular for the slope parameters β_{10} and β_{11}. The situation changes for σ^2 where the between variability is larger than the within variability.

The 'total' covariance matrix, computed as in (5.20) is

$$
\begin{pmatrix}
1.5196 & -1.5005 & -0.1073 & -0.0012 & -0.0421 & -0.0057 \\
-1.5005 & 2.7653 & 0.1061 & -0.0875 & -0.3131 & -0.1002 \\
-0.1073 & 0.1061 & 0.0097 & 0.0001 & 0.0026 & 0.0004 \\
-0.0012 & -0.0875 & 0.0001 & 0.0076 & 0.0222 & 0.0066 \\
-0.0421 & -0.3131 & 0.0026 & 0.0222 & 0.6922 & 0.1116 \\
-0.0057 & -0.1002 & 0.0004 & 0.0066 & 0.1116 & 1.2618
\end{pmatrix}
\quad (5.24)
$$

As was observed in Section 5.8, incompleteness of the data set results in (small) covariances between mean model and covariance model parameters.

The overall estimate for the parameter vector $\boldsymbol{\theta}$ is the average of the 5 estimates in Table 5.17. The precision is estimated from (5.24). The results are displayed in Table 5.18, together with results from a few methods discussed earlier. We performed a second multiple imputation analysis based on $M = 25$ imputations. Even though multiple imputations were created from a model based on the completers, it does not suffer from the biases

TABLE 5.18. *Growth data. Parameter estimates (standard errors) for Model 7 (complete case analysis, ignorable analysis, conditional mean imputation, multiple imputation (M = 5 and M = 25)).*

Par.	CC	Ignorable	Cond.Mean	MI(5)	MI(25)
β_0	18.29(1.38)	17.22(1.22)	16.75(1.24)	16.56(1.23)	16.86(1.40)
β_{01}	-0.12(1.77)	-0.92(1.59)	-0.91(1.61)	-0.86(1.66)	-1.06(1.70)
β_{10}	0.68(0.09)	0.79(0.08)	0.82(0.08)	0.83(0.09)	0.82(0.09)
β_{11}	0.48(0.11)	0.49(0.10)	0.52(0.10)	0.53(0.10)	0.51(0.11)
σ^2	1.75(0.34)	2.02(0.34)	2.13(0.33)	2.55(0.83)	2.47(1.02)
d	2.36(0.94)	3.10(1.00)	3.55(1.12)	3.77(1.12)	3.47(1.19)

seen in the complete case analysis (e.g., overestimated intercepts and underestimated slopes). A similar observation was made about the conditional mean imputation analysis. In fact, the parameter estimates and standard errors are somewhat closer to those obtained under conditional mean imputation than to the ignorable analysis results. Earlier, we argued that the conditional mean imputation is slightly hampered by the fact that the correlation structure among the completers is different from the one in the complete data set (see, e.g., the correlation matrix under Model 1 in Sections 4.4 and 5.4). For conditional mean imputation this implied that the imputed values for age 10 were too close to the corresponding age 8 measurement. For multiple imputation, the imputation model is based on the same model, explaining the relatively close agreement between both single and multiple imputation strategies. The main difference between both is that the standard errors are somewhat larger, which is to be expected since an additional source of uncertainty is taken into account. The most striking difference is that the standard error of σ^2 is very large under multiple imputation, compared to all three other methods. This could be explained by the fact that the distribution of σ^2 is fairly skewed and hence the normality assumption in constructing draws γ^* was not entirely appropriate. This is confirmed by considering the median of the 25 individual estimates under MI($M = 25$), which are 16.940, −1.047, 0.816, 0.507, 2.236, and 3.462 respectively. Finally, MI($M = 5$) and MI($M = 25$) lead to virtually the same conclusions.

In summary, multiple imputation is a valuable technique that combines the ease of a single imputation method with valid precision estimators. Its performance depends on the quality of the imputation model. The example studied in this section can be analyzed in a correct and computationally efficient way using the ignorable analysis method in PROC MIXED. As such, multiple imputation would not be envisaged for a standard analysis of this data set. Arguable, multiple imputation would prove useful in different situations, such as missing covariates. Further, it can be extended to informative non-response (Rubin 1987, pp. 202–243).

5.11   Exploring the Missing Data Process

In the previous sections we argued that an ignorable analysis, performed either using PROC MIXED (Section 5.7), the EM algorithm (Section 5.9), or multiple imputation (Section 5.10), was to be preferred over complete case analysis (Section 5.4), some forms of single imputation (Section 5.5), and available case analysis (Section 5.6), since it is based on the more flexible MAR assumption. The ignorable analysis of PROC MIXED has the further advantages that no explicit assumptions about the missingness process has to be made, and that fitting a model to an incomplete set of data is of no greater complexity than fitting the same model to an equivalent complete data set, provided the sequencing of the repeated measures is correctly passed on to PROC MIXED.

However, this does not preclude that there are situations were the missingness model needs to be considered explicitly. First, scientific interest may be directed to either the missingness model parameters ψ or to the behavior of subjects *conditional on their (non-)response status*. In a selection modeling framework, this implies that the missingness model needs to be considered explicitly. In a pattern-mixture modeling framework, a separate model for each response group will have to be set up and the inestimable parameters identified through appropriate functions, connecting certain parameters of the incomplete subgroup(s) to their counterparts in the complete subgroup (Little 1993, 1995). Here, we will confine attention to the selection modeling framework. Secondly, unless there are good prior grounds to believe otherwise, the presence of an informative response process cannot be excluded. We argue that, even if only for the sake of confirmation, informative dropout models would need to be considered (Baker and Laird 1988, Baker, Rosenberger, and DerSimonian 1992, Diggle and Kenward 1994, Molenberghs, Goetghebeur, and Lipsitz 1997).

We will first study the issue of assessing the non-response mechanism for the growth data set and then briefly discuss issues with informative missingness.

TABLE 5.19. *Growth data. Model fit for logistic non-response models.*

Type	Effects	Deviance	p
MAR	Y_{i1}	19.51	<0.0001
MAR	Y_{i3}	7.43	0.0064
MAR	Y_{i4}	2.51	0.1131
Informative	Y_{i2}	2.55	0.1105

5.11.1 Growth Data

The only prior information we have about the non-response mechanism is that Little and Rubin (1987) conceived it to depend on the measurement at age 8 in such a way that lower values led to higher non-response. Let us assume that the missingness probability follows a logistic model. For example, if dropout would depend solely on the measurement at age 8, a candidate model would be:

$$\ln\left(\frac{P(R_i = 0|\boldsymbol{y}_i)}{1 - P(R_i = 0|\boldsymbol{y}_i)}\right) = \psi_0 + \psi_1 y_{i1},$$

where $R_i = 1$ for complete observations and 0 otherwise, and Y_{i1} is the measurement at age 8. Of course, this model is easily adapted to include a different subset of measurements into the linear predictor. Table 5.19 shows the model fit for a few choices. In each of the four models, missingness depends on a single outcome. When this dependence is on Y_{i2}, the process is informative, while it is MAR otherwise. We used the complete data set to estimate the parameters of the informative model (with linear predictor including Y_{i2}). This is generally not possible. Ways to overcome this problem are discussed on page 256. The only important covariates are the measurements at ages 8 and 12, i.e., the ones adjacent to the possibly missing measurement. A backward logistic regression model retains only Y_{i1}. Its coefficients (standard errors) are estimated as:

$$\ln\left(\frac{P(R_i = 0|y_{i1})}{1 - P(R_i = 0|y_{i1})}\right) = 41.22(18.17) - 1.94(0.85)y_{i1}.$$

This model implies that the missingness probability decreases with increasing Y_{i1}.

It is important to note that omitting a relevant predictor from the non-response model might lead to the wrong conclusions, even about the nature of the non-response mechanism itself. For example, a MCAR mechanism might be classified as informative, if a crucial covariate is omitted from the model. Therefore, it is wise to examine all available information, including covariates, with the greatest care. In the growth example, the only covariate is sex (x_i). Both a model including the age 8 measurement Y_{i1} together with sex x_i as an analysis by sex group lead to a complete separation in the covariate space, resulting in parameter estimates at infinity. Examining the fit carefully, we deduce the following mechanism:

$$\text{boys} \quad : \quad \ln\left(\frac{P(R_i = 0|y_{i1}, x_i = 0)}{1 - P(R_i = 0|y_{i1}, x_i = 0)}\right) = \infty(22 - y_{i1}),$$

$$\text{girls} \quad : \quad \ln\left(\frac{P(R_i = 0|y_{i1}, x_i = 1)}{1 - P(R_i = 0|y_{i1}, x_i = 1)}\right) = \infty(20.75 - y_{i1}).$$

The model for boys is interpreted as follows:

$$P(R_i = 0|y_{i1}, x_i = 0) = \begin{cases} 1 & \text{if } y_{i1} < 22, \\ 0.5 & \text{if } y_{i1} = 22, \\ 0 & \text{if } y_{i1} > 22. \end{cases}$$

This is exactly what is seen in Table 4.11. The same is true for girls, with the sole difference that the cut point lies halfway between two observable outcome values (20.75).

$$P(R_i = 0|y_{i1}, x_i = 1) = \begin{cases} 1 & \text{if } y_{i1} < 20.75, \\ 0 & \text{if } y_{i1} > 20.75. \end{cases}$$

The models are displayed in Figure 5.8. Thus, the missingness mechanism used by Little and Rubin (1987) is in fact *deterministic* (given the outcomes at age 8). This should not be confused with the fact that non-response depends (very clearly) on the observed outcomes and the observed outcomes only, whence it is missing at *random* ! A similar mechanism was employed in Section 5.8.2.

5.11.2   Informative Non-Response

Whenever missing data arise, untestable assumptions have to be made, before one can proceed with an analysis of the data. While it is possible to test the null hypothesis of MCAR *under the alternative hypothesis of MAR* (Diggle 1989), it is by no means standard to test for MAR and thus for ignorability.

Recently, some techniques have been proposed to extend modeling frameworks to informative dropout. Diggle and Kenward (1994) and Diggle *et al* (1994, Chapter 11) extend ignorable analyses in the following way: along with the marginal response model $f(\boldsymbol{y}_i|\boldsymbol{\theta})$, the conditional probability of dropout given the measurements $f(\boldsymbol{r}_i|\boldsymbol{y}_i, \boldsymbol{\psi})$ is modeled. This allows the researcher to entertain informative mechanisms. When the mechanism is

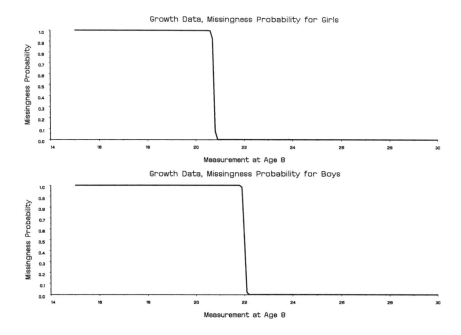

FIGURE 5.8. *Logistic non-response models for growth data.*

MCAR or MAR, both estimation tasks separate since information is disjoint. Measurement and non-response log-likelihoods can be maximized separately. In that case, the measurement part can be fitted using PROC MIXED. Whenever the dropout process is informative, estimation of θ and ψ has to be carried out jointly. Diggle and Kenward (1994) used the simplex algorithm (Nelder and Mead 1965), whereas Molenberghs, Kenward, and Lesaffre (1997) suggest the use of the EM algorithm. The Diggle and Kenward (1994) model is implemented in OSWALD (Version 2.6).

Further approaches are proposed by Schluchter (1988), Laird, Lange, and Stram (1987), Wu and Bailey (1988, 1989), Wu and Carroll (1988). These last authors use random-effects models to describe the censoring or non-response process. Greenlees, Reece, and Zieschang (1982), combine the probit of the dropout probability with the general linear measurement model. Glynn, Laird, and Rubin (1986) use a logistic transform instead. Both approaches are so-called selection models. Glynn *et al* also consider an alternative approach to the analysis of non-ignorable non-response based on mixture modeling and multiple imputation. This approach is easy to implement, is less sensitive to parametric assumptions, and lends itself naturally to the longitudinal data setting.

Brown (1990) constructs an estimator for longitudinal normally distributed data which is valid in case the missing data mechanism only depends on the unobserved values. In a sense it is the mirror image of MAR, and could be termed 'purely informative'. Brown shows how the parameters of a normal distribution can be estimated from the available information. An important feature of this model is that there is no need to estimate the missing data mechanism, reducing the danger of misspecification. Michiels and Molenberghs (1997) present a similar estimator in the case of longitudinal categorical measurements.

Some caution is required with selection modeling approaches for informative missingness. As with all model fitting, the conclusions drawn are conditional on the appropriateness of the assumed model. As suggested earlier, there are aspects of the model that are in a fundamental sense not testable, namely the relationship between non-response and the missing observations. It is assumed in the modeling approach that the relationships among the measurements from a subject are the same whether or not some of these measurements are unobserved due to non-response. It is this assumption that allows us to infer something about the informativeness of the non-response process. Given the dependence of the inferences on this untestable assumption care is needed in the interpretation of the analysis; absence of evidence for informative non-response does not preclude that an informative non-response process is operating in a quite different manner, and in practice it is likely that many such processes are operating simultaneously. We might reasonably expect only to identify a process should it operate approximately in the manner implied by the model and dominate the other non-response mechanisms. Further, evidence supporting informative non-response might have to be interpreted quite differently in the presence of additional information, such as a new covariate associated with both the response and occurrence of non-response. The introduction of an explicit model for the non-response process does allow an exploration of the sensitivity of the results to assumptions about the non-response mechanism, for example by comparing several plausible non-response models. The fitting of informative non-response models can provide useful insights in the analysis of longitudinal data provided that the procedure is treated with sufficient caution (Molenberghs, Kenward, and Lesaffre 1997).

5.11.3   OSWALD for Informative Non-Response

Even though a word of care was issued in the previous section about fitting informative dropout models and applying standard statistical inferential tools to it, such as testing whether the dropout model is informative versus MAR, restricting the model building exercise simply to MAR mechanisms is equally dangerous, since the MAR assumption is itself fundamentally untestable. Often, the choice to restrict model building to MAR is driven by the lack of software for fitting more general models. For instance, PROC MIXED does not allow, at present, the exploration of informative dropout mechanisms.

In this section, we will illustrate how a family of informative dropout models can be fitted with the OSWALD (Smith *et al* 1996) software in S-Plus. It is not natural to use the growth example since its non-response is not of the dropout type. Even though reordering the outcomes (placing the age 10 measurement at the end of the sequence) would turn these data in an example of dropout, we believe it is more satisfactory to study an example with genuine dropout.

In a heart failure study, the primary efficacy endpoint is based upon the ability to do physical exercise. This ability is measured in seconds a subject is able to ride the exercise bike. There are 25 subjects assigned to placebo and 25 to treatment. The treatment consisted of the administration of ace inhibitors. Four measurements were taken at monthly intervals. Table 5.20 presents outcome scores, transformed to normality. We will refer to them as the exercise bike data. All 50 subjects are observed at the first occasion, while there are 44, 41, and 38 subjects seen at the second, the third, and the fourth visit respectively.

To be able to perform a comparison between PROC MIXED and OSWALD, we will restrict attention to a set of models that can be fitted reasonably well with both packages. The measurement models belong to the general class (4.10). We consider it useful to decompose the variability explicitly in three components:

$$\text{var}(\boldsymbol{Y}_i) = Z_i D Z_i' + \tilde{H}_i + \tau^2 I_i.$$

The notation used here is chosen to reflect the OSWALD output and hence deviates slightly from earlier conventions. Recall that $\tilde{H}_i$ represents the serial correlation and τ^2 is the measurement error. For the remainder of this section we will restrict the random effects to a random intercept, and to balanced designs with measurement occasions common to all subjects. As a result, the variance simplifies to

$$\text{var}(\boldsymbol{Y}_i) = \nu^2 J + \tilde{H} + \tau^2 I.$$

Finally, writing $\tilde{H}$ in terms of its correlation matrix yields

$$\text{var}(\boldsymbol{Y}_i) = \nu^2 J + \sigma^2 H + \tau^2 I. \tag{5.25}$$

The symbols ν^2, σ^2, and τ^2 are chosen to reflect the names used in OS-WALD.

TABLE 5.20. *Exercise bike data.*

Placebo				Treatment			
1	2	3	4	1	2	3	4
0.43	0.94	4.32	4.51	-2.54	-0.20	-0.15	3.53
3.10	5.82	5.59	6.32	4.33	5.57	6.86	6.87
0.56	2.21	1.18	1.54	-2.46	.	.	.
-1.18	-0.30	2.48	2.67	2.30	4.64	7.37	7.99
1.24	2.83	1.98	3.21	0.73	3.29	5.23	6.12
-1.87	-0.06	1.16	1.84	0.38	1.25	2.91	4.71
-0.28	1.30	.	.	1.51	4.00	5.98	.
2.93	.	.	.	0.38	0.94	3.28	4.05
-0.20	3.34	3.71	3.69	0.42	2.53	.	.
-0.12	2.01	2.35	2.70	2.41	4.24	4.79	8.14
-1.60	1.42	0.41	0.72	0.12	1.48	3.12	3.69
0.64	.	.	.	-3.46	-0.93	2.78	3.02
-1.14	-1.20	0.09	2.39	-0.55	.	.	.
2.24	2.12	3.00	1.52	0.74	2.40	4.04	5.61
-0.44	0.88	2.83	1.47	2.37	2.79	4.05	5.91
0.39	1.77	3.62	4.35	1.94	5.05	3.06	5.89
-4.37	-2.43	-0.43	-0.13	0.77	2.46	.	.
0.20	2.05	3.18	5.13	1.32	.	.	.
1.31	3.82	2.70	3.59	2.15	4.84	7.70	8.29
-0.38	-1.92	-0.12	-0.40	-0.09	2.02	4.68	5.29
-0.78	.	.	.	2.10	4.91	7.48	8.91
-0.48	0.32	0.66	3.03	1.36	0.62	1.87	.
-0.64	1.53	1.29	.	3.14	5.79	5.95	7.50
0.88	2.10	1.90	3.51	-0.94	-0.08	3.57	3.80
2.02	3.10	4.93	4.76	0.89	1.51	3.14	5.96

The first model we consider is the random intercept Model 7 (see Section 4.4.8). It is given by omitting the H term from (5.25). The next two models are new and, to avoid confusion, they will be assigned numbers 9 and 10. The second model (Model 9) supplements a random intercept with serial correlation. We will choose the serial correlation to be of the AR(1) type. This model is found by omitting the measurement error component $\tau^2 I$ from (5.25) and choosing the elements of H to be $h_{jk} = \rho^{|j-k|} = \exp(-\phi|j-k|)$. Model 10 combines all three sources of variability. SAS code for these models is:

```
proc mixed data = m.bike method = ml covtest;
title 'Exercise Bike, Dropout, Model 7';
class group id;
model y = group time*group / s;
repeated / type = cs subject = id r rcorr;
run;

proc mixed data = m.bike method = ml covtest;
title 'Exercise Bike, Dropout, Model 9';
class group id;
model y = group time*group / s;
repeated / type = ar(1) subject = id r rcorr;
random intercept / type = un subject = id g;
run;

proc mixed data = m.bike method = ml covtest;
title 'Exercise Bike, Dropout, Model 10';
class group id;
model y = group time*group / s;
repeated / type = ar(1) local subject = id r rcorr;
random intercept / type = un subject = id g;
run;
```

The mean and covariance model parameters are summarized in Table 5.21. The parameters supplied by PROC MIXED are supplemented with some additional quantities in order to have both sets of intercepts and slopes for the two treatment groups. Thus, intercept 0 is the sum of intercept 1 and the group 0 effect. Further, ϕ and ρ are connected by $\phi = -\ln(\rho)$. While the mean models are straightforward to interpret from the SAS output, it is necessary to approach the covariance parameters output with some care.

As with the growth data, the random intercept Model 7 is introduced via the 'type=CS' option in the REPEATED statement. Alternatively, we could have chosen to use a random intercept, using the RANDOM statement. The fitted covariance matrix is

$$\tau^2 I + \nu^2 J = \begin{pmatrix} 3.1403 & 2.3781 & 2.3781 & 2.3781 \\ 2.3781 & 3.1403 & 2.3781 & 2.3781 \\ 2.3781 & 2.3781 & 3.1403 & 2.3781 \\ 2.3781 & 2.3781 & 2.3781 & 3.1403 \end{pmatrix}.$$

The SAS summary of the covariance parameters is

```
Covariance Parameter Estimates (MLE)

Cov Parm    Subject       Estimate
```

TABLE 5.21. *SAS output on Models 7, 9, and 10 for the exercise bike data.*

Parameter	Interpretation	Model 7	Model 9	Model 10
intercept	intercept 1	-0.8082	-0.8218	-0.8236
group 0		0.1915	0.1608	0.1606
	intercept 0	-0.6167	-0.6610	-0.6630
time*group 0	slope 0	0.9200	0.9236	0.9230
time*group 1	slope 1	1.6434	1.6449	1.6451
ν^2	random interc.	2.3781	2.1585	2.0938
τ^2	meas. error	0.7622		0.2097
σ^2	serial variance		0.9484	0.8012
ρ	serial corr.		0.3080	0.4440
ϕ	serial corr. (exp.)		1.1778	0.8119
Deviance		564.27	559.69	559.68

```
CS          ID          2.37805794
Residual                0.76223505
```

from which it follows that $\nu^2 = 2.3781$ and $\tau^2 = 0.7622 = 3.1403 - 2.3781$.

Model 9 replaces the independent measurement errors with serially correlated errors. This requires the use of the RANDOM and REPEATED statements simultaneously. The 'r' matrix produced by SAS is now interpreted as

$$\sigma^2 H = \begin{pmatrix} 0.9484 & 0.2921 & 0.0899 & 0.0277 \\ 0.2921 & 0.9484 & 0.2921 & 0.0899 \\ 0.0899 & 0.2921 & 0.9484 & 0.2921 \\ 0.0277 & 0.0899 & 0.2921 & 0.9484 \end{pmatrix}.$$

Observe that this 'r' matrix has a completely different interpretation in these two models, since they refer to different sources of variability. The corresponding correlation matrix is

$$H = \begin{pmatrix} 1.0000 & 0.3080 & 0.0948 & 0.0292 \\ 0.3080 & 1.0000 & 0.3080 & 0.0948 \\ 0.0948 & 0.3080 & 1.0000 & 0.3080 \\ 0.0292 & 0.0948 & 0.3080 & 1.0000 \end{pmatrix}$$

from which we deduce that $\rho = 0.3080$. In addition, the output labelled 'G Matrix' corresponds to the variance of the intercept, $\tau^2 = 2.1585$. The covariance parameters are given in the next panel

```
Covariance Parameter Estimates (MLE)

Cov Parm    Subject      Estimate

UN(1,1)     ID           2.15845062
AR(1)       ID           0.30795893
Residual                 0.94837375
```

of which all components have been discussed. It is slightly misleading that $\sigma^2 = 0.9484$ is labelled 'residual' since it does not refer to measurement error, but rather to the variance of the serially correlated process. This point will be clearer from Model 10. Indeed, this model combines all three components of variability. The full covariance structure output is

```
                    R Matrix for ID 1

Row        COL1          COL2          COL3          COL4

 1     1.01091685    0.35573508    0.15795174    0.07013296
 2     0.35573508    1.01091685    0.35573508    0.15795174
 3     0.15795174    0.35573508    1.01091685    0.35573508
 4     0.07013296    0.15795174    0.35573508    1.01091685

              R Correlation Matrix for ID 1

Row        COL1          COL2          COL3          COL4

 1     1.00000000    0.35189351    0.15624603    0.06937559
 2     0.35189351    1.00000000    0.35189351    0.15624603
 3     0.15624603    0.35189351    1.00000000    0.35189351
 4     0.06937559    0.15624603    0.35189351    1.00000000

                        G Matrix

     Parameter    Subject    Row        COL1

     INTERCEPT    ID 1        1      2.09382622

     Covariance Parameter Estimates (MLE)

          Cov Parm    Subject     Estimate

          UN(1,1)     ID          2.09382622
          Variance    ID          0.80117791
          AR(1)       ID          0.44401509
          Residual                0.20973894
```

This output is easier to understand since the parameters are nicely grouped by source of variability: (1) random intercept, with $\nu^2 = 2.0938$, (2) serial correlation, with $\sigma^2 = 0.8012$ and $\rho = 0.4440$, and (3) measurement error (residual), with $\tau^2 = 0.2097$.

Formal inspection of the deviances shows that Model 7 is too simple and that Model 10 does not improve Model 9 significantly.

Our next goal is to fit the same three models with OSWALD. For a full documentation on OSWALD we refer to Smith et al (1996) or to the Web page:

http://www.maths.lancs.ac.uk:2080/~maa036/Oswald/

The output is presented in the form of a typical S-Plus list object. For Model 7:

```
Longitudinal Data Analysis Model
assuming completely random dropout

Call:
pcmid(formula = bike.bal ~ group * time,
        vparms = c(0, 1.5, 0), correxp = 1)

Analysis Method: Maximum Likelihood (ML)
Correlation structure: exp(- phi * |u| ^ 1 )

Maximised likelihood:
[1] -482.4208

Mean Parameters:
              (Intercept)        group       time group:time
PARAMETER     -0.6166502  -0.1915053 0.92002700  0.7233457
STD.ERROR      0.3792614   0.5374845 0.08554001  0.1232477

Variance Parameters:
 nu.sq sigma.sq    tau.sq phi
     0 2.378172 0.7622228   0
```

Since we want to include only a random intercept and measurement error as components of variability, we would like to omit σ^2 from the model. A way to do this is by specifying initial values for the covariance parameters using the VPARMS argument to the PCMID function. The argument of VPARMS is a vector with three components, containing initial values for ν^2, τ^2, and ϕ respectively. Setting one or more of the initial values equal to 0 prevents these parameters from maximization. However, σ^2 is not included as a component of the initial values vector. A way to circumvent this problem is to set $\phi \equiv 0$. This implies that the serial correlation matrix H reduces to a matrix of ones, $H = J$, whence it takes on the same role as the random intercept component. As a result, ν^2 can be omitted from the model. Thus, the component we are actually interested in needs to be excluded ! Model fit for all three models is summarized in Table 5.22. Comparison with Table 5.21 shows that the fits are virtually identical. The only substantial difference is seen in the deviances. Adding 400.57 to the deviances in Table 5.21 yields the deviances in Table 5.22. Presumably OSWALD uses a slightly different objective function.

Model 9 omits the measurement error, which is simply done by setting the initial value for $\tau^2 \equiv 0$.

```
Longitudinal Data Analysis Model
assuming completely random dropout

Call:
pcmid(formula = bike.bal ~ group * time,
      vparms = c(1, 0, 1), correxp = 1)

Analysis Method: Maximum Likelihood (ML)
Correlation structure: exp(- phi * |u| ^ 1 )

Maximised likelihood:
[1] -480.13

Mean Parameters:
            (Intercept)       group        time group:time
PARAMETER    -0.6609958  -0.1607851  0.92363457  0.7212975
STD.ERROR     0.3923346   0.5559721  0.09760774  0.1403651

Variance Parameters:
    nu.sq  sigma.sq tau.sq       phi
 2.158405 0.9483919      0  1.177751
```

Finally, the unrestricted Model 10 produces the following output.

```
Longitudinal Data Analysis Model
assuming completely random dropout

Call:
pcmid(formula = bike.bal ~ group * time,
```

```
vparms = c(2, 0.2, 1), correxp = 1,
reqmin = 1e-012)
```

```
Analysis Method: Maximum Likelihood (ML)
Correlation structure: exp(- phi * |u| ^ 1 )
```

```
Maximised likelihood:
[1] -480.1222
```

```
Mean Parameters:
            (Intercept)      group       time group:time
PARAMETER   -0.6629645 -0.1606256 0.92304454  0.7221020
STD.ERROR    0.3932421  0.5572348 0.09842758  0.1415133
```

```
Variance Parameters:
    nu.sq  sigma.sq    tau.sq        phi
 2.094417 0.8016666 0.2087339 0.8139487
```

In all of the above models, CORREXP=1 ensures that an AR(1) serial correlation structure is used. OSWALD accepts any value between 1 and 2 as arguments to CORREXP (the latter corresponds to Gaussian decay). The model formula is equivalent to a SAS model

```
model y = group time group*time
```

and follows standard model formulating conventions of S-Plus. The object BIKE.BAL is a member of the BALANCED class, designed within OS-WALD for collections of time series with a common set of measurement times. For unbalances designs, a different class (LDA.MAT) is conceived.

All models considered in this section have a simple random-effects structure. Indeed, Models 7, 9, and 10 include only a random intercept. Clearly, more elaborate random-effects models can be fitted with PROC MIXED using the RANDOM statement. In OSWALD Version 2.6 the function PCMID does not allow more complex structures. The predecessor of the function PCMID (the function REML.FIT) allows the user to specify several random effects, but constrains its variance-covariance matrix D to be diagonal. A future release of OSWALD will include more elaborate random-effects models using PCMID.

All analyses done on the exercise bike data so far assumed ignorable non-response, in the spirit of Section 5.7. This means that they are valid under MAR (and not only under MCAR, in spite of the claim printed in the OSWALD output). Of great potential value is the feature of OSWALD to be able to go beyond an ignorable analysis and to fit a specific class

TABLE 5.22. *S-Plus (OSWALD) output on Models 7, 9, and 10 for Exercise bike data.*

Parameter	Interpretation	Model 7	Model 9	Model 10
intercept	intercept 0	-0.6167	-0.6610	-0.6630
group		-0.1915	-0.1608	-0.1606
	intercept 1	-0.8082	-0.8218	-0.8236
time	slope 0	0.9200	0.9236	0.9230
group:time		0.7233	0.7213	0.7221
	slope 1	1.6434	1.6449	1.6451
ν^2	random interc.		2.1584	2.0944
τ^2	measurem. error	0.7622		0.2087
σ^2	serial variance	2.3782	0.9484	0.8017
ρ	serial corr.		0.3080	0.4431
ϕ	expon. param.		1.1778	0.8139
Deviance		964.84	960.26	960.24

of informative models. We will exemplify this power using the exercise bike data. Illustration will be on the basis of the most general Model 10, even though the slightly simpler Model 9 fits the data equally well. The analysis featured by OSWALD couples a linear mixed-effects model for the measurements with a logistic model for dropout, with predictors given by the current outcome as well as a set of previous responses. Details of the model are to be found in Diggle and Kenward (1994). For instance, assuming that the dropout probability at occasion j depends on both the current outcome Y_{ij} and the previous one $Y_{i,j-1}$, leads to the following model:

$$\ln \left(\frac{P(R_{ij} = 0|\boldsymbol{y}_i)}{1 - P(R_{ij} = 0|\boldsymbol{y}_i)} \right) = \psi_0 + \psi_1 y_{ij} + \psi_2 y_{i,j-1}. \quad (5.26)$$

Such an analysis is done in OSWALD through the DROP.PARMS, DROP-MODEL, and DROP.COV.PARMS arguments of the PCMID function. Explicitly, DROP.PARMS specifies starting values for a number of time points, starting from the current one, to be included in the dropout model. In model (5.26), this number is 2 (ψ_1 and ψ_2). A starting value for the intercept ψ_0 is given by means of the DROP.COV.PARMS statement. A very important feature of this argument is that it can be used to include *covariate* effects as well. In that case, model (5.26) is extended to

$$\ln \left(\frac{P(R_{ij} = 0|\boldsymbol{y}_i)}{1 - P(R_{ij} = 0|\boldsymbol{y}_i)} \right) = \psi_0 + \boldsymbol{x}_i \boldsymbol{\psi}_c + \psi_1 y_{ij} + \psi_2 y_{i,j-1}, \quad (5.27)$$

where $\boldsymbol{x}_i$ is a vector of covariates and $\boldsymbol{\psi}_c$ is an additional vector of parameters. The actual form of the dropout model is specified in the DROP-MODEL argument, using standard S-Plus model building conventions. An illustration will be given in the sequel. As before, setting one or more of the initial values equal to zero prevents their inclusion in the maximization process. This is a useful feature, since it allows the user to estimate the dropout parameters under MCAR and MAR assumptions, not only under informative assumptions. For example, model (5.26) corresponds to an MAR process by setting the initial value for $\psi_1 \equiv 0$.

Let us discuss OSWALD analyses for dropout model (5.26), in the MCAR, MAR, and informative contexts respectively. The MCAR analysis output is as follows.

```
Longitudinal Data Analysis Model
assuming random dropout based on 0 previous observations

Call:
pcmid(formula = bike.bal ~ group * time,
      vparms = c(2, 0.2, 1), drop.parms = c(0),
      drop.cov.parms = c(-2), dropmodel =  ~ 1,
      correxp = 1, maxfn = 1600, reqmin = 1e-012)

Analysis Method: Maximum Likelihood (ML)
Correlation structure: exp(- phi * |u| ^ 1 )

Maximised likelihood:
[1] -520.6167

Mean Parameters:
            (Intercept)       group      time group:time
PARAMETER    -0.6629601 -0.1606322 0.9230446  0.7221012
STD.ERROR     0.3859817  0.5470223 0.1009714  0.1451370

Variance Parameters:
    nu.sq  sigma.sq    tau.sq        phi
 2.094412 0.8016692 0.2087333 0.8139474

Dropout parameters:
 (Intercept) y.d
    -2.32728   0

Iteration converged after 993 iterations.
```

The indication that the dropout model is random with a dependence on 0 previous observations effectively refers to a MCAR process. The mechanism is turned into MCAR by specifying DROP.PARMS=c(0) and by setting DROP.COV.PARMS=c(-2). We increased the maximum number of iterations MAXFN to 1600, since more complex dropout models tend to require more iterations. As is seen from the output, a bit under 1000 iterations were actually needed. In addition, the tolerance of the relative gradient was set equal to 10^{-12} by means of the REQMIN argument.

The MAR program and output are similar:

```
Longitudinal Data Analysis Model
assuming random dropout based on 1 previous observations

Call:
pcmid(formula = bike.bal ~ group * time,
      vparms = c(2, 0.2, 1), drop.parms = c(0, -0.1),
      drop.cov.parms = c(-2), dropmodel =  ~ 1,
      correxp = 1, maxfn = 3000, reqmin = 1e-012)

Analysis Method: Maximum Likelihood (ML)
Correlation structure: exp(- phi * |u| ^ 1 )

Maximised likelihood:
[1] -520.3494

Mean Parameters:
            (Intercept)       group       time group:time
PARAMETER    -0.6629684  -0.1606169  0.9230426  0.7221043
STD.ERROR     0.3859815   0.5470220  0.1009713  0.1451369

Variance Parameters:
    nu.sq  sigma.sq     tau.sq         phi
  2.09441 0.8016771  0.2087185  0.8139738

Dropout parameters:
  (Intercept) y.d         y.d-1
    -2.166139    0 -0.09920587

Iteration converged after 1203 iterations.
```

Note that the number of iterations has increased somewhat, even though the extra dropout parameter, ψ_2, appears to be very small. In fact, the likelihood has increased only marginally over the MCAR analysis.

Finally, we allow for informative dropout.

```
Longitudinal Data Analysis Model
assuming informative dropout
based on 1 previous observations

Call:
pcmid(formula = bike.bal ~ group * time,
      vparms = c(2, 0.4, 0.5), drop.parms = c(2, -2),
      drop.cov.parms = c(-3), dropmodel =  ~ 1,
      correxp = 1, maxfn = 10000, reqmin = 1e-012)

Analysis Method: Maximum Likelihood (ML)
Correlation structure: exp(- phi * |u| ^ 1 )

Maximised likelihood:
[1] -520.2316

Mean Parameters:
            (Intercept)        group        time group:time
PARAMETER    -0.6666244   -0.1740098   0.9377247  0.7317099
STD.ERROR            NA           NA          NA         NA

Variance Parameters:
    nu.sq   sigma.sq      tau.sq         phi
 2.106741  0.8348588   0.1577192   0.9310764

Dropout parameters:
 (Intercept)        y.d       y.d-1
   -2.731573  0.3279598  -0.3869054

Iteration converged after 5034 iterations.
```

The number of iterations has increased considerably, which is a typical feature of informative dropout models. The likelihood has changed only marginally, and the dropout parameters are all somewhat larger, even though this is no scientific judgment by the lack of precision estimates. Note also that no standard errors for the mean parameters are provided, in contrast to the other PCMID analyses. This is a very sensible decision since, unlike with ignorable analyses, standard errors are not obtained as simple by-products of the maximization process and require in general considerable extra code. A few methods are listed on page 234.

Results for the three dropout models are summarized in Table 5.23, under the headings MCAR, MAR, and Inf. respectively. Also included is the earlier ignorable analysis. Since MCAR and MAR are ignorable, whether or not the dropout model parameters are estimated explicitly, the first three

TABLE 5.23. *Informative models, fitted to the Exercise bike data. Model 10.*

Parameter	Ign.	Dropout Modeled		
		MCAR	MAR	Inf.
intercept	-0.6630	-0.6630	-0.6630	-0.6666
group	-0.1606	-0.1606	-0.1606	0.1740
time	0.9230	0.9230	0.9230	0.9377
group:time	0.7221	0.7221	0.7221	0.7317
ν^2	2.0944	2.0944	2.0944	2.1067
σ^2	0.8017	0.8017	0.8017	0.8349
τ^2	0.2087	0.2087	0.2087	0.1577
ϕ	0.8139	0.8139	0.8139	0.9311
ψ_0		-2.3273	-2.1661	-2.7316
ψ_1				0.3280
ψ_2			-0.0992	-0.3869
deviance	960.24	1041.23	1040.70	1040.46

models in Table 5.23 yield exactly the same values for the mean and co-variance parameter estimates, as they should. Note that the deviance from the ignorable model is not comparable to the other deviances, since the dropout parameters are not estimated. Comparing the parameters in these models to the informative dropout models shows some shifts, although they are very modest.

We may now want to compare the dropout models. The likelihood ratio test statistic to compare MAR with MCAR is 0.53 on 1 degree of freedom ($p = 0.4666$). This means that MCAR would be acceptable *provided MAR were the correct alternative hypothesis* and the actual parametric form for the MAR process were correct. In addition, a comparison between the informative and random dropout models yields a likelihood ratio test statistic of 0.24 ($p = 0.6242$). Of course, for reasons outlined at the end of Section 5.11.2 (page 258) one should use informative dropout models with caution, since they rely on assumptions that are at best only partially verifiable.

In spite of these limitations, neglecting to address the question whether the missingness model goes beyond ignorability puts a strong belief on MAR, probably too strong to be warranted. Such a practice is as bad as blindly making inferences from fitting informative dropout models. There-fore, allowing for informative dropout should be seen as a sensitivity anal-ysis, which, if no strong evidence for informative dropout is found, will strengthen the researcher's faith in the MAR mechanism. In the opposite

TABLE 5.24. *Informative models, fitted to the Exercise bike data. Model 10. Treatment assignment (group) included into the dropout model.*

Parameter	MAR	Inf.
intercept	-0.6630	-0.6214
group	-0.1606	-0.2288
time	0.9231	0.9032
group:time	0.7221	0.7252
ν^2	2.0944	2.0438
σ^2	0.8017	0.7859
τ^2	0.2087	0.2931
ϕ	0.8139	0.6289
ψ_0	-2.4059	-2.1036
ψ_1		0.3036
ψ_2	-0.1289	0.1238
group	0.5395	0.7979
deviance	1039.96	1039.83

case where informative dropout seems plausible, one can compare relevant quantities (such as mean and covariance model parameters and their standard errors) under MAR and informative assumptions, to assess their robustness.

To conclude, let us illustrate the capability of OSWALD to incorporate covariates into the dropout model, as in model (5.27). Including the treatment assignment (group) into the MAR and informative models of Table 5.23 yields

```
Longitudinal Data Analysis Model
assuming random dropout based on 1 previous observations

Call:
pcmid(formula = demo2.bal ~ group * time,
      vparms = c(2, 0.2, 0.8), drop.parms = c(0, -0.1),
      drop.cov.parms = c(-2, 0.1),
      dropmodel = ~ 1 + group,
      correxp = 1, maxfn = 5000, reqmin = 1e-012)

Analysis Method: Maximum Likelihood (ML)
Correlation structure: exp(- phi * |u| ^ 1 )
```

```
Maximised likelihood:
[1] -519.9814
```

Mean Parameters:

	(Intercept)	group	time	group:time
PARAMETER	-0.6629779	-0.1606298	0.9230512	0.7220979
STD.ERROR	0.3859810	0.5470213	0.1009712	0.1451367

Variance Parameters:

nu.sq	sigma.sq	tau.sq	phi
2.094418	0.8016748	0.2087164	0.8139889

Dropout parameters:

(Intercept)	group	y.d	y.d-1
-2.405863	0.5395115	0	-0.1289393

```
Iteration converged after 2983 iterations.
```

and

```
Longitudinal Data Analysis Model
assuming informative dropout
based on 1 previous observations

Call:
pcmid(formula = demo2.bal ~ group * time,
      vparms = c(2, 0.2, 0.8),
      drop.parms = c(0.3, -0.3),
      drop.cov.parms = c(-2, 0.1),
      dropmodel =  ~ 1 + group,
      correxp = 1, maxfn = 10000, reqmin = 1e-012)

Analysis Method: Maximum Likelihood (ML)
Correlation structure: exp(- phi * |u| ^ 1 )

Maximised likelihood:
[1] -519.9143
```

Mean Parameters:

	(Intercept)	group	time	group:time
PARAMETER	-0.6213682	-0.228779	0.9032322	0.7251818
STD.ERROR	NA	NA	NA	NA

Variance Parameters:

```
    nu.sq  sigma.sq    tau.sq        phi
2.043767 0.7858604 0.2930629 0.6288833
```

```
Dropout parameters:
 (Intercept)      group        y.d      y.d-1
   -2.103619 0.7979308 -0.303576 0.1238007
```

Iteration converged after 5930 iterations.

The model fit is summarized in Table 5.24.

Again, the main effect and variance parameters in the MAR column have not changed relative to their ignorable counterparts in Table 5.23. In contrast, the informative dropout model parameters are all different, compared to the informative model in Table 5.23.

Appendix A

Inference for Fixed Effects

In this appendix, we will describe some standard inferential tools for the fixed effects of the general linear mixed model. Recall that this model assumes the form

$$Y = X\beta + Zb + \varepsilon, \tag{A.1}$$

with Y the vector of responses, X and Z the design matrices for the fixed effects β and random effects b, and ε the vector of measurement errors. It is further assumed that b and ε are independently normally distributed with zero mean vectors and covariance matrices D and Σ respectively.

Appendix A.1 describes likelihood based estimation of the fixed effects β. Hypothesis testing and related topics are discussed in Appendices A.2–A.4.

A.1 Estimation

It follows from the general linear mixed model (A.1) that Y is marginally normally distributed with mean $X\beta$ and covariance matrix $V = \text{Var}(Y) = ZDZ' + \Sigma$.

The associated log-likelihood function is

$$\ell(\beta, V) = -\frac{N}{2} \log 2\pi - \frac{1}{2} \log |V| - \frac{1}{2}(Y - X\beta)'V^{-1}(Y - X\beta).$$

Assuming V known, the likelihood equations to obtain maximum likelihood estimators for β are

$$\ell_\beta(\beta, V) \equiv -\frac{1}{2}\frac{\partial}{\partial\beta}(Y - X\beta)'V^{-1}(Y - X\beta) = 0$$

or equivalently

$$X'V^{-1}X\beta = X'V^{-1}Y.$$

Since the existence of the inverse $X'V^{-1}X$ is in general not guaranteed, we use a generalized inverse of $X'V^{-1}X$ to obtain

$$\widehat{\beta}_{\text{GLS}} = (X'V^{-1}X)^- X'V^{-1}Y$$

as a solution for the system of likelihood equations. Here, A^- denotes a generalized inverse of A. For general matrices A there are always matrices A^- satisfying $AA^-A = A$. Each such A^- is called a generalized inverse of A. For A a full rank square matrix there is a unique generalized inverse that coincides with the inverse of A, i.e., $A^- = A^{-1}$.

Another interpretation (explaining the use of GLS as index) is as follows: minimization of $(\boldsymbol{Y} - X\boldsymbol{\beta})'V^{-1}(\boldsymbol{Y} - X\boldsymbol{\beta})$ with respect to $\boldsymbol{\beta}$ gives $\hat{\boldsymbol{\beta}}_{\mathrm{GLS}}$. This approach is the generalized least squares (GLS) method.

The variance-covariance matrix of $\hat{\boldsymbol{\beta}}_{\mathrm{GLS}}$ equals

$$
\begin{aligned}
D(\hat{\boldsymbol{\beta}}_{\mathrm{GLS}}) &= (X'V^{-1}X)^- X'V^{-1}D(\boldsymbol{Y})V^{-1}X(X'V^{-1}X)^- \\
&= (X'V^{-1}X)^-.
\end{aligned}
$$

The fact that $\hat{\boldsymbol{\beta}}_{\mathrm{GLS}}$ and $D(\hat{\boldsymbol{\beta}}_{\mathrm{GLS}})$ do contain the dispersion matrix V, which so far was assumed to be known, makes the expressions obtained above not useful in practice. With $\hat{V}$ the matrix obtained by replacing the parameters in V by estimators (e.g., the REML estimators), we obtain

$$
\hat{\boldsymbol{\beta}} = (X'\hat{V}^{-1}X)^- X'\hat{V}^{-1}\boldsymbol{Y}
$$

as estimator for $\boldsymbol{\beta}$ and $(X'\hat{V}^{-1}X)^-$ as approximate variance-covariance matrix. Here we assume the existence of $\hat{V}^{-1}$. The estimator $(X'\hat{V}^{-1}X)^-$ is biased downwards since the variability introduced by working with estimated variance components in V, rather than with the true but unknown variance components, is not taken into account in our approximation for $(X'V^{-1}X)^-$. Of course, this will also affect the distribution of test statistics based on this expression.

As already mentioned above, an important problem in linear (mixed) model theory is that, in cases of overparameterization, the matrix $X'V^{-1}X$ in the likelihood equations, is not of full rank and therefore does not have an inverse. We therefore are forced to use a (non-unique) generalized inverse. From a practical point of view, it would appear that this is not acceptable. However, this issue can be solved in two different but equivalent ways. First, one can reformulate the model such that the overparameterization is avoided. For example, consider a simple one-way ANOVA model with overall mean μ and group effects τ_i $(i = 1, \ldots, a)$. Clearly, this model is overparameterized since adding an arbitrary constant c to μ and subtracting it from all τ_i leaves the a group means $\mu + \tau_i$ invariant. The model can be reparameterized in the following ways: (1) by setting $\mu = 0$; (2) by setting $\tau_a = 0$; (3) by imposing $\sum_{i=1}^{a} \tau_i = 0$. The first and the second constraints can be achieved by deleting a single column in the design matrix X. Alternatively, one can keep the original overspecified design matrix. The consequence is that the parameter estimates are not uniquely determined and only certain linear combinations can be estimated uniquely. Such a linear combination is called **estimable**. Let us reconsider the above ANOVA example. The mean for group i can be expressed as $\mu + c + \tau_i - c = \mu + \tau_i$ and is independent of the arbitrary constant c. Similarly, the difference between the means of groups i and j reduces to $\tau_i - \tau_j$, independent of c. It turns out that in practice many relevant parameters are estimable. For more details on estimable functions see Section 8.7 in Searle (1987).

A.2   Hypothesis Testing

Consider general linear hypotheses of the fixed effects, i.e., testing problems of the form

$$H_0 : H'\beta = 0 \qquad \text{versus} \qquad H_1 : H'\beta \neq 0,$$

with β a $(p \times 1)$ vector and H a $(p \times q)$ matrix $(q \leq p)$ of full rank $(\text{rank}(H) = q)$. With $h_j = (h_{1j}, \ldots, h_{pj})'$ the j-th column of the H matrix, we assume $h_j'\beta$ estimable, for $j = 1, \ldots, q$. As estimator for $H'\beta$ we use $H'\widehat{\beta}$ and, since

$$D(H'\widehat{\beta}) = H'D(\widehat{\beta})H = H'(X'V^{-1}X)^- H,$$

we use $H'(X'\widehat{V}^{-1}X)^- H$ as estimated dispersion matrix. It can be shown that the statistic

$$\frac{(H'\widehat{\beta})'(H'(X'\widehat{V}^{-1}X)^- H)(H'\widehat{\beta})}{\text{rank}(H)}$$

approximately follows an F-distribution with $\text{rank}(H)$ as degrees of freedom for the numerator. It belongs to the general class of Wald-type test statistics. The denominator degrees of freedom (ddf) have to be approximated. The procedures available to this end within PROC MIXED, are described in Section A.3. Further details on approximate F-tests for general linear hypotheses using moment approximations are in Fai and Cornelius (1996).

A.3   Determination of Degrees of Freedom

Only for balanced data sets and for a number of hypotheses the determination of the denominator degrees of freedom is simple. In that case, the background variability against which to test corresponds to a single variance component, and the associated number of degrees of freedom should be used in the F-test. If the data are unbalanced, the denominator degrees of freedom for the approximate t- and F-statistics should be calculated from the data. As default PROC MIXED uses the so-called containment method to determine degrees of freedom, but using the 'ddfm=' option the user can select from a set of procedures. Depending on specific design features one method might be more tractable than other methods. We now briefly explain the different options. For a more detailed discussion see Littell *et al* (1996).

The 'ddfm=residual' option takes for each fixed effects factor the degrees of freedom of the residual error variance. This number typically overestimates the optimal denominator degrees of freedom. Therefore, this option is not recommended.

The 'ddfm=bw' option only applies to models with repeated measures data or to models with only one additional random effects factor apart from the error term.

The 'ddfm=contain' option uses the containment method to determine the denominator degrees of freedom. Assume FACT is a fixed-effects factor, for which the denominator degrees of freedom for testing 'equality of the mean response at all levels' must be determined. In the containment method, the random-effects list is searched for effects that syntactically contain FACT. For instance RAND*FACT or RAND(FACT), with RAND a random effect, contain FACT. Technically, the degrees of freedom corresponding to each of these terms is computed, and the lowest value is assigned as the denominator degrees of freedom for the approximate F-statistic.

If no terms in the random effects list are found that contain the fixed effects, the denominator degrees of freedom is set equal to the degrees of freedom of the error variance.

If the 'ddfm=contain' option is used, the resulting degrees of freedom depend on the parameterization of the model, as it is based on a syntactical rule. If the random-effects factor is not specified as an interaction term in which the fixed-effects factor is present, such as RAND*FACT, but rather as a separate factor with its own name, the containment method will no longer use the degrees of freedom of this random effects factor as the denominator degrees of freedom for FACT, although the matrix corresponding to the user specified random effects factor and the interaction RAND*FACT is exactly the same.

The denominator degrees of freedom derived by the containment method are correct if the data are balanced. For unbalanced data different variance components contribute to the background variability. Therefore the denominator degrees of freedom assigned by the containment method are not always optimal as they correspond to the degrees of freedom associated with a single random effect, whereas a better choice would lie between the lowest and highest value of degrees of freedom associated with the various random-effects factors.

The final option, Satterthwaite's procedure, is discussed in the next section.

A.4   Satterthwaite's Procedure

The denominator degrees of freedom can also be approximated by the slightly more computer intensive Satterthwaite procedure, which can be obtained from the MIXED procedure of SAS by specifying 'ddfm=satterth'. An advantage is that it is using the matrices of the random and fixed effects factors itself to determine the denominator degrees of freedom, so that only the matrix and not the syntactical name matters to determine the denominator degrees of freedom. This is in contrast to the containment method, discussed in Appendix A.3.

Inspired by quadratic form ideas (mean squares typically are quadratic forms) Satterthwaite's method uses a $\chi^2(\nu)$ distribution to approximate the distribution function of

$$S_h^2 = \frac{\nu h'(X'\widehat{V}^{-1}X)^- h}{E(h'(X'\widehat{V}^{-1}X)^- h)}.$$

Note that $E(S_h^2) = \nu$. So S_h^2 has the same mean as a $\chi^2(\nu)$ distribution. To obtain the approximate degrees of freedom we match the variances of the two distributions, i.e.,

$$\text{Var}(S_h^2) = \frac{\nu^2 \text{Var}(h'(X'\widehat{V}^{-1}X)^- h)}{(E(h'(X'\widehat{V}^{-1}X)^- h))^2} \approx 2\nu$$

or

$$\nu \approx \frac{2(E(h'(X'\widehat{V}^{-1}X)^- h))^2}{\text{Var}(h'(X'\widehat{V}^{-1}X)^- h)}.$$

We now want an approximation for $\text{Var}(h'(X'\widehat{V}^{-1}X)^- h)$. Therefore note that, as illustrated in Example 2.6, the incidence matrix Z can be partitioned into submatrices $Z_1, \ldots, Z_{k-1}$ where Z_j is the incidence matrix for the j-th random effect (and $k - 1$ is the number of random effects). The random error can also be seen as a random effect. Indeed the linear mixed model equation

$$Y = X\beta + (Z_1 \mid Z_2 \mid \ldots \mid Z_{k-1})b + \varepsilon$$

can also be written as

$$Y = X\beta + (Z_1 \mid Z_2 \mid \ldots \mid Z_{k-1} \mid I_N)\begin{pmatrix} b \\ \varepsilon \end{pmatrix}.$$

In terms of Z_j, $j = 1, \ldots, k$ (with $Z_k \equiv I_N$) and using a Taylor series expansion, Giesbrecht and Burns (1985) show that

$$\mathrm{Var}(h'(X'\widehat{V}^{-1}X)^- h) \approx \sum_{i=1}^{k} \sum_{j=1}^{k} \mathrm{Cov}(\widehat{\sigma}_i^2, \widehat{\sigma}_j^2) M_i M_j, \qquad (\mathrm{A.2})$$

where

$$M_j = h'(X'\widehat{V}^{-1}X)^- X'\widehat{V}^{-1}Z_j Z_j' \widehat{V}^{-1}X(X'\widehat{V}^{-1}X)^- h$$

and $\mathrm{Cov}(\widehat{\sigma}_i^2, \widehat{\sigma}_j^2)$ are the asymptotic variances and covariances obtained from the Hessian matrix. The right hand side of (A.2) gives a stochastic approximation for $\mathrm{Var}(h'(X'\widehat{V}^{-1}X)^- h)$.

Satterthwaite (1946) and Neter *et al* (1996) indicate that, if the quadratic form $h'(X'\widehat{V}^{-1}X)^- h$ can be written as a linear combination of mean squares, i.e., $a_1 MS_1 + \ldots + a_s MS_s$ in which $a_1, \ldots, a_s$ are constants and MS_j is the mean squares due to source $j = 1, \ldots, s$ (s the total number of sources), then the Satterthwaite procedure simplifies. In this case the degrees of freedom for the t-distribution are given by

$$\nu = \frac{(a_1 MS_1 + \ldots + a_s MS_s)^2}{\dfrac{(a_1 MS_1)^2}{df_1} + \ldots + \dfrac{(a_s MS_s)^2}{df_s}},$$

with df_j the degrees of freedom for MS_j, $j = 1, \ldots, s$. See Neter *et al* (1996, pp. 971–975) for a nice introductory discussion.

Appendix B

Variance Components and Standard Errors

Testing for the significance of random effects is a non-standard problem since null hypotheses that include zero values for one or more variance parameters lie on the boundary of the parameter space. It was highlighted in Section 3.9.1 that the well-known large sample results, such as asymptotic chi-squared null distribution for the likelihood ratio, Wald, and score test statistics, are invalid in these circumstances. The results of Self and Liang (1987) and Stram and Lee (1994) establish indeed that these null distributions are, for example, mixtures of chi-squared distributions.

In the light of this, it was misleading that the SAS procedure PROC MIXED (Version 6.11) showed Z-statistics and associated p-values for all covariance parameters in the 'Covariance Parameter Estimates' panel. Let us consider this panel for Model 10 on page 261:

Covariance Parameter Estimates (MLE)

Cov Parm	Ratio	Estimate	Std Error	Z	Pr > |Z|
INTERCEPT UN(1,1)	9.98301123	2.09382622	0.85883760	2.44	0.0148
DIAG Diagonal	3.81988152	0.80117791	0.64622805	1.24	0.2151
AR(1)	2.11698926	0.44401509	1.10443712	0.40	0.6877
Residual	1.00000000	0.20973894	1.18122451	0.18	0.8591

In this case, the p-values for all parameters except for the 'AR(1)' correlation, are incorrect.

Throughout the book, we have avoided the display and use of such incorrect p-values and of the Z-statistics on which they are based. Where feasible, the corrections proposed by Stram and Lee (1994) were used. However, we did at times report standard errors even though they should be approached with care. First, the distribution of many covariance parameters is highly skewed, a fact which standard errors fail to convey. Secondly, one could argue that the covariance parameters in random-effects models are but a by-product of the random-effects structure. Therefore, assessing the need of random effects should be done on other grounds than merely conducting mechanical model selection on the variance-covariance parameters. The reader is referred to Section 3.9 for a discussion on this matter.

In view of this, it is wise that SAS Version 6.12 does not by default display measures of precision and associated tests. The panel displayed earlier has changed to

```
Covariance Parameter Estimates (MLE)

Cov Parm   Subject      Estimate

UN(1,1)    ID           2.09382622
Variance   ID           0.80117791
AR(1)      ID           0.44401509
Residual                0.20973894
```

In case one would be interested in the asymptotic standard errors the 'cov-test' option should be added to the PROC MIXED statement. This generates the following output:

```
Covariance Parameter Estimates (MLE)

Cov Parm   Subject      Estimate     Std Error       Z  Pr > |Z|

UN(1,1)    ID           2.09382622   0.85883760   2.44    0.0148
Variance   ID           0.80117791   0.64622805   1.24    0.2151
AR(1)      ID           0.44401509   1.10443712   0.40    0.6877
Residual                0.20973894   1.18122451   0.18    0.8591
```

Not only the standard errors, but also the Z-values and the p-values are produced by means of this option.

Finally, should the ratio between a variance parameter and the residual variance be of interest, then the 'ratio' option can be added as well. The following output, which very closely resembles the Version 6.11 output, is then found:

```
Covariance Parameter Estimates (MLE)

Cov Parm   Subject       Ratio     Estimate    Std Error     Z  Pr > |Z|

UN(1,1)    ID        9.98301123   2.09382622  0.85883760  2.44   0.0148
Variance   ID        3.81988152   0.80117791  0.64622805  1.24   0.2151
AR(1)      ID        2.11698926   0.44401509  1.10443712  0.40   0.6877
Residual             1.00000000   0.20973894  1.18122451  0.18   0.8591
```

However, we believe that this ratio will in most practical situations be of limited value.

Appendix C

Details on Table 2.10: Expected Mean Squares

To illustrate how the expected mean squares in Table 2.10 on page 44 are obtained we give the details for $E(SS_{\text{plate}})$ and $E(SS_{\text{gsf}})$ (the expected sum of squares for the sources 'plate' and 'growth stimulating factor'). Recall that

factor	#levels
plate	9
gsf	2
drug	2

Use $\overline{Y}_{..k} - \overline{Y}_{...} = (p_k + \overline{c}_{.k} + \overline{\varepsilon}_{..k}) - (\overline{p}_. + \overline{c}_{..} + \overline{\varepsilon}_{...})$ to obtain

$$SS_{\text{plate}} \stackrel{def}{=} 4 \sum_{k=1}^{9} (\overline{Y}_{..k} - \overline{Y}_{...})^2$$

$$= 4 \sum_{k=1}^{9} (p_k + \overline{c}_{.k} + \overline{\varepsilon}_{..k} - \overline{p}_. - \overline{c}_{..} - \overline{\varepsilon}_{...})^2$$

$$= 4 \sum_{k=1}^{9} (p_k - \overline{p}_.)^2 + 4 \sum_{k=1}^{9} (\overline{c}_{.k} - \overline{c}_{..})^2 + 4 \sum_{k=1}^{9} (\overline{\varepsilon}_{..k} - \overline{\varepsilon}_{...})^2.$$

Since

$$E\left(\sum_{k=1}^{9} (p_k - \overline{p}_.)^2\right) = 8\sigma_p^2,$$

$$E\left(\sum_{k=1}^{9} (\overline{c}_{.k} - \overline{c}_{..})^2\right) = 4\sigma_c^2,$$

$$E\left(\sum_{k=1}^{9} (\overline{\varepsilon}_{..k} - \overline{\varepsilon}_{...})^2\right) = 2\sigma^2,$$

we have

$$E(SS_{\text{plate}}) = 8(4\sigma_p^2 + 2\sigma_c^2 + \sigma^2).$$

Therefore the expected mean squares for the factor 'plate' is

$$E(MS_{\text{plate}}) = E\left(\frac{SS_{\text{plate}}}{8}\right) = 4\sigma_p^2 + 2\sigma_c^2 + \sigma^2.$$

Use

$$\overline{Y}_{i..} - \overline{Y}_{...} = (\alpha_i - \overline{\alpha}_.) + (\overline{\alpha\beta})_{i.} - (\overline{\alpha\beta})_{..}) + (\overline{c}_{i.} - \overline{c}_{..}) + (\overline{\varepsilon}_{i..} - \overline{\varepsilon}_{...})$$

to obtain

$$SS_{\text{gsf}} \stackrel{def}{=} 18 \sum_{i=1}^{2} (\overline{Y}_{i..} - \overline{Y}_{...})^2$$

$$= \phi(\text{gsf}) + 18 \sum_{i=1}^{2} (\overline{c}_{i.} - \overline{c}_{..})^2 + 18 \sum_{i=1}^{2} (\overline{\varepsilon}_{i..} - \overline{\varepsilon}_{...})^2$$

with

$$\phi(\text{gsf}) = 18 \sum_{i=1}^{2} \left((\alpha_i - \overline{\alpha}_.) + ((\overline{\alpha\beta})_{i.} - (\overline{\alpha\beta})_{..})\right)^2.$$

Since

$$E\left(\sum_{i=1}^{2} (\overline{c}_{i.} - \overline{c}_{..})^2\right) = \frac{\sigma^2}{9},$$

$$E\left(\sum_{i=1}^{2} (\overline{\varepsilon}_{i..} - \overline{\varepsilon}_{...})^2\right) = \frac{\sigma^2}{18},$$

it is immediate that

$$E(SS_{\text{gsf}}) = \phi(\text{gsf}) + 2\sigma_c^2 + \sigma^2.$$

This is the expected mean squares since the factor 'gsf' has only one degree of freedom.

Appendix D

Example 2.8: Cell Proliferation

We give the explicit form of the model elements of Example 2.8 (page 28, see also Example 2.5, page 20).

$$
Y = \begin{pmatrix} Y_{111} \\ Y_{121} \\ Y_{211} \\ Y_{221} \\ Y_{112} \\ Y_{122} \\ Y_{212} \\ Y_{222} \\ Y_{113} \\ Y_{123} \\ Y_{213} \\ Y_{223} \\ \vdots \\ Y_{119} \\ Y_{129} \\ Y_{219} \\ Y_{229} \end{pmatrix}, \beta = \begin{pmatrix} \mu \\ \alpha_1 \\ \alpha_2 \\ \beta_1 \\ \beta_2 \\ (\alpha\beta)_{11} \\ (\alpha\beta)_{12} \\ (\alpha\beta)_{21} \\ (\alpha\beta)_{22} \end{pmatrix}, b = \begin{pmatrix} p_1 \\ p_2 \\ p_3 \\ p_4 \\ p_5 \\ p_6 \\ p_7 \\ p_8 \\ p_9 \\ c_{11} \\ c_{21} \\ c_{12} \\ c_{22} \\ c_{13} \\ c_{23} \\ \vdots \\ c_{19} \\ c_{29} \end{pmatrix}, \varepsilon = \begin{pmatrix} \varepsilon_{111} \\ \varepsilon_{121} \\ \varepsilon_{211} \\ \varepsilon_{221} \\ \varepsilon_{112} \\ \varepsilon_{122} \\ \varepsilon_{212} \\ \varepsilon_{222} \\ \varepsilon_{113} \\ \varepsilon_{123} \\ \varepsilon_{213} \\ \varepsilon_{223} \\ \vdots \\ \varepsilon_{119} \\ \varepsilon_{129} \\ \varepsilon_{219} \\ \varepsilon_{229} \end{pmatrix}.
$$

The design matrix X is of form

$$
X = \begin{pmatrix}
1 & 1 & 0 & 1 & 0 & 1 & 0 & 0 & 0 \\
1 & 1 & 0 & 0 & 1 & 0 & 1 & 0 & 0 \\
1 & 0 & 1 & 1 & 0 & 0 & 0 & 1 & 0 \\
1 & 0 & 1 & 0 & 1 & 0 & 0 & 0 & 1 \\
1 & 1 & 0 & 1 & 0 & 1 & 0 & 0 & 0 \\
1 & 1 & 0 & 0 & 1 & 0 & 1 & 0 & 0 \\
1 & 0 & 1 & 1 & 0 & 0 & 0 & 1 & 0 \\
1 & 0 & 1 & 0 & 1 & 0 & 0 & 0 & 1 \\
1 & 1 & 0 & 1 & 0 & 1 & 0 & 0 & 0 \\
1 & 1 & 0 & 0 & 1 & 0 & 1 & 0 & 0 \\
1 & 0 & 1 & 1 & 0 & 0 & 0 & 1 & 0 \\
1 & 0 & 1 & 0 & 1 & 0 & 0 & 0 & 1 \\
 & & & & \vdots & & & & \\
1 & 1 & 0 & 1 & 0 & 1 & 0 & 0 & 0 \\
1 & 1 & 0 & 0 & 1 & 0 & 1 & 0 & 0 \\
1 & 0 & 1 & 1 & 0 & 0 & 0 & 1 & 0 \\
1 & 0 & 1 & 0 & 1 & 0 & 0 & 0 & 1
\end{pmatrix}.
$$

Finally, $Z = (Z_1 | Z_2)$, with

$$
Z_1 = \begin{pmatrix}
1 & 0 & 0 & 0 & 0 & 0 & 0 & 0 & 0 \\
1 & 0 & 0 & 0 & 0 & 0 & 0 & 0 & 0 \\
1 & 0 & 0 & 0 & 0 & 0 & 0 & 0 & 0 \\
1 & 0 & 0 & 0 & 0 & 0 & 0 & 0 & 0 \\
0 & 1 & 0 & 0 & 0 & 0 & 0 & 0 & 0 \\
0 & 1 & 0 & 0 & 0 & 0 & 0 & 0 & 0 \\
0 & 1 & 0 & 0 & 0 & 0 & 0 & 0 & 0 \\
0 & 1 & 0 & 0 & 0 & 0 & 0 & 0 & 0 \\
0 & 0 & 1 & 0 & 0 & 0 & 0 & 0 & 0 \\
0 & 0 & 1 & 0 & 0 & 0 & 0 & 0 & 0 \\
0 & 0 & 1 & 0 & 0 & 0 & 0 & 0 & 0 \\
0 & 0 & 1 & 0 & 0 & 0 & 0 & 0 & 0 \\
 & & & & \vdots & & & & \\
0 & 0 & 0 & 0 & 0 & 0 & 0 & 0 & 1 \\
0 & 0 & 0 & 0 & 0 & 0 & 0 & 0 & 1 \\
0 & 0 & 0 & 0 & 0 & 0 & 0 & 0 & 1 \\
0 & 0 & 0 & 0 & 0 & 0 & 0 & 0 & 1
\end{pmatrix}
$$

and

$$
Z_2 = \begin{pmatrix}
1 & 0 & 0 & 0 & 0 & 0 & 0 & 0 & 0 & 0 & 0 & 0 & 0 & 0 & 0 & 0 & 0 & 0 \\
1 & 0 & 0 & 0 & 0 & 0 & 0 & 0 & 0 & 0 & 0 & 0 & 0 & 0 & 0 & 0 & 0 & 0 \\
0 & 1 & 0 & 0 & 0 & 0 & 0 & 0 & 0 & 0 & 0 & 0 & 0 & 0 & 0 & 0 & 0 & 0 \\
0 & 1 & 0 & 0 & 0 & 0 & 0 & 0 & 0 & 0 & 0 & 0 & 0 & 0 & 0 & 0 & 0 & 0 \\
0 & 0 & 1 & 0 & 0 & 0 & 0 & 0 & 0 & 0 & 0 & 0 & 0 & 0 & 0 & 0 & 0 & 0 \\
0 & 0 & 1 & 0 & 0 & 0 & 0 & 0 & 0 & 0 & 0 & 0 & 0 & 0 & 0 & 0 & 0 & 0 \\
0 & 0 & 0 & 1 & 0 & 0 & 0 & 0 & 0 & 0 & 0 & 0 & 0 & 0 & 0 & 0 & 0 & 0 \\
0 & 0 & 0 & 1 & 0 & 0 & 0 & 0 & 0 & 0 & 0 & 0 & 0 & 0 & 0 & 0 & 0 & 0 \\
0 & 0 & 0 & 0 & 1 & 0 & 0 & 0 & 0 & 0 & 0 & 0 & 0 & 0 & 0 & 0 & 0 & 0 \\
0 & 0 & 0 & 0 & 1 & 0 & 0 & 0 & 0 & 0 & 0 & 0 & 0 & 0 & 0 & 0 & 0 & 0 \\
0 & 0 & 0 & 0 & 0 & 1 & 0 & 0 & 0 & 0 & 0 & 0 & 0 & 0 & 0 & 0 & 0 & 0 \\
0 & 0 & 0 & 0 & 0 & 1 & 0 & 0 & 0 & 0 & 0 & 0 & 0 & 0 & 0 & 0 & 0 & 0 \\
 & & & & & & & & \vdots & & & & & & & & & \\
0 & 0 & 0 & 0 & 0 & 0 & 0 & 0 & 0 & 0 & 0 & 0 & 0 & 0 & 0 & 0 & 1 & 0 \\
0 & 0 & 0 & 0 & 0 & 0 & 0 & 0 & 0 & 0 & 0 & 0 & 0 & 0 & 0 & 0 & 1 & 0 \\
0 & 0 & 0 & 0 & 0 & 0 & 0 & 0 & 0 & 0 & 0 & 0 & 0 & 0 & 0 & 0 & 0 & 1 \\
0 & 0 & 0 & 0 & 0 & 0 & 0 & 0 & 0 & 0 & 0 & 0 & 0 & 0 & 0 & 0 & 0 & 1
\end{pmatrix}.
$$

References

Akaike, H. (1974) A new look at the statistical model identification. *IEEE Transactions on automatic control*, **19**, 716–723.

Altham, P.M.E. (1984) Improving the precision of estimation by fitting a model. *Journal of the Royal Statistical Society, Series B*, **46**, 118–119.

Baker, S.G. (1992) A simple method for computing the observed information matrix when using the EM algorithm with categorical data. *Journal of Computational and Graphical Statistics*, **1**, 63–76.

Baker, S.G. (1994) Regression analysis of grouped survival data with incomplete covariates: non-ignorable missing-data and censoring mechanisms. *Biometrics*, 50, 821–826.

Baker, S.G., and Laird, N.M. (1988) Regression analysis for categorical variables with outcome subject to non-ignorable non-response. *Journal of the American Statistical Association*, **83**, 62–69.

Baker, S.G., Rosenberger, W.F., and DerSimonian, R. (1992) Closed-form estimates for missing counts in two-way contingency tables. *Statistics in Medicine*, **11**, 643–657.

Bartlett, M.S. (1937) Some examples of statistical methods of research in agriculture and applied botany. *Journal of the Royal Statistical Society, Series B*, **4**, 137–170.

Beckman, R.J., Nachtsheim, C.J., and Cook, R.D. (1987) Diagnostics for mixed-model analysis of variance. *Technometrics*, **29**, 413–426.

Box, G.E.P. and Tiao, G.C. (1992) *Bayesian Inference in Statistical Analysis*. Wiley Classics Library edition. John Wiley & Sons, New York.

Brant, L.J., Pearson, J.D., Morrell, C.H., and Verbeke, G. (1992) Statistical methods for studying individual change during aging. *Collegium Antropologicum*, **16**, 359–369.

Breslow, N.E. and Clayton, D.G. (1993) Approximate inference in generalized linear mixed models. *Journal of the American Statistical Association*, **88**, 9–25.

Brown, C.H. (1990) Protecting against nonrandomly missing data in longitudinal studies. *Biometrics*, **46**, 143–155.

Buck, S.F. (1960) A method of estimation of missing values in multivariate data suitable for use with an electronic computer. *Journal of the Royal Statistical Society, Series B*, **22**, 302–306.

Butler, S.M. and Louis, T.A. (1992) Random effects models with nonparametric priors. *Statistics in Medicine*, **11**, 1981–2000.

Carlin, B.P. and Louis, T.A. (1996) *Bayes and Empirical Bayes Methods for Data Analysis*, Chapman and Hall.

Carter, H.B. and Coffey, D.S. (1990) The prostate : An increasing medical problem. *The Prostate*, **16**, 39–48.

Carter, H.B., Morrell, C.H., Pearson, J.D., Brant, L.J., Plato, C.C., Metter, E.J., Chan, D.W., Fozard, J.L., and Walsh, P.C. (1992a) Estimation of prostate growth using serial prostate-specific antigen measurements in men with and without prostate disease. *Cancer Research*, **52**, 3323–3328.

Carter, H.B., Pearson, J.D., Metter, E.J., Brant, L.J., Chan, D.W., Andres, R., Fozard, J.L., and Walsh, P.C. (1992b) Longitudinal evaluation of prostate-specific antigen levels in men with and without prostate disease. *Journal of the American Medical Association*, **267**, 2215–2220.

Chatterjee, S. and Hadi, A.S. (1988) *Sensitivity Analysis in Linear Regression*. John Wiley & Sons, New York.

Chi, E.M. and Reinsel, G.C. (1989) Models for longitudinal data with random effects and AR(1) errors. *Journal of the American Statistical Association*, **84**, 452–459.

Christensen, R., Pearson, L.M., and Johnson, W. (1992) Case-deletion diagnostics for mixed models. *Technometrics*, **34**, 38–45.

Cook, R.D. (1977a) Detection of influential observations in linear regression. *Technometrics*, **19**, 15–18.

Cook, R.D. (1977b) Letter to the editor. *Technometrics*, **19**, 348.

Cook, R.D. (1979) Influential observations in linear regression. *Journal of the American Statistical Association*, **74**, 169–174.

Cook, R.D. (1986) Assessment of local influence. *Journal of the Royal Statistical Society, Series B*, **48**, 133–169.

Cook, R.D. and Weisberg, S. (1982) *Residuals and Influence in Regression*, Chapman and Hall, London.

Cox, D.R. and Hinkley, D.V. (1974) *Theoretical Statistics*. Chapman and Hall, London.

Cox, D.R. and Hinkley, D.V. (1990) *Theoretical Statistics*. Chapman and Hall, London.

Crépeau, H., Koziol, J., Reid, N. and Yuh, Y.S. (1985) Analysis of incomplete multivariate data from repeated measurements experiments. *Biometrics*, **41**, 505–514.

Cressie, N.A.C. (1991) *Statistics for Spatial Data*. John Wiley & Sons, New York.

Crowder, M.J. and Hand, D.J. (1990) *Analysis of Repeated Measures*. Chapman and Hall, London.

Davidian, M. and Giltinan, D.M. (1995) *Nonlinear Models for Repeated Measurement Data*. Chapman and Hall, London.

DeGruttola, V., Lange, N., and Dafni, U. (1991) Modeling the progression of HIV infection. *Journal of the American Statistical Association*, **86**, 569–577.

DeGruttola, V., Ware, J.H., and Louis, T.A. (1987) Influence analysis of generalized least squares estimators. *Journal of the American Statistical Association*, **82**, 911–917.

Dempster, A.P., Laird, N.M., and Rubin, D. B. (1977) Maximum likelihood from incomplete data via the EM algorithm (with discussion). *Journal of the Royal Statistical Society, Series B*, **39**, 1–38.

Dempster, A.P. and Rubin, D.B. (1983) Overview, in *Incomplete Data in Sample Surveys, Vol. II: Theory and Annotated Bibliography* (W.G. Madow, I. Olkin, and D.B. Rubin, Eds.). Academic Press, New York, 3–10.

Dempster, A.P., Rubin, R.B., and Tsutakawa, R.K. (1981) Estimation in covariance components models. *Journal of the American Statistical Association*, **76**, 341–353.

Diem, J.E. and Liukkonen, J.R. (1988) A comparative study of three methods for analysing longitudinal pulmonary function data. *Statistics in Medicine*, **7**, 19–28.

Diggle, P.J. (1983) *Statistical Analysis of Spatial Point Patterns*. Mathematics in Biology. Academic Press, London.

Diggle, P.J. (1988) An approach to the analysis of repeated measures. *Biometrics*, **44**, 959–971.

Diggle, P.J. (1989) Testing for random dropouts in repeated measurement data. *Biometrics*, **45**, 1255–1258.

Diggle, P.J. (1992) On informative and random dropouts in longitudinal studies. Letter to the Editor. *Biometrics*, **48**, 947.

Diggle, P.J. (1993) Estimation with missing data. Reply to a Letter to the Editor. *Biometrics*, **49**, 580.

Diggle, P.J. and Kenward, M.G. (1994) Informative drop-out in longitudinal data analysis (with discussion). *Applied Statistics*, **43**, 49–93.

Diggle, P.J., Liang, K.-Y., and Zeger, S.L. (1994) *Analysis of Longitudinal Data*. Oxford Science Publications, Clarendon Press, Oxford.

Edlefsen, L.E. and Jones, S.D. *GAUSS*. Aptech Systems Inc., P.0. Box 6487, Kent, WA 98064, USA.

Edwards, A.W.F. (1972) *Likelihood*. Cambridge University Press, Cambridge.

Efron, B. (1994) Missing data, imputation, and the bootstrap (with discussion). *Journal of the American Statistical Association*, **89**, 463–479.

Efron, B. and Hinkley, D.V. (1978) Assessing the accuracy of the maximum likelihood estimator: observed versus expected Fisher information. *Biometrika*, **65**, 457–487.

Fahrmeir, L., Tutz, G. (1994) *Multivariate Statistical Modelling Based on Generalized Linear Models*. Springer-Verlag, Heidelberg.

Fai, A.H. and Cornelius, P.L. (1996) Approximate F-tests of multiple degree of freedom hypotheses in generalized least squares analyses of unbalanced split-plot experiments. *Journal of Statistical Computing and Simulation*, **54**, 363–378.

Fitzmaurice, G.M., Laird, N.M., and Lipsitz, S.R. (1994) Analysing incomplete longitudinal binary responses: A likelihood-based approach. *Biometrics*, **50**, 601–612.

Gelman, A., Carlin, J.B., Stern, H.S., and Rubin, D.B. (1995) *Bayesian Data Analysis*, Texts in Statistical Science, Chapman and Hall, London.

Ghosh, J.K. and Sen, P.K. (1985) On the asymptotic performance of the log likelihood ratio statistic for the mixture model and related results. In: *Proceedings of the Berekely Conference in Honor or Jerzy Neyman and Jack Kiefer*, **2**, L.M. Le Cam and R.A. Olshen (Eds.), copyright ©by Wadsworth, Inc., pp. 789–806.

Giesbrecht, F.G. and Burns, J.C. (1985) Two-stage analysis based on a mixed model: Large-sample asymptotic theory and small-sample simulation results. *Biometrics*, **41**, 477–486.

Glynn, R.J., Laird, N.M., and Rubin, D.B. (1986) Selection modelling versus mixture modelling with non-ignorable nonresponse. In: *Drawing Inferences from Self Selected Samples*, H. Wainer (Ed.), Springer-Verlag, New York, pp. 115–142.

Goldstein, H. (1979) *The Design and Analysis of Longitudinal Studies.* Academic Press, London.

Greenlees, W.S., Reece, J.S., and Zieschang, K.D. (1982) Imputation of missing values when the probability of response depends on the variable being imputed. *Journal of the American Statistical Association*, **77**, 251–261.

Gregoire, T. (1997) *Proceedings of the Nantucket Conference on Modelling Longitudinal and Spatially Correlated Data: Methods, Applications, and Future Directions.* Lecture Notes in Statistics, Springer-Verlag, New York.

Hand, D.J., Daly, F., Lunn, A.D., McConway, K.J., and Ostrowski, E. (1994) *A Handbook of Small Data Sets.* First Edition, Chapman and Hall, London.

Harville, D.A. (1974) Bayesian inference for variance components using only error contrasts. *Biometrika*, **61**, 383–385.

Harville, D.A. (1977) Maximum likelihood approaches to variance component estimation and to related problems. *Journal of the American Statistical Association*, **72**, 320–340.

Heitjan, D.F. (1993) Estimation with missing data. Letter to the Editor. *Biometrics*, **49**, 580.

Heitjan, D.F. (1994) Ignorability in general incomplete-data models. *Biometrika*, **81**, 701–708.

Helms, R.W. (1992) Intentionally incomplete longitudinal designs: Methodology and comparison of some full span designs. *Statistics in Medicine*, **11**, 1889–1913.

Henderson, C.R. (1953) Estimation of variance and covariance components. *Biometrics*, **9**, 226–252.

Jennrich, R.I. and Schluchter, M.D. (1986) Unbalanced repeated measures models with structured covariance matrices. *Biometrics*, **42**, 805–820.

Johnson, R.A. and Wichern, D.W. (1992) *Applied Multivariate Statistical Analysis.* Third Edition, Prentice-Hall, Englewood Cliffs.

Kackar, R.N. and Harville, D.A. (1984) Approximations for standard errors of estimators of fixed and random effects in mixed linear models. *Journal of the American Statistical Assocation,* **79**, 853–862.

Kenward, M.G., Molenberghs, G. and Lesaffre, E. (1994) An application of maximum likelihood and estimating equations to the analysis of ordinal data from a longitudinal study with cases missing at random. *Biometrics,* **50**, 945–953.

Kenward, M.G. and Molenberghs, G. (1997) Likelihood based frequentist inference when data are missing at random. *Submitted for publication.*

Krzanowski, W.J. (1988) *Principles of Multivariate Analysis.* Clarendon Press, Oxford.

Laird, N.M. (1978) Nonparametric maximum likelihood estimation of a mixing distribution. *Journal of the American Statistical Association,* **73**, 805–811.

Laird, N.M. (1988) Missing data in longitudinal studies. *Statistics in Medicine,* **7**, 305–315.

Laird, N.M., Lange, N., and Stram, D. (1987) Maximum likelihood computations with repeated meausres: application of the EM algorithm. *Journal of the American Statistical Association,* **82**, 97–105.

Laird, N.M. and Ware, J.H. (1982) Random effects models for longitudinal data. *Biometrics,* **38**, 963–974.

Lange, N. and Ryan, L. (1989) Assessing normality in random effects models. *The Annals of Statistics,* **17**, 624–642.

Lesaffre, E. and Verbeke, G. (1997) Local influence in linear mixed models. *Submitted for publication.*

Liang, K.-Y. and Zeger, S. L. (1986) Longitudinal data analysis using generalized linear models. *Biometrika,* **73**, 13–22.

Lindley, D.V. and Smith, A.F.M. (1972) Bayes estimates for the linear model. *Journal of the Royal Statistical Society, Series B,* **34**, 1–41.

Lindstrom, M.J. and Bates, D.M. (1988) Newton-Raphson and EM algorithms for linear mixed-effects models for repeated-measures data. *Journal of the American Statistical Association,* **83**, 1014–1022.

Littell, R.C., Milliken, G.A., Stroup, W.W., and Wolfinger, R.D. (1996) *SAS System for Mixed Models.* SAS Institute Inc, Cary, NC, USA.

Little, R.J.A. (1976) Inference about means for incomplete multivariate data. *Biometrika*, **63**, 593–604.

Little, R.J.A. (1993) Pattern-mixture models for multivariate incomplete data. *Journal of the American Statistical Association*, **88**, 125–134.

Little, R.J.A. (1995) Modeling the drop-out mechanism in repeated measures studies. *Journal of the American Statistical Association*, **90**, 1112–1121.

Little, R.J.A. and Rubin, D.B. (1987) *Statistical Analysis with Missing Data*. John Wiley & Sons, New York.

Longford, N.T. (1993) *Random Coefficient Models*. Oxford University Press, Oxford.

Louis, T.A. (1982) Finding the observed information matrix when using the EM algorithm. *Journal of the Royal Statistical Society, Series B*, **44**, 226-233.

Mansour, H., Nordheim, E.V., and Rutledge, J.J. (1985) Maximum likelihood estimation of variance components in repeated measures designs assuming autoregressive errors. *Biometrics*, **41**, 287–294.

McCullagh, P. and Nelder, J.A. (1989) *Generalized Linear Models*. Chapman & Hall, London.

McLachlan, G.J. and Basford, K.E. (1988) *Mixture models. Inference and Applications to Clustering*. Marcel Dekker, New York.

McLachlan, G.J. and Krishnan, T. (1997) *The EM Algorithm and Extensions*. Wiley & Sons, New York.

McLean, R.A. and Sanders, W.L. (1988) Approximating degrees of freedom for standard errors in mixed linear models. *Proceedings of the statistical computing section, American Statistical Association, New Orleans*, 50–59.

Meilijson, I. (1989) A fast improvement to the EM algorithm on its own terms. *Journal of the Royal Statistical Society, Series B*, **51**, 127–138.

Meng, X.-L. and Rubin, D.B. (1991) Using EM to obtain asymptotic variance covariance matrices: the SEM algorithm. *Journal of the American Statistical Association*, **86**, 899–909.

Michiels, B. and Molenberghs, G. (1997) Protective estimation of longitudinal categorical data with nonrandom dropout. *Communications in Statistics, Theory and Methods*, **26**, 000–000.

Miller, J.J. (1977) Asymptotic properties of maximum likelihood estimates in the mixed model of the analysis of variance. *The Annals of Statistics*, **5**, 746–762.

Molenberghs, G., Goetghebeur, E., and Lipsitz, S.R. (1997) Non-random missingness in categorical data: strengths and limitations. *Submitted for publication.*

Molenberghs, G., Michiels, B., Kenward, M.G., and Diggle, P.J. (1997) Missing data mechanisms and pattern-mixture models. *Submitted for publication.*

Molenberghs, G., Kenward, M. G., and Lesaffre, E. (1997) The analysis of longitudinal ordinal data with non-random dropout. *Biometrika*, **84**, 000–000.

Morrell, C.H. and Brant, L.J. (1991) Modelling hearing thresholds in the elderly. *Statistics in Medicine*, **10**, 1453–1464.

Morrell, C.H., Pearson, J.D., and Brant, L.J. (1997) Linear transformations of linear mixed-effects models. *The American Statistician*, In Press.

Murray, G.D. and Findlay, J.G. (1988) Correcting for the bias caused by drop-outs in hypertension trials. *Statististics in Medicine*, **7**, 941-946.

Nabugoomu, F. and Allen, O.B. (1994) The estimation of fixed effects in a mixed linear model. *Proceedings of the 1993 Kansas State University Conference on Applied Statistics in Agriculture*, 111–121.

Nelder, J.A. (1954) The interpretation of negative components of variance. *Biometrika*, **41**, 544–548.

Nelder, J.A. and Mead, R. (1965) A simplex method for function minimisation. *The Computer Journal*, **7**, 303–313.

Neter, J., Wasserman, W., and Kutner, M.H. (1990) *Applied Linear Statistical Models. Regression, Analysis of Variance and Experimental Designs*. Third Edition, Richard D. Irwin, Inc., Homewood, IL.

Neter, J., Kutner, M.H., Nachtsheim, C.J., and Wasserman, W. (1996) *Applied Linear Statistical Models. Regression, Analysis of Variance and Experimental Designs*. Fourth Edition, Richard D. Irwin, Inc., Homewood, IL.

Nevens, F., Van Steenbergen, W., Yap, S.H., and Fevery, J. (1996) Assessment of variceal pressure by continuous non-invasive endoscopic registration : A placebo controlled evaluation of the effect of terlipressin and octreotide. *Gut*, **38**, 129–134.

Núñez-Antón, V. and Woodworth, G.G. (1994) Analysis of longitudinal data with unequally spaced observations and time-dependent correlated errors. *Biometrics*, **50**, 445–456.

Patel, H.I. (1991) Analysis of incomplete data from clinical trials with repeated measurements. *Biometrika*, **78**, 609-619.

Patterson, H.D. and Thompson, R. (1971) Recovery of inter-block information when block sizes are unequal. *Biometrika*, **58**, 545–554.

Pearson, J.D., Kaminski, P., Metter, E.J., Fozard, J.L., Brant, L.J., Morrell, C.H., and Carter, H.B. (1991) Modeling longitudinal rates of change in prostate specific antigen during aging. *Proceedings of the Social Statistics Section of the American Statistical Assciation, Washington D.C.*, 580–585.

Pearson, J.D., Morrell, C.H., Landis, P.K., Carter, H.B., and Brant, L.J. (1994) Mixed-effects regression models for studying the natural history of prostate disease. *Statistics in Medicine*, **13**, 587–601.

Peixoto, J.L. (1987) Hierarchical variable selection in polynomial regression models. *The American Statistician*, **41**, 311–313.

Peixoto, J.L. (1990) A property of well-formulated polynomial regression models. *The American Statistician*, **44**, 26–30.

Potthoff, R.F. and Roy, S.N. (1964) A generalized multivariate analysis of variance model useful especially for growth curve problems. *Biometrika*, **51**, 313–326.

Prasad, N.G.N. and Rao, J.N.K. (1990) The estimation of mean squared error of small-area estimators. *Journal of the American Statistical Association*, **85**, 163–171.

Rang, H.P. and Dale, M.M. (1990) *Pharmacology*. Churchill Livingstone, Edinburgh.

Rao, C.R. (1971a) Estimation of variance and covariance components - MINQUE theory. *Journal of Multivariate Analysis*, **1**, 257–275.

Rao, C.R. (1971b) Minimum variance quadratic unbiased estimation of variance components. *Journal of Multivariate Analysis*, **1**, 445–456.

Rao, C.R. (1973) *Linear Statistical Inference and Its Applications*. Second edition. John Wiley & Sons, New York.

Ripley, B.D. (1981) *Spatial Statistics*. John Wiley & Sons, New York.

Robins, J.M., Rotnitzky, A., and Zhao, L.P. (1995) Analysis of semiparametric regression models for repeated outcomes in the presence of missing data. *Journal of the American Statistical Association*, **90**, 106–121.

Rochon, J. (1992) ARMA covariance structures with time heteroscedasticity for repeated measures experiments. *Journal of the American Statistical Association*, **87**, 777–784.

Roger, J.H. (1993) A new look at the facilities in PROC MIXED. *Proceedings SEUGI*, **93**, 521–532.

Roger, J.H. and Kenward, M.G. (1993) Repeated measures using proc mixed instead of proc glm. in *Proceedings of the First Annual South-East SAS Users Group conference, Cary, NC, U.S.A. : SAS Institute*, 199–208.

Rubin, D.B. (1976) Inference and missing data. *Biometrika*, 581–592.

Rubin, D.B. (1978) Multiple imputations in sample surveys – a phenomenological Bayesian approach to nonresponse. In: *Imputation and Editing of Faulty or Missing Survey Data*, U.S. Department of Commerce, pp. 1–23.

Rubin, D.B. (1987) *Multiple Imputation for Nonresponse in Surveys*. John Wiley & Sons, New York.

Rubin, D.B. and Schenker, N. (1986) Multiple imputation for interval estimation from simple random samples with ignorable nonresponse. *Journal of the American Statistical Association*, **81**, 366–374.

SAS Institute Inc., Cary, NC: SAS Institute Inc. (1989) *SAS/STAT User's guide, Version 6, Volume 1*, Fourth Edition.

SAS Institute Inc., Cary, NC: SAS Institute Inc. (1991) *SAS System for Linear Models*, Third Edition.

SAS Institute Inc., Cary, NC: SAS Institute Inc. (1992) *SAS Technical Report P-229, SAS/STAT Software: Changes and Enhancements, Release 6.07*.

SAS Institute Inc., Cary, NC: SAS Institute Inc. (1996) *SAS/STAT Software: Changes and Enhancements through Release 6.11*.

Satterthwaite, F.E. (1941) Synthesis of variance. *Psychometrika*, **6**, 309–316.

Satterthwaite, F.E. (1946) An approximate distribution of estimates of variance components. *Biometrics Bulletin*, **2**, 110–114.

Schluchter, M. (1988) Analysis of incomplete multivariate data using linear models with structured covariance matrices. *Statistics in Medicine*, **7**, 317–324.

Schwarz, G. (1978) Estimating the dimension of a model. *The Annals of Statistics*, **6**, 461–464.

Searle, S.R. (1982) *Matrix Algebra Useful for Statitics*. John Wiley & Sons, New York.

Searle, S.R. (1987) *Linear Models for Unbalanced Data*. John Wiley & Sons, New York.

Searle, S.R., Casella, G., and McCulloch, C.E. (1992) *Variance Components*. John Wiley & Sons, New York.

Seber, G.A.F. (1984) *Multivariate Observations*. John Wiley & Sons, New York.

Self, S.G. and Liang, K.Y. (1987) Asymptotic properties of maximum likelihood estimators and likelihood ratio tests under nonstandard conditions. *Journal of the American Statistical Association*, 605–610.

Serfling, R.J. (1980) *Approximation Theorems of Mathematical Statistics*. John Wiley & Sons, New York.

Sharples, K. and Breslow, N.E. (1992) Regression analysis of correlated binary data: some small sample results for the estimating equation approach. *Journal of Statistical Computation and Simulation*, **42**, 1–20.

Smith, A.F.M. (1973) A general Bayesian linear model. *Journal of the Royal Statistical Society, Series B*, **35**, 67–75.

Smith, D.M., Robertson, B., and Diggle, P.J. (1996) *Object-oriented Software for the Analysis of Longitudinal Data in S*. Technical Report MA 96/192. Department of Mathematics and Statistics, University of Lancaster, LA1 4YF, United Kingdom.

Sprott, D.A. (1975) Marginal and conditional sufficiency. *Biometrika*, **62**, 599–605.

Stram, D.O. and Lee, J.W. (1994) Variance components testing in the longitudinal mixed effects mode. *Biometrics*, **50**, 1171–1177.

Stram, D.A. and Lee, J.W. (1995) Correction to: Variance components testing in the longitudinal mixed effects model. *Biometrics*, **51**, 1196.

Strenio, J.F., Weisberg, H.J., and Bryk, A.S. (1983) Empirical bayes estimation of individual growth-curve parameters and their relationship to covariates. *Biometrics*, **39**, 71–86.

Tanner, M.A. and Wong, W.H. (1987) The calculation of posterior distributions by data augmentation. *Journal of the American Statistical Association*, **82**, 805–811.

Thompson, W.A. Jr. (1962) The problem of negative estimates of variance components. *Annals of Mathematical Statistics*, **33**, 273–289.

Verbeke, G. (1995) *The linear mixed model. A critical investigation in the context of longitudinal data analysis*, PhD thesis, Catholic University of Leuven, Faculty of Science, Department of Mathematics.

Verbeke, G. and Lesaffre, E. (1996a) A linear mixed-effects model with heterogeneity in the random-effects population. *Journal of the American Statistical Association*, **91**, 217–221.

Verbeke, G. and Lesaffre, E. (1996b) Large sample properties of the maximum likelihood estimators in linear mixed models with misspecified random-effects distributions. Technical report, Biostatistical Centre for Clinical Trials, Catholic University of Leuven, Belgium [Report # 1996.1].

Verbeke, G. and Lesaffre, E. (1997a) The effect of misspecifying the random effects distribution in linear mixed models for longitudinal data. *Computational Statistics and Data Analysis*, **23**, 541–556.

Verbeke, G. and Lesaffre, E. (1997b) The linear mixed model. A critical investigation in the context of longitudinal data. In: *Proceedings of the Nantucket conference on Modelling Longitudinal and Spatially Correlated Data: Methods, Applications, and Future Directions*, Gregoire, T. (Ed.), Lecture Notes in Statistics, Springer-Verlag, New York, pp. 000–000.

Verbeke, G., Lesaffre, E., and Brant L.J. (1997) The detection of residual serial correlation in linear mixed models. *Submitted for publication.*

Waternaux, C., Laird, N.M., and Ware, J.H. (1989) Methods for analysis of longitudinal data : Bloodlead concentrations and cognitive development. *Journal of the American Statistical Association*, **84**, 33–41.

Weiner, D.L. (1981) Design and analysis of bioavailability studies. In: *Statistics in the pharmaceutical industry*, C.R. Buncher and J.-Y. Tsay (Eds.) Marcel Dekker, New York, pp. 205–229.

Westfall, P.H. and Young, S.S. (1993) *Resampling-Based Multiple Testing: Examples and Methods for p-Value Adjustment.* John Wiley & Sons, New York.

White, H. (1980) Nonlinear regression on cross-section data. *Econometrica,* **48**, 721–746.

White, H. (1982) Maximum likelihood estimation of misspecified models. *Econometrica,* **50**, 1–25.

Wu, M.C. and Bailey, K.R. (1988) Analysing changes in the presence of informative right censoring caused by death and withdrawal. *Statistics in Medicine,* **7**, 337–346.

Wu, M.C. and Bailey, K.R. (1989) Estimation and comparison of changes in the presence of informative right censoring: conditional linear model. *Biometrics,* **45**, 939–955.

Wu, M.C. and Carroll, R.J. (1988) Estimation and comparison of changes in the presence of informative right censoring by modeling the censoring process. *Biometrics,* *44*, 175–188.

Yates, F. (1933) The analysis of replicated experiments when the field results are incomplete. *Empirical Journal of Experimental Agriculture,* **1**, 129–142.

Index

Lecture Notes in Statistics

For information about Volumes 1 to 70,
please contact Springer-Verlag

Vol. 71: E.M.R.A. Engel, A Road to Randomness in
Physical Systems. ix, 155 pages, 1992.

Vol. 72: J.K. Lindsey, The Analysis of Stochastic Processes
using GLIM. vi, 294 pages, 1992.

Vol. 73: B.C. Arnold, E. Castillo, J.-M. Sarabia,
Conditionally Specified Distributions. xiii, 151 pages, 1992.

Vol. 74: P. Barone, A. Frigessi, M. Piccioni, Stochastic
Models, Statistical Methods, and Algorithms in Image
Analysis. vi, 258 pages, 1992.

Vol. 75: P.K. Goel, N.S. Iyengar (Eds.), Bayesian Analysis
in Statistics and Econometrics. xi, 410 pages, 1992.

Vol. 76: L. Bondesson, Generalized Gamma Convolutions
and Related Classes of Distributions and Densities. viii, 173
pages, 1992.

Vol. 77: E. Mammen, When Does Bootstrap Work?
Asymptotic Results and Simulations. vi, 196 pages, 1992.

Vol. 78: L. Fahrmeir, B. Francis, R. Gilchrist, G. Tutz
(Eds.), Advances in GLIM and Statistical Modelling:
Proceedings of the GLIM92 Conference and the 7th
International Workshop on Statistical Modelling, Munich,
13-17 July 1992. ix, 225 pages, 1992.

Vol. 79: N. Schmitz, Optimal Sequentially Planned Decision
Procedures. xii, 209 pages, 1992.

Vol. 80: M. Fligner, J. Verducci (Eds.), Probability Models
and Statistical Analyses for Ranking Data. xxii, 306 pages,
1992.

Vol. 81: P. Spirtes, C. Glymour, R. Scheines, Causation,
Prediction, and Search. xxiii, 526 pages, 1993.

Vol. 82: A. Korostelev and A. Tsybakov, Minimax Theory
of Image Reconstruction. xii, 268 pages, 1993.

Vol. 83: C. Gatsonis, J. Hodges, R. Kass, N. Singpurwalla
(Editors), Case Studies in Bayesian Statistics. xii, 437 pages,
1993.

Vol. 84: S. Yamada, Pivotal Measures in Statistical
Experiments and Sufficiency. vii, 129 pages, 1994.

Vol. 85: P. Doukhan, Mixing: Properties and Examples. xi,
142 pages, 1994.

Vol. 86: W. Vach, Logistic Regression with Missing Values
in the Covariates. xi, 139 pages, 1994.

Vol. 87: J. Müller, Lectures on Random Voronoi
Tessellations.vii, 134 pages, 1994.

Vol. 88: J. E. Kolassa, Series Approximation Methods in
Statistics. Second Edition, ix, 183 pages, 1997.

Vol. 89: P. Cheeseman, R.W. Oldford (Editors), Selecting
Models From Data: AI and Statistics IV. xii, 487 pages,
1994.

Vol. 90: A. Csenki, Dependability for Systems with a
Partitioned State Space: Markov and Semi-Markov Theory
and Computational Implementation. x, 241 pages, 1994.

Vol. 91: J.D. Malley, Statistical Applications of Jordan
Algebras. viii, 101 pages, 1994.

Vol. 92: M. Eerola, Probabilistic Causality in Longitudinal
Studies. vii, 133 pages, 1994.

Vol. 93: Bernard Van Cutsem (Editor), Classification and
Dissimilarity Analysis. xiv, 238 pages, 1994.

Vol. 94: Jane F. Gentleman and G.A. Whitmore (Editors),
Case Studies in Data Analysis. viii, 262 pages, 1994.

Vol. 95: Shelemyahu Zacks, Stochastic Visibility in
Random Fields. x, 175 pages, 1994.

Vol. 96: Ibrahim Rahimov, Random Sums and Branching
Stochastic Processes. viii, 195 pages, 1995.

Vol. 97: R. Szekli, Stochastic Ordering and Dependence in
Applied Probability. viii, 194 pages, 1995.

Vol. 98: Philippe Barbe and Patrice Bertail, The Weighted
Bootstrap. viii, 230 pages, 1995.

Vol. 99: C.C. Heyde (Editor), Branching Processes:
Proceedings of the First World Congress. viii, 185 pages,
1995.

Vol. 100: Wlodzimierz Bryc, The Normal Distribution:
Characterizations with Applications. viii, 139 pages, 1995.

Vol. 101: H.H. Andersen, M.Højbjerre, D. Sørensen,
P.S.Eriksen, Linear and Graphical Models: for the
Multivariate Complex Normal Distribution. x, 184 pages,
1995.

Vol. 102: A.M. Mathai, Serge B. Provost, Takesi Hayakawa,
Bilinear Forms and Zonal Polynomials. x, 378 pages, 1995.

Vol. 103: Anestis Antoniadis and Georges Oppenheim
(Editors), Wavelets and Statistics. vi, 411 pages, 1995.

Vol. 104: Gilg U.H. Seeber, Brian J. Francis, Reinhold
Hatzinger, Gabriele Steckel-Berger (Editors), Statistical
Modelling: 10th International Workshop, Innsbruck, July
10-14th 1995. x, 327 pages, 1995.

Vol. 105: Constantine Gatsonis, James S. Hodges, Robert E.
Kass, Nozer D. Singpurwalla(Editors), Case Studies in
Bayesian Statistics, Volume II. x, 354 pages, 1995.

Vol. 106: Harald Niederreiter, Peter Jau-Shyong Shiue
(Editors), Monte Carlo and Quasi-Monte Carlo Methods in
Scientific Computing. xiv, 372 pages, 1995.

Vol. 107: Masafumi Akahira, Kei Takeuchi, Non-Regular
Statistical Estimation. vii, 183 pages, 1995.